Gene Transfer and Expression Protocols

Methods in Molecular Biology

John M. Walker, SERIES EDITOR

Methods in Molecular Biology • 7

Gene Transfer and Expression Protocols

Edited by

E. J. Murray

Roche Products Ltd.
Welwyn Garden City, Hertfordshire, UK

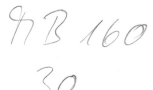
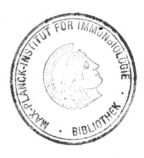

 Humana Press • **Clifton, New Jersey**

© 1991 The Humana Press Inc.
Crescent Manor
PO Box 2148
Clifton, New Jersey 07015

Printed in the United States of America

Library of Congress Cataloging in Publication Data
Main entry under title:

Methods in molecular biology.

        (Biological methods)
        Vol. 5-6 edited by Jeffrey W. Pollard and John M.
    Walker; v. 7 edited by E.J. Murray.
        Vol. 7 lacks series statement.
        Includes bibliographies and indexes.
        Contents: v. 1. Proteins—v. 2. Nucleic
acids— [etc.] — v. 7. Gene transfer and expression
protocols.
        1. Molecular biology—Technique. I. Walker,
John M., 1948–   .   II. Pollard, Jeffrey W.
QH506.M45   1984   574.8'8'078   84-15696
ISBN 0-89603.062-8 (v. 1)
ISBN 0-89603.178-0 (v. 7 hardcover)
ISBN 0-89603.216-7 (v. 7 softcover)

Preface

Biology is the study of living things. The classical approach might be described as holistic and descriptive, whereas the modern molecular approach aims to be investigative, reductionist, and mechanistic.

Genes contain all the information for the structure of all living things; thus, the understanding of how genes are regulated is an important step toward understanding the nature of living things. The study of gene regulation has been made more tractable by the design of simple experimental models in which a single gene can be isolated from the milieu of the organism. The new science of molecular biology has introduced techniques that permit the design of such experimental models. In essence, the genome of the organism is dissected in such a manner that specific genes may now be introduced into an appropriate cell line. Subsequent analysis of the proteins expressed from the genes under study results in the identification of the regulatory DNA sequences.

The design of the chapters in this book follows the successful formula found in previous volumes in this series. Each chapter describes a single particular technique. An Introduction explains the significance of the protocol and provides background information. The Materials section lists all the requirements necessary to carry out the technique (buffers, storage stability, and so on). The Methods section details the procedure in a step-by-step protocol. Finally, the Notes section highlights pitfalls likely to be encountered in using the method, along with alternative or substitute procedures that may then be resorted to without hazarding the successful conclusion of the experiment. This type of information is rarely seen in the literature, but is invaluable to anyone trying a technique for the first time.

The purpose of this book is to detail most of the techniques used to introduce an isolated gene into a cell line, using a variety of transfection techniques. This variety is not redundant, since different cell lines respond in different ways to each transfection technique. The second section describes the use of viral vectors, which represents a more efficient method of gene transfer. Sections 3 and 4 demonstrate the use of a variety of reporter genes to define important regulatory features of the gene under study, either using transient expression protocols or via the generation of cell lines that contain the isolated gene as a stable genetic unit integrated in the host cell genome. Section 5 demonstrates how to analyze the steady-state level of transcription in the transfected cell line generated in the previous sections. This is followed by Section 6 which describes the assay for newly initiated transcriptional complexes. Section 7 explains the use of immunocy-tological techniques to examine the expression of the transfected gene product using conjugated antibodies for either cell staining or FACS analysis. Section 8 provides a description of a variety of techniques used to assay the structure and replication state of the transfected gene. Also included in this section is the polymerase chain reaction (PCR) as a means to establish whether ho-mologous integration of the transfected gene has occurred. Finally, most of the preceding techniques are brought into focus in Section 9, which details the overall strategy of defining the regulatory sequences required for the expression of the erythroid-specific human beta-globin gene.

This volume is directed toward final-year graduate students engaged in research projects, as well as postgraduates and/or postdoctorate scientists who wish to pursue a research interest in the study of gene regulation.

Finally, I would like to acknowledge the patient consideration of Roche Products Ltd. for permitting time to finish this compilation of protocols, and also that of the series editor, John M. Walker, for valuable editorial help.

E. J. Murray

Contents

Section 8. Southern Blot Analysis of Transfected Cell Lines

Section 9
Use of Cell Lines for Studying Tissue-Specific Gene Expression

Contributors

MICHAEL ANTONIOU • *Laboratory of Gene Structure and Expression, National Institute for Medical Research, Mill Hill, London, UK*

RÉMY AUBIN • *Molecular Genetics and Carcinogenesis Laboratory, W. W. Cross Cancer Institute, Edmonton, Alberta, Canada*

MARK J. BAILEY • *Institute of Virology and Environmental Microbiology, Mansfield Road, Oxford, UK*

KEITH BALLINGALL • *The Moredun Research Institute, Edinburgh, UK*

ALISON C. BREWER • *King's College, University of London, London, UK*

RAYMOND BUJDOSO • *Department of Veterinary Pathology, University of Edinburgh, Edinburgh, UK*

CLAUDIA CHEN • *Laboratory of Cell Biology, National Institute of Mental Health, Bethesda, MD; Research Institute for Microbial Diseases, Osaka University, Osaka, Japan*

KEVIN D. DIETRICH • *Molecular Genetics and Carcinogenesis Laboratory, W. W. Cross Cancer Institute, Edmonton, Alberta, Canada*

PHILIP L. FELGNER • *Vical, Inc., San Diego, CA*

STEVEN FIERING • *Department of Genetics, Stanford University, Stanford, CA*

MITCHELL H. FINER • *Cell Genesys Inc., Foster City, CA*

RONALD M. FOURNEY • *Molecular Genetics and Carcinogenesis Laboratory, W. W. Cross Cancer Institute, Edmonton, Alberta, Canada*

VINCENT GIGUÈRE • *Division of Endocrinology, Hospital for Sick Children, Toronto, Canada*

PETER N. GOODFELLOW • *Imperial Cancer Research Fund, London, UK*

FRANK L. GRAHAM • *Departments of Biology and Pathology, McMaster University, Hamilton, Ontario, Canada*

BRIAN W. GRINNELL • *Department of Molecular Biology, Lilly Research Laboratories, Indianapolis, IN*

PETER GRUSS • *Abteilung Molekulare Zellbiologie, Max-Planck-Institut für biophysikalische Chemie, Gottingen, FRG*

MARIE-LOUISE HAMMARSKJÖLD • *Departments of Microbiology and Oral Biology, State University of New York, Buffalo, NY*

JANET HARWOOD • *Imperial Cancer Research Fund, Clare Hall Laboratories, South Mimms, Hertfordshire, UK*

LEONARD A. HERZENBERG • *Department of Genetics, Stanford University, Stanford, CA*

MASAHIRO ISHIURA • *National Institute for Basic Biology, Myodaijicho, Okazaki, Aichi, Japan*

ROBB KRUMLAUF • *National Institute for Medical Research, Mill Hill, London, UK*

RICHARD A. LAKE • *Imperial Cancer Research Fund Laboratories, St. Bartholomew's Hospital, London, UK*

HARTMUT LAND • *Imperial Cancer Research Fund, London, UK*

MARK W. LEONARD • *King's College, University of London, London UK*

GRANT R. MACGREGOR • *Institute for Molecular Genetics, Howard Hughes Medical Institute, Baylor College of Medicine, Houston, TX*

MICHAEL MACKETT • *Paterson Institute for Cancer Research, Christie Hospital and Holt Radium Institute, Withington, Manchester, UK*

MARK MEUTH • *Imperial Cancer Research Fund, Clare Hall Laboratories, South Mimms, Hertfordshire, UK*

JAY P. MORGENSTERN • *Imperial Cancer Research Fund, London, UK*

ROGER MORRIS • *Laboratory of Neurobiology, National Institute for Medical Research, Mill Hill, London, UK*

GARRY P. NOLAN • *Department of Genetics, Stanford University, Stanford, CA*

HIROTO OKAYAMA • *Laboratory of Cell Biology, National Institute of Mental Health, Bethesda, MD; Research Institute for Microbial Diseases, Osaka University, Osaka, Japan*

MICHAEL J. OWEN • *Imperial Cancer Research Fund Laboratories, St. Bartholomew's Hospital, London, UK*

MALCOLM C. PATERSON • *Molecular Genetics and Carcinogenesis Laboratory, W. W. Cross Cancer Institute, Edmonton, Alberta, Canada*

ROGER K. PATIENT • *King's College, University of London, London, UK*

ROBERT D. POSSEE • *Institute of Virology and Environmental Microbiology, Mansfield Road, Oxford, UK*

LUDVIK PREVEC • *McMaster University, Hamilton, Ontario, Canada*

MARIO ROEDERER • *Department of Genetics, Stanford University, Stanford, CA*

ANDREW SANDERSON • *Department of Zoology, University of Edinburgh, Edinburgh, UK*

ROBERT F. SANTERRE • *Department of Molecular Biology, Lilly Research Laboratories, Indianapolis, IN*

DAVID SARGAN • *Department of Veterinary Pathology, University of Edinburgh, Edinburgh, UK*

DENISE SHEER • *Human Cytogenics Laboratory, Imperial Cancer Research Fund, London, UK*

JANET M. SHIPLEY • *Human Cytogenics Laboratory, Imperial Cancer Research Fund, London, UK*

SARAH C. SPENCER • *Clinical Research Centre, Harrow, Middlesex, UK*

DAVID STOTT • *Laboratory of Eukaryotic Molecular Genetics, National Institute for Medical Research, Mill Hill, London, UK*

MICHAEL A. TAINSKY • *University of Texas, M. D. Anderson Cancer Center, Houston, TX*

JENNA D. WALLS • *Department of Molecular Biology, Lilly Research Laboratories, Indianapolis, IN*

MAGGIE E. WALMSLEY • *King's College, University of London, London, UK*

MICHAEL WEINFELD • *Molecular Genetics and Carcinogenesis Laboratory, W. W. Cross Cancer Institute, Edmonton, Alberta, Canada*

ANGUS C. WILSON • *King's College, University of London, London, UK*

NICHOLAS C. WRIGHTON • *National Institute for Medical Research, The Ridgeway, Mill Hill, London, UK*

ANDREAS ZIMMER • *Abteilung molekulare Zellbiologie, Max-Planck-Institut für biophysikalische Chemie, Gottingen, FRG*

SECTION 1
DNA TRANSFECTION TECHNIQUES

CHAPTER 1

Preparation of Recombinant Plasmid DNA for DNA-Mediated Gene Transfer

*Rémy Aubin, Michael Weinfeld,
and Malcolm C. Paterson*

1. Introduction

Recombinant plasmid constructs are frequently employed in transfection experiments. With the availability of a wide spectrum of specialized and versatile eucaryotic cloning/expression vectors, investigators have been given powerful tools to expedite the elucidation of mechanisms governing gene expression, and to facilitate the identification of genes participating in diverse cellular processes (namely, metabolism, the immune response, differentiation and development, the repair of DNA damage, and malignant transformation).

The success of a particular gene transfer experiment depends largely on the quality of the donor DNA preparation. Indeed, the requirement for highly purified form I (covalently closed circular supercoiled) plasmid molecules, to ensure both consistency and optimal levels of gene expression in "transient" assays, as well as reproducible frequencies of stable transfection, is well documented.

Many plasmid purification schemes exist, but the Triton lysis/CsCl "double banding" procedure is the one most frequently quoted as providing transfection-grade DNA. The technique, however, does require a considerable amount of time (3–5 d) and relies on specialized ultracentrifugation

From: *Methods in Molecular Biology, Vol. 7: Gene Transfer and Expression Protocols*
Edited by: E. J. Murray © 1991 The Humana Press Inc., Clifton, NJ

equipment. As a result, only a limited number of large-scale plasmid preparations can be processed at once. A detailed description of this protocol was recently published by Gorman *(1)* and is presented here with only minor modifications.

By way of an alternative, this chapter also describes how milligram quantities of comparably pure form I plasmid DNA (i.e., free of contaminating bacterial chromosomal DNA, RNA, and other host cell components) can be obtained by incorporating the acidified-phenol extraction scheme of Zasloff and coworkers *(2)* as a final step to the preparative alkaline lysis procedure of Birnboim *(3)*. The method is rapid (1–2 d) and lends itself to the preparation of multiple plasmid stocks. Briefly, plasmid molecules are first extracted from bacteria at alkaline pH (in the range of 12.0–12.6) in the presence of detergent. Under these conditions, linear (chromosomal) DNA will denature, whereas intact plasmid duplexes will not. Neutralization of the lysate at high ionic strength allows essentially all of the chromosomal DNA and most of the host cellular RNA and protein to precipitate, while the plasmid remains in solution. Complete removal of residual RNA and protein is then accomplished through a sequence of LiCl precipitation, RNAse and proteinase K digestion, phenol extractions, and ethanol precipitations. At this stage, a plasmid preparation consisting of >90% form I molecules is routinely obtained. Extraction with acidified phenol is then used to remove selectively linear and open circular duplexes from the preparation in one step. The mechanism appears to exploit differences in the hydrophilic character of the different DNA species *(4)*. At pH 4.0 in the presence of 75 m*M* NaCl, open circular and linear molecules are converted to their single-stranded forms and are therefore less hydrophilic than the form I duplexes, because the bases are not shielded from the aqueous environment. In addition, the protonation of the nucleotide bases contributes to reduce significantly the overall charge of the DNA. As a result, open circular and linear DNA species are partitioned to the acidified phenolic phase, whereas intact form I plasmid molecules are retained in the upper aqueous layer. One round of acid-phenol extraction is usually sufficient to obtain a preparation consisting of essentially 100% form I plasmid DNA. A schematic outline of the alkaline lysis/acid-phenol purification method is presented in Fig. 1.

2. Materials

All stock solutions and buffers should be prepared using "nanopure" (double distilled and deionized) water and chemicals of the highest purity available (i.e., certified as molecular biology grade). In addition, and unless stated otherwise, buffers as well as all glass and plasticware should be autoclaved to inactivate contaminating deoxyribonucleases.

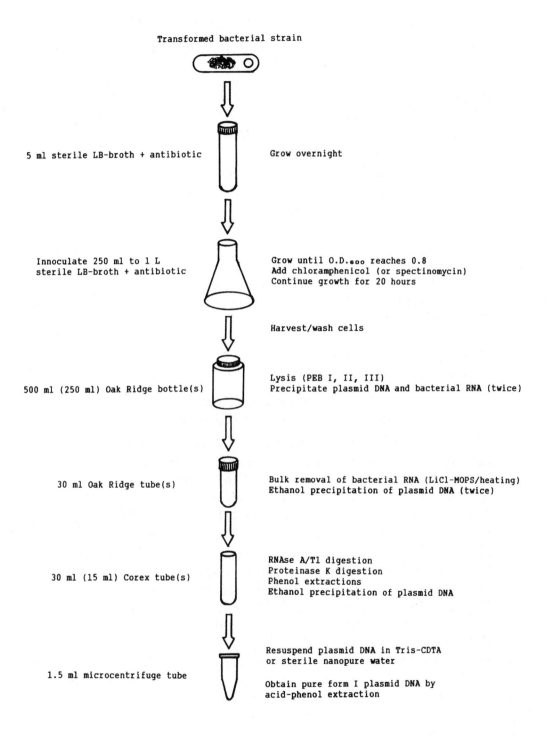

Fig. 1. Schematic outline of the alkaline lysis/acid-phenol plasmid purification procedure.

2.1. Triton Lysis/CsCl Double Banding Method

1. Superbroth: Superbroth is prepared from stock solutions A and B. To prepare solution A, mix 120 g of tryptone, 240 g of yeast extract, and 50 mL glycerol in 9000 mL of water. Prepare solution B by mixing 125 g of K_2HPO_4 and 38 g of KH_2PO_4 in a total vol of 1 L. Sterilize each solution separately in the autoclave. Prepare 1 L of Superbroth by combining 900 mL of solution A and 100 mL of solution B. The final pH should be 7.2.
2. TE: 10 mM Tris-HCl, pH 7.9; 1 mM EDTA, pH 8.0.
3. TES: 50 mM Tris-HCl, pH 7.5; 40 mM EDTA; 25% (w/v) sucrose. Sterilize by filtration (0.22 μm).
4. 0.25M EDTA, pH 8.0.
5. Triton solution: Mix together 1 mL of 10% Triton X-100; 31.5 mL 0.25M EDTA, pH 8.0; 5 mL of 1M Tris-HCl, pH 7.9; and 62.5 mL of water. Sterilize the solution by filtration (0.22 μm) and store at 4°C.
6. Ethidium bromide: 10 mg/mL in 10 mM Tris-HCl, pH 7.5. This solution does not require sterilization.
7. 5M NaCl.
8. HPLC-grade ethanol (95%).
9. Isopropanol.

2.2. Large-Scale Isolation of Plasmid DNA by Alkaline Lysis

1. LB (Luria-Bertani) broth: Dissolve 10 g of tryptone, 5 g of yeast extract, and 10 g of NaCl in 900 mL of water and adjust the pH to 7.5. Complete to 1 L with water and sterilize immediately in the autoclave.
2. NTE buffer: 10 mM Tris-HCl, 100 mM NaCl, 1 mM EDTA (pH 7.5).
3. PEB I: 50 mM D-glucose, 25 mM Tris-HCl, 10 mM CDTA (pH 8.0). Sterilize the solution by filtration (0.22 μm) and store at 4°C. Do not autoclave. PEB I is stable indefinitely if stored under aseptic conditions.
4. PEB II: 0.2N NaOH, 1.0% SDS. Clarify the solution by filtration (0.22 μm). Do not autoclave. Store at room temperature. PEB II is stable for at least 3 mo.
5. PEB III: 3M potassium acetate, 1.8M formic acid. Clarify the solution by filtration (0.22 μm) and store at room temperature. Do not autoclave. PEB III is stable for at least 3 mo.
6. Acetate-MOPS: 100 mM sodium acetate; 50 mM MOPS, pH 8.0. Clarify the solution by filtration (0.22 μm) before sterilizing in the autoclave.
7. LiCL-MOPS: 5M LiCl; 50 mM MOPS, pH 8.0. This solution tends to be turbid even if high-purity LiCl is used. Clarify the solution by filtration (0.45 μm) before sterilizing in the autoclave.

8. RNAse buffer: 50 m*M* Tris-HCl, 10 m*M* NaCl, 10 m*M* EDTA (pH 7.5).
9. RNAse A (DNAse-free): Dissolve lyophylized RNase A to a final concentration of 1 mg/mL in sterile 5 m*M* Tris-HCl, pH 7.5. Hold the preparation at 80°C for 15 min to inactivate traces of contaminating deoxyribonucleases, and allow to cool at room temperature for 20 min. Dispense 100-µL vol in sterile microcentrifuge tubes and store at –20°C. Individual tubes may be thawed and refrozen repeatedly without significant loss of enzyme activity.
10. RNAse T1: Concentrated RNase T1 (125,000 U/mL) is diluted to a final concentration of 500 U/mL in sterile 5 m*M* Tris-HCl, pH 7.5, and stored at 4°C.
11. 10% SDS: Dissolve 10 g of molecular biology grade sodium dodecyl sulfate (SDS) in 100 mL of autoclaved nanopure water. Clarify the solution by filtration (0.22 µm) and store at room temperature. Do not autoclave.
12. Proteinase K: Dissolve lyophylized proteinase K to a final concentration of 20 mg/mL in autoclaved nanopure water. Dispense 100-µL vol in sterile microcentrifuge tubes and store at –20°C. Individual tubes may be thawed and refrozen repeatedly without significant loss of potency.
13. Tris-buffered phenol (pH 8.0): The use of high-purity (redistilled) phenol is critical. Begin by melting crystallized phenol in a 65°C water bath. Add an equal vol of 1 *M* Tris-HCl, pH 8.0/0.2% β-mercaptoethanol. Shake vigorously to create an emulsion, and allow the phases to separate by gravity. Remove the upper aqueous layer by aspiration and equilibrate the phenol twice with an equal vol of 0.1 *M* Tris-HCl, pH 8.0/0.2% β-mercaptoethanol. Store the buffered phenol in the dark at 4°C under a film of 0.1 *M* Tris-HCl, pH 8.0/0.2% β-mercaptoethanol. The preparation remains stable for at least 3 mo under these conditions. CAUTION: Phenol is a strong oxidant and can cause severe burns. Always wear gloves and exercise due care in handling. Phenol is also light-sensitive. Always prepare and store in an amber glass bottle.
14. Phenol:chloroform (1:1): Add 1 vol of Tris-buffered phenol to an equal vol of chloroform:isoamyl alcohol (24:1) *(see below)* in an amber glass bottle. Store in the dark at 4°C under a film of 0.1 *M* Tris-HCl, pH 8.0/0.2% β-mercaptoethanol.
15. Chloroform:isoamyl alcohol (24:1): Mix 240 mL of chloroform and 10 mL of isoamyl alcohol in a glass amber bottle. Store in the dark at 4°C.
16. 2.5 *M* sodium acetate, pH 5.5.
17. Tris-CDTA: 10 m*M* Tris-HCl; 1 m*M* CDTA, pH 8.0.
18. HPLC-grade ethanol (95%).

19. Lyzozyme (lyophylized).
20. Chloramphenicol: Prepare a 34-mg/mL stock solution using 95% ethanol just prior to use.
21. Spectinomycin: Spectinomycin is usually present at 66% potency. Prepare as required at a stock concentration of 30 mg/mL in nanopure water. Sterilize by filtration (0.22 µm) before use.

2.3. Purification of Form I Plasmid DNA by Acid-Phenol Extraction

1. 50 m*M* sodium acetate/75 m*M* NaCl, pH 4.0: To 400 mL of autoclaved nanopure water, add 10 mL of 2.5*M* sodium acetate, pH 5.5, and 7.5 mL of a 5*M* NaCl stock solution. Adjust the final pH exactly to 4.0 with glacial acetic acid, and complete the vol to 500 mL. Sterilize the solution by filtration (0.22 µm) *only* and store at room temperature.
2. 50 m*M* sodium acetate, pH 4.0: To 400 mL of autoclaved nanopure water, add 10 mL of 2.5*M* sodium acetate, pH 5.5. Adjust the final pH to 4.0 with glacial acetic acid and complete the vol to 500 mL. Sterilize the solution by filtration (0.22 µm) *only* and store at room temperature.
3. Acidified phenol: Melt high-purity (redistilled) phenol in a 65°C water bath. Add an equal vol of 50 m*M* sodium acetate, pH 4.0, and shake vigorously to create an emulsion. Allow the phases to separate by gravity and remove the upper aqueous layer by aspiration. Repeat this procedure twice. Store acidified phenol in the dark at 4°C under a film of 50 m*M* sodium acetate (pH 4.0). This product has a short shelf-life and should be prepared either as required or on a biweekly basis.

3. Methods

3.1. Isolation of Form I Plasmid DNA by Triton Lysis Followed by CsCl Banding

1. Initiate a 5-mL culture from a single colony (or frozen stock) of bacteria containing the plasmid at 37°C overnight. Use the entire culture to seed 800 mL of Superbroth, and incubate for 36 h at 37°C with vigorous shaking.
2. Collect the bacteria by centrifigation at 5000*g* for 10 min (4°C), using a Sorvall GS-3 rotor (or its equivalent; DuPont).
3. Resuspend the bacteria in 100 mL of TE. Centrifuge again to pellet the material. The sample may be stored frozen (–20°C) at this stage.
4. Resuspend the pellet thoroughly in 9 mL of ice-cold TES.
5. Add 0.9 mL of 10 mg/mL lysozyme (freshly prepared in TES) and hold on ice for 5 min.

6. Add 3.7 mL of 0.25 M EDTA, pH 8.0, mix thoroughly, and hold on ice for another 5 min.
7. Add 14.5 mL of ice-cold Triton lysis solution, mix thoroughly, and hold on ice for 10 min.
8. Remove the debris by centrifugation (25,000 rpm in a Beckman SW27 rotor or its equivalent) for 30 min at 4°C.
9. Decant the supernatant into a 50-mL polypropylene tube and adjust the weight of the liquid to 30.17 g with TE. Add 28.14 g of solid CsCl and mix thoroughly until completely dissolved. Add 4.5 mL of ethidium bromide solution and mix by inversion. CAUTION: Ethidium bromide is a very strong mutagen. Always wear gloves while handling it.
10. Transfer the mixture to a Beckman polyallomer Quick Seal® ultracentrifuge tube, and seal the vessel according to the supplier's instructions. A single preparation can be accommodated by the Beckman VTi 50 or Ti 60 rotor. The VTi 50 rotor should be spun for at least 18 h at 45,000 rpm (20°C), whereas the Ti 60 unit will require a run time of at least 60 h at 35,000 rpm (20°C). NOTE: The new generation of Beckman rotors and benchtop ultracentrifuges allows for smaller plasmid preparations to be banded in much shorter time periods.
11. Following centrifugation, view the tubes under medium-wave (302-nm) UV light. CAUTION: Ultraviolet light is both mutagenic and carcinogenic. Wear adequate protection (i.e., use a UV-protective face shield [eye goggles will not protect the rest of your face or neck], ensure that your lab-coat sleeves cover your forearms, and wear latex gloves). Secure the tube and insert a 19-gage syringe needle at the top to create an air inlet. Puncture the side of the tube at a point just below the lowermost band (form I plasmid; the upperband consists of open circular and linear molecules) using a 20-mL hypodermic syringe equipped with a 19-gage needle. Collect the banded material in a total vol of 4–5 mL.
12. Either reband the plasmid sample (*see* step 13) or remove the ethidium bromide with isopropanol saturated with CsCl solution at the concentration used for banding. Dialyse extensively against a large vol of TE to remove the CsCl. Add 1/10 vol of 5 M NaCl and 2 vol of ethanol. Allow the plasmid to precipitate overnight at –20°C, and collect the material by centrifugation at 10,000g for 15 min at 4°C. Drain away the ethanol carefully and air-dry the pellet to remove all traces of ethanol.
13. It is often necessary to reband the plasmid preparation. To do this, prepare a 1.08 g/mL CsCl solution in TE. Add 0.17 mL of ethidium bromide solution for each mL of TE used. Add the DNA sample obtained in step 12 to the solution, mix thoroughly, centrifuge, and process as in steps 10–21.

3.2. Large-Scale Isolation
of Plasmid DNA by Alkaline Lysis

1. Revive a stock of plasmid-bearing bacteria in 5 mL of LB broth containing the antibiotic(s) required for plasmid selection. Incubate overnight at 37°C with shaking. The next morning, transfer 2.5 mL of the saturated culture to two 2-L Erlenmeyer flasks (each containing 500 mL of sterile antibiotic/LB broth), and grow the bacteria at 37°C with vigorous shaking (250 rpm) until the OD_{600} reaches 0.8. Add 2.5 mL of the 34 mg/mL chloramphenicol stock (final concentration, 170 µg/mL) to each flask and allow plasmid amplification to proceed over 20 h at 37°C with shaking. Plasmids containing a transcriptionally active chloramphenicol acetyl transferase cassette can be amplified using 150 µg/mL spectinomycin.

2. Harvest the bacteria by centrifugation at 500*g* for 8 min (4°C) in 500-mL Oak Ridge bottles using a Sorvall GS-3 rotor or its equivalent. Discard the supernatant into a receptacle containing germicidal detergent or liquid bleach.

3. Resuspend each bacterial pellet in 50 mL of ice-cold NTE buffer. Pool the material in a single 250-mL Oak Ridge bottle and recover the washed cells by centrifugation at 5000*g* for 8 min at 4°C using a Sorvall GS-A rotor or its equivalent. Discard the supernatant as in step 2.

4. Using a sterile 1-mL plastic pipet as a stirring rod, gently dissolve the pellet in 1 mL of ice-cold PEB I buffer. A homogeneous slurry should be obtained. Add 9 mL of ice-cold PEB I buffer supplemented with 10 mg of lysozyme, and mix thoroughly with the plastic pipet. Allow cell lysis to proceed for 30 min in ice water (*see* Note 2).

5. Add 20 mL of room-temperature PEB II and stir the mixture thoroughly but gently with the plastic pipet. The lysate should become very viscous and translucent. Hold in ice water for 15 min and stir occasionally.

6. Add 15 mL of room-temperature PEB III and stir the mixture vigorously with the plastic pipet for several min until a coarse white precipitate forms and the viscosity disappears. Hold in ice water for 30 min and collect the debris by centrifugation at 10,000*g* for 10 min (4°C).

7. Transfer the supernatant to a new 250-mL Oak Ridge bottle and add 2 vol (90 mL) of chilled (–20°C) ethanol. Mix well and precipitate the nucleic acids at –70°C for 30 min. Collect the material by centrifugation at 10,000*g* for 10 min (4°C).

8. Using a sterile pipet, gently dissolve the pellet in 5.0–7.5 mL of acetate-MOPS buffer. Transfer the solution to a sterile 30-mL Oak Ridge or Corex® tube and precipitate the nucleic acids at –70°C for 30 min. Collect the material by

centrifugation at 10,000g for 10 min (4°C) using a Sorvall HB-4 or SS-34 rotor.

9. Decant the ethanol carefully and resuspend the pellet in 5.0–7.5 mL of autoclaved nanopure water. Measure the vol of the sample and add an *equal vol* of LiCl-MOPS buffer. Mix well and place in ice water for 15 min. Centrifuge at 10,000g for 10 min (4°C). This step will precipitate the bulk of the coextracted RNA and leave the plasmid DNA (with residual low-mol-wt RNA species) in solution.

10. Using a sterile pipet, transfer the supernatant to a new Oak Ridge or Corex® tube. Hold at 60°C for 10 min, and collect any residual precipitate by centrifugation as in step 9 (*see* Note 3).

11. Divide the supernatant between two 30-mL Corex® tubes and add 2 vol of chilled ethanol. Hold at –70°C for about 1 h and recover the nucleic acids by centrifugation at 10,000g for 10 min (4°C).

12. Resuspend each pellet in 5.0–7.5 mL of acetate-MOPS buffer and combine the material in one of the Corex® tubes. Precipitate the sample with 2 vol of chilled ethanol as outlined in step 8. Repeat the precipitation once. Decant the ethanol carefully and air-dry the pellet for 10–15 min.

13. Dissolve the pellet in 5.0–7.5 mL of RNase buffer. Add 10 µL/mL RNase A stock (final concentration 10 µg/mL) and 10 µL/mL RNase T1 stock (final concentration 5 U/mL). Incubate at 37°C for 90 min.

14. Add 50 µL/mL 10% SDS stock (final concentration 0.5%) and 2.5 µL/mL proteinase K stock (final concentration 50 µg/mL). Incubate for 2 h at 37°C.

15. Extract the aqueous mixture as follows: once with Tris-buffered phenol, twice with phenol:chloroform (1:1), and once with chloroform:isoamyl alcohol (24:1). Disposable polypropylene culture tubes (sterile; 17 × 100 mm) are very practical for this purpose. For each extraction step, add an equal vol of the organic solvent, create an emulsion by shaking (do not use a mechanical vortex), and separate the phases by centrifugation at 5000g for 5 min (25°C). A Sorvall HB-4 rotor allows sharp phase separation. Transfer the upper aqueous phase to a new tube following each extraction step.

16. To the final aqueous phase, add 1/10 vol of 2.5M sodium acetate, pH 5.5, and 2 vol of chilled ethanol. Precipitate the plasmid DNA for 20 min at –70°C and centrifuge as described in step 8.

17. Clean the plasmid DNA twice by acetate-MOPS/ethanol precipitation as described in step 12. Dry the DNA pellet briefly under vacuum and dissolve in 1 mL of sterile Tris-CDTA buffer. Avoid using a mechanical vortex to assist solubilization. Determine the concentration of the plasmid DNA stock by taking the absorbance of a 1/20 dilution at 260 nm

and assuming that 1.0 OD_{260} unit is equivalent to a concentration of 50 µg DNA/mL. For example, mix 25 µL of the DNA preparation in 475 µL of Tris-CDTA. Using a 0.5 mL *quartz* cuvet (glass cuvets absorb significantly in the UV spectrum), "zero" the spectrophotometer using Tris-CDTA. Take the OD reading of the DNA and calculate its concentration as follows:

$$\text{(reading at 260 nm)} \times 20^{(1)} \times 50^{(2)} = \text{[DNA] in µg/mL}$$

where [1] is the dilution factor and [2] is the conversion factor.

The sample should also be scanned within the 200- to 300-nm range in order to obtain a rough measure of the purity of the preparation. The scan should show two peaks, the first around 205 nm (attributed to the Tris-CDTA) and the other at 260 nm (contributed by DNA). A high-purity DNA preparation should show no evidence of a shoulder beyond 260 nm, and the 260 nm/280 nm ratio should be >1.8.

If care is taken throughout the procedure to pipet gently and minimize the use of a mechanical vortex, form I plasmid DNA is routinely obtained at >90% yield for plasmids of 15 kbp or less, as verified by agarose gel electrophoresis.

3.3. Purification of Form I Plasmid DNA by Acidified-Phenol Extraction

1. Transfer the DNA stock to a sterile 1.5-mL microcentrifuge tube. Add 1/10 vol 2.5*M* sodium acetate, pH 5.5, mix well, and add 2 vol of chilled ethanol. Precipitate the DNA at –70°C for 30 min and recover by centrifugation at 10,000*g* for 10 min (4°C). Air-dry the pellet for 15 min at room temperature.

2. Gently redissolve the sample to a final concentration *not exceeding* 250 µg/mL in 50 m*M* sodium acetate/75 m*M* NaCl, pH 4.0. A total vol of 400–500 µL is practical (*see* Notes 4 and 5).

3. Add an equal vol of acidified phenol and shake vigorously by hand (DO NOT VORTEX) for 2–3 min. Separate the phases by centrifugation at 10,000*g* for 60 s at room temperature.

4. Transfer the upper aqueous layer to a sterile 1.5-mL microcentrifuge tube and precipitate the plasmid DNA as outlined in Step 1. Redissolve the pellet in 250 µL of acetate-MOPS buffer and precipitate the DNA with 2 vol of chilled ethanol. Repeat this step once. Resuspend the DNA sample in 0.5 mL of Tris-CDTA. Determine the concentration and verify the integrity of the preparation by spectrophotometry and agarose gel electrophoresis, respectively. One round of acid-phenol extraction is generally sufficient to achieve a high degree (i.e., > 98% form I) of plasmid purification.

4. Notes

1. The preparative alkaline extraction scheme will provide between 0.8 and 2 mg of plasmid DNA from 1 L of amplified bacterial culture, depending on the plasmid construct and the host strain. Alternatively, between 0.3 and 0.8 mg of material can be isolated from 250 mL of saturated (nonamplified) cultures. The latter provides adequate yields and is very practical for processing multiple samples. Because bacterial growth is inhibited during plasmid amplification, the vols of the PEB extraction buffers should not be scaled down when 250-mL cultures are used for extraction. If this is done, the high viscosity of the lysate will reduce plasmid recovery.

2. The recovery of plasmid DNA will depend greatly on the efficiency of cell lysis. For this reason, ensure that the bacterial pellet is completely resuspended in the PEB I buffer prior to the addition of lysozyme.

3. Many bacterial strains produce endonucleases. Heating the plasmid in the LiCl-MOPS solution also ensures inactivation of these potential contaminants.

4. Effective and quantitative recovery of form I DNA by acidified-phenol extraction is critically dependent on pH and ionic strength. For this reason, acidified phenol stocks and equilibration buffers should be prepared carefully. Phenol stocks previously equilibrated to pH 8.0 with Tris buffer should *never* be used as starting material.

5. RNA will not be removed by acid-phenol treatment.

6. Purified DNA stocks destined for use in gene-transfer experiments should be stored frozen (–20°C), in small aliquots. Once thawed, samples should not be refrozen, but rather stored under aseptic conditions at 4°C. The integrity of the donor DNA should be verified periodically by agarose gel electrophoresis. We do not recommend storing DNA over a drop of chloroform, since this solvent will prove cytotoxic to recipient cells even in small amounts.

References

1. Gorman, C. (1985) High efficiency gene transfer into mammalian cells, in *DNA Cloning,* vol. II. (Glover, D. M., ed.), IRL, Oxford, pp. 143–190.
2. Zasloff, M., Ginder, G. D., and Felsenfeld, G. (1978) A new method for the purification and identification of covalently closed circular DNA molecules. *Nucleic Acids Res.* **5**, 1139.
3. Birnboim, H. C. (1983) A rapid alkaline extraction method for the isolation of plasmid DNA. *Methods Enzymol.* **100**, 243.
4. Muller, M., Hofer, B., Koch, A., and Koster, H. (1983) Aspects of the mechanism of acid phenol extraction of nucleic acids. *Biochem. Biophys. Acta* **740**, 1.

CHAPTER 2

Calcium Phosphate Mediated Gene Transfer into Established Cell Lines

Hiroto Okayama and Claudia Chen

1. Introduction

DNA transfection is one of the most important techniques in molecular genetics. It is this technique that has made possible the dissection of complex eukaryotic genes and the characterization of the function of their components *(1–7)* as well as the isolation of particular genes on the basis of their expression in cultured cells *(8–11)*.

The most widely used transfection method involves the use of calcium phosphate *(12)*, as a facilitator for adsorption onto the cell surface and subsequent uptake of transfected DNA. When calcium chloride, DNA, and a buffer containing phosphate are mixed at a neutral pH, visible precipitates of a calcium phosphate–DNA complex are formed. Following the addition to culture cells, the calcium phosphate–DNA complex forms a sediment on the surface of the cells, and is then actively taken up by endocytosis. The complex taken up into the phagosome is transported to various cellular organella, including the nucleus. Most of the DNA within the nucleus is retained as extrachromosomal DNA for only a short period of time (transient expression) and is gradually degraded, then subsequently lost from the nucleoplasm of the proliferating host cells. However, some DNA will integrate into the host chromosome by nonspecific recombination, leading to stable transformation of the cells to the new phenotype encoded by the DNA.

From: *Methods in Molecular Biology, Vol. 7: Gene Transfer and Expression Protocols*
Edited by: E. J. Murray © 1991 The Humana Press Inc., Clifton, NJ

The calcium phosphate method was originally developed by Graham and van der Eb in 1973 *(12)*. Subsequently, various modifications of this method have been made in an attempt to improve the transfection efficiency. These modifications center around the posttransfection treatment of the cells with various chemicals, including glycerol *(13)*, DMSO *(14)*, tubulin inhibitors *(15)*, and lysosomal inhibitors *(16)*, and result in a 10–100-fold increase in the efficiency for some cell lines. Although they generally work well for transient expression (>10% of the cell population), these modified methods are still inefficient for stable transformation. Only a small fraction of transfected cells (0.001–1%) are stably transformed.

Recently, Chen and Okayama found that the *in situ* formation of calcium phosphate–DNA complex in culture medium during incubation with the cells greatly enhances stable transformation frequencies of various fibroblastic and epithelial cell lines *(17)*. Using this method, commonly used cell lines L, NIH3T3, BHK, HeLa, CV1, NRK, C127, and CHO are stably transformed at efficiencies of 10–50% with pcD*neo* *(17,18)*.

Two calcium phosphate methods are described here. The first is the standard calcium phosphate method developed by van der Eb *(12)*, with the modification of the use of the posttransfection glycerol treatment *(16)*. In this method, calcium phosphate–DNA precipitates are formed in the test tube by mixing calcium chloride, a HEPES buffer of pH 7.1, containing sodium phosphate and DNA. The precipitate is then added to the culture dishes containing rapidly growing cells. After 4–6 h of incubation with the precipitate, cells are given an osmotic shock with 15% glycerol.

The second method is the *in situ* precipitation method developed by Chen and Okayama *(17,18)*. This method uses a sodium phosphate containing buffer of pH 6.95. Because of the slightly acidic pH, calcium phosphate–DNA precipitates are not formed in the test tube. Instead, after addition of the mixture to the culture dishes, the precipitates slowly develop in the medium before being actively taken up by the cells during the next 16–24 h incubation.

For stable transformation, both methods work equally well for genomic DNA, but the second method is 5–30-fold more efficient for circular plasmid DNA. For transient expression, both are almost identical. A variety of established cell lines can be used as a host for these methods. However, anchorage growth-independent cells, such as immune cells, are generally a poor host for calcium phosphate mediated transfection.

2. Materials

2.1. In Vitro Precipitation Method

1. 2.5 M CaCl$_2$: Filter-sterilize and store at –20°C.
2. 2X HBS: 280 mM NaCl, 1.5 mM Na$_2$HPO$_4$, 50 mM HEPES (pH 7.1)

(HEPES: N-2-Hydroxyethylpiperazine-N'-2-ethanesulfonic acid). Adjust the pH to 7.1 with 1 M NaOH at 25°C. Filter-sterilize and store at –20°C.

3. TE: 10 mM Tris-HCl, pH 7.5; 1 mM EDTA.

4. 15% glycerol:glycerol, 15 mL; distilled water to 100 mL. Filter-sterilize and store at –20°C.

5. Trypsin(/EDTA) solution: NaCl, 8 g; KCl, 0.2 g; Na_2HPO_4, 1.15 g; KH_2PO_4, 0.2 g; (EDTA.2Na.2H$_2$O, 0.2 g for trypsin/EDTA solution); trypsin, 5 g; distilled water to 1 L. Filter-sterilize and store at –20°C.

6. PBS: KCl, 0.2 g; KH_2PO_4, 0.2 g; NaCl, 8 g; Na_2HPO_4, 1.15 g; distilled water to 1 L. Autoclave and store at –20°C.

7. DNA: 1 mg/mL in TE.

2.2. In Situ *Precipitation Method*

Follow the in vitro precipitation method, but substitute 2× HBS for 2× BBS.

1. 2× BBS (280 mM NaCl, 1.5 mM Na_2HPO_4, 50 mM BES [pH 6.95]): NaCl, 16.3 g; BES, N-,N-bis(2-hydroxy-ethyl)-2-amino-ethane-sulfonic acid, 10.6 g; Na_2HPO_4, 0.21 g; distilled water to 1 L. Adjust the pH to 6.95 with 1 M NaOH at 25°C. Filter-sterilize, aliquot, and store at –20°C.

3. Methods

3.1. The In Vitro Precipitation Method (Note 1)

1. Aspirate the medium (Dulbecco's Modified Eagle's Medium, αMEM, RPMI) from the dish containing rapidly growing anchorage-dependent cells (*see* Note 2). Rinse twice with 10 mL of PBS. Trypsinize cells with 1 mL of trypsin solution (or trypsin/EDTA) at room temperature for 1–3 min, until cells are about to detach from dish (*see* Note 3).

2. Seed 5×10^5 cells in a 10-cm culture dish containing 10 mL of fresh growth medium. Incubate overnight at 37°C in 5–7% CO_2.

3. Dilute 2.5 M CaCl$_2$ tenfold with sterile distilled water. Take 0.5 mL of 0.25 M CaCl$_2$ into a sterile 15-mL Falcon tube. DNA (1 mg/mL in TE) is then added to the CaCl$_2$ solution (*see* Notes 1 and 4). Add 0.5 mL of 2× HBS dropwise to the mixture with constant swirling, and leave it at room temperature for 20 min.

4. Add the mixture dropwise to the dish containing the growing cells, swirl the dish to mix well, and incubate for 4–6 h (for genomic DNA transfection, 15–24 h) at 37°C in 5–7% CO_2. Aspirate the medium and rinse the cells with 10 mL of PBS.

5. Add 2 mL of 15% glycerol to the dish, swirling the dish to spread glycerol evenly on the cells. Incubate for 1 min at room temperature (*see* Note 1). Aspirate the glycerol, and rinse the cells twice with 10 mL of PBS and twice with 10 mL of growth medium. (This step is for plasmid DNA transfection only.)
6. Refeed the cells with fresh growth medium. Incubate at 37°C for 24 h in 5–7% CO_2.
7. Trypsinize and split the cells at an appropriate ratio (>1:10). Incubate the cells for another 24 h under the regular growth conditions before starting selection (*see* Notes 4 and 5; Chapter 19). For assaying the transient expression of transfected DNA, incubate the cells for 48 h before harvest without splitting.

3.2. The In Situ *Precipitation Method (Note 6)*

1. Aspirate the medium (Dulbecco's Modified Eagle's Medium, αMEM, RPMI) from the dish containing rapidly growing anchorage-dependent cells (*see* Note 2). Rinse twice with 10 mL of PBS. Trypsinize cells with 1 mL of trypsin solution at room temperature for 1–3 min, until cells are about to detach from dish (*see* Note 3).
2. Seed 5×10^5 cells in a 10 cm culture dish containing 10 mL of fresh growth medium (Dulbecco's Modified Eagle's Medium plus 10% fetal bovine serum). Incubate overnight at 35°C in 5% CO_2.
3. Make $0.25M$ $CaCl_2$ by diluting $2.5M$ $CaCl_2$ stock solution tenfold with sterile distilled water. Take 0.5 mL of $0.25M$ $CaCl_2$ into a sterile 15 mL Falcon tube. Add the optimum amount (generally between 10–30 μg) of DNA to the $CaCl_2$ solution. Add 0.5 mL of 2× BBS to the mixture, and leave it at room temperature for 10 min.
4. Add the mixture dropwise to the dish containing the growing cells, and swirl it to mix well. Incubate for 15–24 h at 35°C in 3% CO_2.
5. Aspirate the medium, and rinse the cells with 10 mL of growth medium. Refeed with fresh growth medium, and incubate at 35°C for 24 h in 5–7% CO_2.
6. Trypsinize and split cells at an appropriate ratio (>1:10). Refeed and incubate for another 24 h under regular growth conditions before selection (*see* Notes 4 and 5). For assaying transient expression of transfected DNA, incubate the cells for 48 h without splitting.

4. Notes

1. The in vitro precipitation method is relatively insensitive to the amount of DNA and the culture conditions used, and generally yields nearly the same number of transformants or a level of expression

between 10 and 40 µg DNA. Glycerol is toxic to cells. The optimum duration of glycerol treatment may differ and should be found for each cell line. When genomic DNA is used as carrier DNA, use the protocol for genomic DNA transfection.

2. Unhealthy cells, such as mycoplasma-infected cells, or cells grown either to confluency or under suboptimal conditions, generally give poor results.

3. Some cells are sensitive to EDTA, and some others are difficult to detach from the dish with trypsin only. Test trypsin and trypsin/EDTA on your cells, and use the regimen that gives better survival.

4. Transfection vectors also greatly influence transformation frequencies. Use of a vector that expresses the marker gene weakly, or use of a marker gene that requires harsh selection conditions, generally results in poor transformation. For many epithelial or fibroblastic cells, the *neo* marker gene yields approx 10× more transformants than the Eco*gpt (19)*, hygromycin *(20)*, or *hprt* markers *(17)*. For the best results, use the minimum selectable concentration of G418 (the smallest dose that will kill all the cells within 10–14 d) for each cell line, and split cells at a ratio of >1:20. *See* Chapter 19 for further details. pcD*neo* is 5–10× as efficient as pSV2*neo (17)*.

5. During selection of transformants, the composition of growth medium is not so critical: 10% fetal bovine serum can be substituted with 5% fetal bovine serum plus 10% newborn bovine serum for most of the commonly used cell lines.

6. The *in situ* precipitation method is very sensitive to the quality and amount of DNA, the pH of 2× BBS, and the CO_2 level of incubator during transfection. Plasmid DNA used for transfection should be clean and free of contamination by *E. coli* proteins. DNA purified through a Dowex column is generally contaminated by a chemical highly toxic to cells. The optimum amount of DNA often changes with host cells and preparations of 2× BBS, growth medium, and DNA. When one of these is newly prepared or a new host cell is used, the DNA amount should be reoptimized. The optimum DNA amount is roughly determined by observing the properties of the calcium phosphate precipitate formed after overnight incubation with the cells. At a suboptimum DNA amount, the precipitate is coarse and forms clumps. At a supraoptimum DNA amount, the precipitate is very fine and barely visible under the microscope at a low magnification power. At the optimum DNA amount, precipitates are always fine but visible, and homogeneous in size *(17)*. Transfection conditions are optimized for Dulbecco's Modified Eagle's Medium plus 10% fetal bovine serum, and are proven to work well for αMEM and RPMI. If your cells require a special medium, the DNA amount and the pH of 2× BBS may have to be reoptimized.

References

1. Banerji, J., Olson, L., and Schaffner, W. (1983) A lymohocyte-specific cellular enhancer is located downstream of the joining region in immunoglobulin heavy chain genes. *Cell* **33,** 727–740.
2. Benoist, C. and Chambon, P. (1981) In vivo sequence requirements of the SV40 early region. *Nature* **290,** 304–309.
3. Fromm, M. and Berg, P. (1982) Deletion mapping of DNA regions required for SV40 early promoter function *in vivo. J. Mol. Appl. Genet.* **1,** 457–481.
4. Ghosh, P. K., Lebowitz, P., Frisque, R. J., and Gluzman, Y. (1981) Identification of a promoter component involved in positioning the 5' termini of simian virus 40 early mRNAs. *Proc. Natl. Acad. Sci. USA* **78,** 100–104.
5. Queen, C. and Baltimore, D. (1983) Immunoglobulin gene transcription is activated by downstream sequence elements. *Cell* **33,** 741–748.
6. Schechter, A. L., Stern, D. F., Vaidyanathan, L., Decker, S. J., Drebin, J. A., Greene, M. I., and Weinberg, R. A. (1984) The nue oncogene: An erb-B-related gene encoding a 185,000-M_r tumour antigen. *Nature* **321,** 513–616.
7. Shih, C. and Weinberg, R. A. (1982) Isolation of a transforming sequence from a human bladder carcinoma cell line. *Cell* **29,** 161–169.
8. Shimizu, K., Goldfarb, M., Perucho, M., and Wigler, M. (1983) Isolation and preliminary characterization of the transforming gene of a human neuroblastoma cell line. *Proc. Natl. Acad. Sci. USA* **80,** 383–387.
9. Westerveld, A., Hoeijimakers, H. J., van Duin, M., deWit, J., Odijk, H., Pastink, A., R. D. Wood, R. D., and Bootsma, D. (1984) Molecular cloning of a human DNA repair gene. *Nature* **310,** 425–429.
10. Jolly, D. J., Esty, A. C., Bernard, H. U., and Friedman, T. (1982) Isolation of a genomic clone partially encoding human hypoxanthine phosphoribosyl transferase. *Proc. Natl. Acad. Sci. USA* **79,** 5038–5041.
11. Noda,M., Kitayama, H., Matsuzaki, T., Sugimoto, Y., Okayama, H., Bassin, R. H., and Ikawa, Y. (1989) Detection of genes with a potential for suppressing the transformed phenotype associated with activated *ras* genes. *Proc. Natl. Acad. Sci. USA* **86,** 162–166.
12. Graham, F. L. and van der Eb, A. J. (1973) A new technique for the assay of infectivity of human adenovirus 5. *Virology* **52,** 456–467.
13. Parker, B. A. and Strak, G. R. (1979) Regulation of simian virus 40 transcription: Sensitive analysis of the RNA species present early in infections by virus or viral DNA. *J. Virol.* **31,** 360–369.
14. Lewis, W. H., Strinivasan, P. R., Stokoe, N., and Siminovitch, L. (1980) Parameters governing the transfer of the genes for the thymidine kinase and dihydrofolate reductase into mouse cells using metephase chromosomes or DNA. *Somatic Cell Genet.* **6,** 333–348.
15. Faber, F. E. and Eberle, R. (1976) Effects of cytochalasin and alkaloid drugs on the biological expression of herpes simplex virus type 2 DNA. *Exp. Cell Res.* **103,** 15–22.
16. Luthman, H. and Magnusson, G. (1983) High efficiency polyoma DNA transfection of chloroquine treated cells. *Nucleic Acids Res.* **11,** 1295–1307.
17. Chen, C. and Okayama, H. (1987) High-efficiency transformation of mammalian cells by plasmid DNA. *Mol. Cell. Biol.* **7,** 2745–2752.
18. Chen, C. A. and Okayama, H. (1988) Calcium phosphate-mediated gene transfer: A highly efficient transfection system for stably transforming cells with plasmid DNA. *Biotechniques* **6,** 632–638.

19. Mulligan, R. C. and Berg, P. (1981) Selection for animal cells that express the *Escherichia coli* gene coding for xanthine-guanine phosphoribosyltransferase. *Proc. Natl. Acad. Sci. USA* **78,** 2072–2076.
20. Kaster, K. R., Burgett, S. G., Nagaraja, R., and Ingolia, T. D. (1983) Analysis of a bacterial hygromycin B resistance gene by transcriptional and translational fusion and by DNA sequencing. *Nucleic Acids Res.* **11,** 6895–6911.

CHAPTER 3

Transfection of the Chloramphenicol-Acetyltransferase Gene into Eukaryotic Cells Using Diethyl-Aminoethyl (DEAE)-Dextran

Richard A. Lake and Michael J. Owen

1. Introduction

The study of gene regulation in eukaryotic cells involves a practical requirement for two distinct techniques: first, a transfection system, or more simply, a way of getting DNA into a cell; and second, a reporter system, which, as the name suggests, is a means of finding out what the transfected DNA does from its new location inside the cell. These two requirements are amply met by transfecting cells, in the presence of the polycation diethyl aminoethyl-dextran (DEAE-dextran), with a plasmid vector that has regulatory sequences adjacent to the chloramphenicol acetyl transferase (CAT) gene. This type of gene transfer is often referred to as a transient expression system. Production of the CAT enzyme peaks at around 40–48 h and thereafter the level falls as the plasmid DNA is diluted out in a growing population of cells. The general strategy of subcloning putative regulatory regions followed by transfection and quantification of CAT activity is outlined in a flow diagram (Fig. 1).

From: *Methods in Molecular Biology, Vol. 7: Gene Transfer and Expression Protocols*
Edited by: E. J. Murray ©1991 The Humana Press Inc., Clifton, NJ

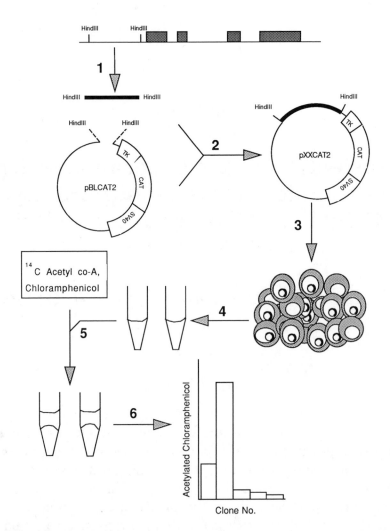

Fig. 1. Flow diagram showing the key steps in transient transfection analysis. (1) Putative regulatory regions are excised from genomic DNA by restriction enzyme digestion. Fragments are (2) subcloned into the CAT vector and (3) transfected into eukaryotic cells using DEAE dextran. (4) About 40 h after transfection, the cells are lysed and the lysates incubated with chloramphenicol and radiolabeled acetyl coenzyme A. (5) Radiolabeled chloramphenicol is extracted from the mixture and (6) the level of radioactivity related to the function of the subcloned fragment.

In 1965, DEAE-dextran was shown to increase the infectivity of poliovirus RNA for cells in culture: subsequently, a similar increase in infectivity was shown for the DNA from SV40 *(1)*. Interestingly, DEAE-dextran reduced the infectivity of intact virus. It seems likely that the key interaction is coulombic. Thus, DNA, which has a net negative charge, forms a complex with the positively charged DEAE-dextran; the complex binds to the cell surface, from where it is internalized by endocytosis. The transfected DNA enters the nucleus, but it is not integrated into chromatin during the period of the assay. DEAE-dextran is a suitable transfection vehicle for most cell types. Both adherent cells and those that grow in suspension can be transfected by this method. Cell lines are differentially susceptible to the toxic effects of increasing concentrations of DEAE-dextran. This, coupled with the variation of the optimum ratio of DEAE-dextran to plasmid DNA for transfection between cell lines, means that it is essential to titrate the DEAE-dextran for each cell line.

There are a number of plasmid vectors that are suitable for transfection analyses. We routinely use the constructions pBLCAT2 and pBLCAT3 *(2)* because both have multiple unique restriction sites, both 5' and 3' of the CAT gene (Fig. 2). In general, plasmid vectors must contain an origin of replication and an antibiotic resistance marker. These sequences allow the amplification and selection of the plasmid in a bacterial host. Eukaryotic control elements must also be present to achieve efficient expression in transfected cells: pBLCAT2 and pBLCAT3 contain the small t intron and polyadenylation signals from SV40. In addition, the promoter of the thymidine kinase (*tk*) gene from herpes simplex virus has been appropriately inserted in pBLCAT2. No transcriptional activity from the CAT gene can be detected after transfection of pBLCAT3 into eukaryotic cells. We have noted only minimal activity from the *tk* promoter of pBLCAT2 in the absence of an enhancer element after transfection into a range of different cells.

Several properties of the CAT enzyme make it the reporter protein of choice for many systems. CAT is not normally expressed by eukaryotic cells. Furthermore, its presence within the cytoplasm is not toxic to the host cell. Until recently, however, quantification of CAT activity necessitated a laborious separation procedure involving thin-layer chromatography, followed by scraping plates and scintillation counting *(3)*. Here we give detailed modifications of a procedure originally described by Sleigh *(4)*. The assay is simple, cheap, reliable, and reproducible, and it has a sensitivity (0.001 IU) that compares well with the chromatographic method.

Transient expression systems can be used to define minimal functional regions around a gene; in other words, they are used to locate both promoters and enhancers. By cloning putative regulatory elements in tandem or at either side of the CAT gene, it becomes possible to investigate not only the properties of isolated elements within a compound structure, but also the tissue specificity of the different elements. Deletion studies across an enhancer can reveal both positive and negative regulatory elements that define within a cell type the level of expression of a given gene. Most cellular genes require enhancer elements for efficient transcription. Enhancers are de-

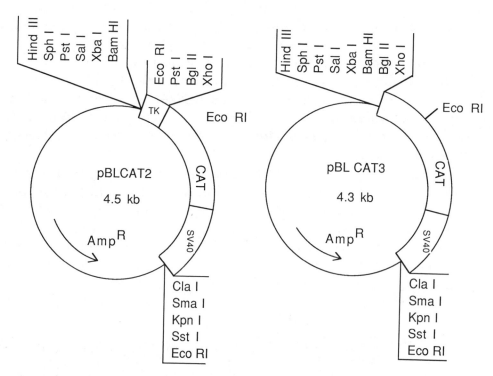

Fig. 2. Vectors for the functional analysis of eukaryotic regulatory elements. The CAT gene, the small t intron, and the polyadenylation signal from SV40 were inserted into pUC18. The herpes simplex virus thymidine kinase (*tk*) promoter is situated 5' of the CAT gene in pBLCAT2 (*see* ref. 2).

fined operationally by their ability to function over large distances upstream or downstream of a gene and in either orientation. It is now clear that many enhancers are composite structures of individual motifs that serve to bind transacting factors that, in turn, regulate transcription. Thus, tissue-specific gene expression depends crucially on the differential presence in cells of transcriptional activators (5).

It is important to be aware that the interaction of an enhancer with a heterologous promoter (e.g., *tk* in pBLCAT2) may well be different from that of the homologous pair. Thus, it is advisable to confirm and extend an analysis of enhancer specificity, using the homologous promoter. One recent study in transgenic mice underlined this problem clearly. A globin gene under the control of its own promoter and the *CD2* enhancer was expressed in *both* T-cells and erythroblasts (6). In conclusion, it seems likely that tissue specific gene expression can result from both promoter and enhancer elements individually, as well as their cognate interaction (*reviewed* in 7).

2. Materials

2.1. Materials for Transfection

1. Cells for transfection.
2. Medium for cell growth: We use a commercial RPMI 1640 containing penicillin (100 U/mL) and streptomycin (100 μg/mL), and supplemented with glutamine (2 mM). Complete growth medium additionally contains 10% fetal calf serum (FCS). Cells are grown at 37°C in a water-saturated atmosphere of 5% CO_2 in air.
3. Trypsin, 0.025% in isotonic saline: for subculture of adherent cells. Use only tissue-culture-grade material. Some cells are detached more readily using trypsin and EDTA (2 g/L); both solutions can be bought as (×10) liquid concentrates.
4. Plasmid DNA (1 mg/mL) (Note 1).
5. DEAE-dextran (average M_r 500,000; transfection-grade material): Make a stock solution of 100 mg/mL in distilled water. This should be filtered (0.22 μm) and is then stable at 4°C.
6. Dimethyl sulfoxide (DMSO, AnalaR grade).
7. Tris-buffered saline, pH 7.4 (TBS): 25 mM Tris-HCl pH 7.4, 137 mM NaCl, 5 mM KCl, 0.7 mM CaCl$_2$, 0.5 mM MgCl$_2$, 0.6 mM NaH$_2$PO$_4$. TBS can be autoclaved or sterilized by filtration, and is then stable at room temperature.

2.2. Materials for CAT Assay

1. Phosphate-buffered saline, pH 7.2 (PBS): 137 mM NaCl, 2.7 mM KCl, 8 mM Na$_2$HPO$_4$, 1.47 mM KH$_2$PO$_4$.
2. Hypotonic Tris buffer, pH 7.4 (TNE): 10 mM Tris-HCl, pH 7.4, 100 mM NaCl, 1 mM EDTA.
3. Chloramphenicol: stock solution, 0.1 M in ethyl alcohol (stable at least 6 mo at −20°C).
4. Acetyl coenzyme A, sodium salt: stock solution, 4 mM (stable at least 6 mo at −20°C; store at −70°C if possible).
5. [1-^{14}C] Acetyl coenzyme A, 50–60 mCi/mM. Store in aliquots as above.
6. Ethyl acetate (AnalaR grade).
7. 0.25 M Tris-HCl, pH 7.8.
8. Chloramphenicol acetyl transferase (CAT). Store aliquots at −20°C.

3. Methods

3.1. Transfection Method (Nonadherent Cells)

1. Work at ambient temperature (17–20°C).

2. Harvest cells from mid-log phase by centrifugation (200*g*/10 min). The importance of the state of the cells cannot be overemphasized, since use of an effete population will result in poor expression of CAT (Fig. 3). For reproducible results, seed the cells at 25% of their maximum density 18 h before transfection. For weakly adherent cells, harvest at 50% or lower confluence and use only the most gentle treatments to separate the cells from the plate (*see* Notes 2 and 7). Alternatively, it is quite reasonable to carry out the whole procedure *in situ (see below)*.

3. Wash the cells twice in serum-free RPMI 1640, and then once more in TBS (*see* Note 3).

4. Resuspend the cells in TBS at 10^6 cells/mL. Take 10 mL of this suspension in a 15 mL Falcon tube for each transfection. Pellet the cells (200*g*/10 min).

5. Resuspend the cells in a transfection cocktail that consists of 20 μg plasmid DNA in 375 μL TBS and 125 μL of DEAE-dextran (1mg/mL) (*see* Note 4).

6. Leave the cells at room temperature for 15 min. Resuspend them by gentle agitation of the tube and leave them for a further 15 min.

7. Add 0.5 mL of 20% DMSO (in TBS) to each tube and mix by gentle agitation (*see* Note 5).

8. After 2 min add 10 mL of RPMI 1640 containing 10% FCS (complete growth medium) to each tube, mix by inversion, and pellet the cells.

9. Wash the cells one more time and seed them in 10 mL of fresh complete growth medium (*see* Note 6).

10. Return the cells to 37°C for 40–48 h.

3.2. Transfection Method (Adherent Cells)

1. Seed the cells at between 1 and 5×10^6 cells/9-cm dish in 10 mL of complete growth medium 18 h before transfection (*see* Note 7).

2. Wash the cells twice in serum-free RPMI 1640 by simply aspirating old medium and adding 10 mL of fresh medium. Swirl the fresh medium over the cells 3 or 4 times before aspirating.

3. In similar manner, wash the cells twice in TBS.

4. Add 5mL of transfection cocktail, which contains 20 μg plasmid DNA and 250 μg DEAE-dextran (*see* Note 4).

5. Leave the plates at room temperature for 30 min. Aspirate the transfection cocktail and add 5 mL of 10% DMSO in TBS.

6. After 2 min wash the cells twice using 10 mL of complete growth medium and seed them in 10 mL of fresh medium.

7. Return the plates to 37°C for 40–48 h.

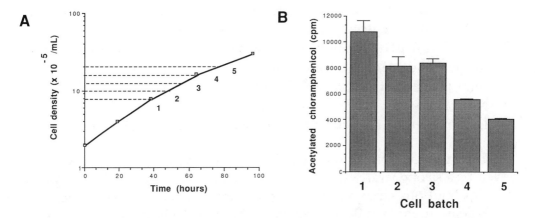

Fig. 3. Jurkat cells in logarithmic growth phase express CAT most efficiently after transfection. A population of actively growing Jurkat cells (8×10^5 /mL) was divided into five aliquots (50 mL each), and 0, 25, 50, 100, or 150 mL of fresh medium was added to each culture. After the cells were grown for 40 h, they were subjected to transfection with 20 µg of pRSVCAT. The cell density was determined, and each batch was then transfected in triplicate. (A) The cell counts were used to reconstruct a growth curve. (B) The transfection efficiency in each different cell batch was quantified as described.

3.3. Preparation of Cell Lysates

1. Work at 4°C or on ice.
2. Harvest the cells and wash them twice in PBS.
3. Resuspend the cell pellet in 1 mL of TNE. Leave on ice for 5 min (*see* Note 8).
4. Pellet the cells and resuspend them in 120 µL of 0.25 *M* Tris-HCl, pH 7.8 (*see* Note 9).
5. Completely lyse the cells by subjecting them to three cycles of freezing and thawing. Snap-freeze on dry ice (5–10 min) or in liquid nitrogen (3–4 min), then thaw at 37°C (3–4 min). Vortex the mixture after each cycle.
6. Heat-inactivate CAT inhibitors at 65°C for 10 min (*see* Note 10).
7. Cool the tubes on ice and pellet the cell debris in a microfuge (12,000g/10 min). Store the supernatants at –20°C.

3.4. CAT Assay

1. Dilute the stock reagents. The best way to do this is to make a cocktail. Thus, for 10 reactions, mix 16 µL chloramphenicol (0.1 *M*), 22.5 µL acetyl coenzyme A (4 m *M*), 20 µL 1-^{14}C Acetyl coenzyme A (1 µCi), and 341.5 µL distilled water. Add 40 µL of cocktail to each 60 µL of cell lysate, mix, and incubate at 37°C in a water bath for 1 h.

2. Cool the tubes on ice. Add 200 µL of ethyl acetate to each tube. Vortex for 30 s, and then centrifuge the tubes (12,000g/3 min).
3. Transfer 170 µL of the organic (upper) phase to a scintillation vial. Add a further 200 µL of fresh ethyl acetate to the original tubes and reextract. This time, take 200 µL of the organic phase and add it to the first portion (*see* Note 11).
4. Determine the radioactivity in each tube by liquid scintillation counting.

Each transfection should include, as a positive control, the CAT gene driven by a strong viral promoter and enhancer. We use pRSVCAT, which contains the Rous sarcoma virus long terminal repeat. The construction is highly active in many different cell lines. We also include standards of CAT enzyme. The assay is sensitive to <0.001U of enzyme. Results can then be given either as the absolute amount of CAT produced per unit number of cells or, probably more meaningfully, as a percentage of the activity of pRSVCAT in similarly transfected cells.

It is important to know that differences in the measured CAT activity of two constructions are a function of the regulatory sequence under investigation and not trivially resulting from differences in the amount of plasmid DNA that gets into the cells. We cotransfect with a marker plasmid (*see* Chapters 16–18) or use Southern analysis *(8)* to accommodate any such variability.

4. Notes

1. All DNA preparations should be pure; double banding through cesium chloride gradients *(8)* or a preparation of equivalent high quality is essential (*see also* Chapter 1).
2. Use a rubber policeman to scrape the cells from the plastic surface. These can be bought individually and asceptically wrapped, or you can construct your own. Take some thin walled silicon rubber tubing, cut it into 3- to 4-mm² pieces, and wash these thoroughly, using detergents. Store the pieces in 70% alcohol and use them with forceps. They are reusable.
3. The washing procedure may seem overly laborious, but, clearly, any protein present during the transfection could interfere with the uptake of DNA, and there is some evidence that phosphates reduce the transfection efficiency *(9)*. In any case, it is convenient to count a portion of the cells and to prepare the transfection cocktail during these washing cycles.
4. The most effective concentrations of DNA and DEAE-dextran must be empirically determined. The concentrations listed are, in our experience, median values; transfection efficiency can be improved severalfold by

Table 1
Variation of Transfection Efficiency[a]

DNA concentration, μg/mL	Acetylated chloramphenicol, cpm DEAE-dextran concentration		
	500 μg/mL	250 μg/mL	125 μg/mL
2	677	1688	1480
20	1682	12,307	29,368
200	20,670	125,640	2207

[a]Jurkat cells were transfected with pRSVCAT as described. The concentrations of pRSVCAT and DEAE-dextran were varied independently, and the results are expressed as the mean of duplicate counts of acetylated chloramphenicol from a typical experiment.

titrating the DEAE-dextran over a range of doubling dilutions. Table 1 shows an example of this type of checkerboard titration. Although it is possible to get higher levels of expression by using more DNA, 20 μg is a reasonable compromise amount. Furthermore, the given assay conditions allow for a maximum possible conversion of around 200,000 cpm: values that approach this maximum are less likely to be related in a linear fashion to the amount of CAT enzyme.

5. There are many reports in the literature of manipulations designed to improve the efficiency of expression of transfected DNA. We have found that a 10% DMSO shock, as described by Sussman and Milman (9), is both easy to administer and reproducible in its effects. Others report enhanced expression after a 15% glycerol shock (10) or by treatment with sodium butyrate (11). Similarly, exposure of cells to chloroquine after DEAE-dextran-mediated transfection of polyoma DNA increased the transformation efficiency sixfold (12).

6. The cells, depending on type, often aggregate after transfection. They can be dispersed before final seeding by gently pipeting them up and down.

7. Subculture of adherent cells requires their removal from the plate and reseeding at a lower density. Add 1 mL of trypsin/EDTA solution per 9-cm dish and swirl to ensure good contact of the medium. After 1–2 min, the cells viewed under a microscope should be rounded. They can be dislodged by gentle rotation of the plate. Fetal calf serum contains trypsin inhibitor and should be added (as complete growth medium) as soon as the cells are detached.

8. This hypotonic solution causes the cells to swell, so that their subsequent lysis is complete.

9. This volume is sufficient for a duplicate CAT assay. We routinely cotransfect with a marker plasmid (β-galactosidase) to monitor transfection efficiency in different tubes, and therefore make the cell lysate to 150 μL; 2 × 60 μL for CAT assay and 1 × 30 μL for the β-galactosidase assay (Chapter 17).

10. Sleigh (*4*) reports a marked loss of CAT activity if this step is not followed. The heat-sensitive CAT-degrading factor is probably a protease.

11. Take considerable care throughout this procedure. Any contamination with the aqueous phase will result in a spuriously high value. It is better to take less organic phase and reextract than to risk such contamination. Differences between the duplicates almost always result from problems at this step.

Acknowledgments

We would like to thank our colleagues at the ICRF laboratories at Dominion House for their helpful advice. Figure 1 is an adaptation of an idea originally created by David Wotton.

References

1. McCutchan, J. H. and Pagano, J. S. (1968) Enhancement of the infectivity of Simian Virus 40 Deoxyribonucleic acid with Diethylaminoethyl-Dextran. *J. Natl. Can. Inst.* **41**, 351–356.

2. Luckow, B. and Schutz, G. (1987) CAT constructions with multiple unique restriction sites for the functional analysis of eukaryotic promoters and regulatory elements. *Nucleic Acids Res.* **15(13)**, 5490.

3. Gorman, C. M., Moffat, L. M., and Howard, B. H. (1982) Recombinant genomes which express chloramphenicol acetyltransferase in mammalian cells. *Mol. Cell. Biol.* **2(9)**, 1044–1051.

4. Sleigh, M. J. (1986) A nonchromatographic assay for the expression of the chloramphenicol acetyltransferase gene in eukaryotic cells. *Anal. Biochem.* **156**, 251–256.

5. Ptashne, M. (1988) How eukaryotic transcriptional activators work. *Nature* **335**, 683–689.

6. Greaves, D. R., Wilson, F. D., Lang, G., and Kioussis, D. (1989) Human CD2 3' flanking sequences confer high level, T-cell specific, position independent gene expression in transgenic mice. *Cell* **56**, 979–986.

7. Maniatis, T., Goodbourn, S., and Fisher, J. A. (1987) Regulation of inducible and tissue specific gene expression. *Science* **236**, 1237–1245.

8. Maniatis, T., Fritsch, E. F., and Sambrook, J. (1982) *Molecular Cloning (A Laboratory Manual)* (Cold Spring Harbor Laboratory, Cold Spring Harbor, New York).

9. Sussman, D. J. and Milman, G. (1984) Short term, high efficiency expression of transfected DNA. *Mol. Cell. Biol.* **4(8)**, 1641–1643.

10. Lopata, M. A., Cleveland, D. W., and Sollner-Webb, B. (1984) High level transient expression of a chloramphenicol acetyl transferase gene by DEAE-dextran mediated transfection coupled with dimethyl sulphoxide or glycerol shock treatment *Nucleic Acids Res.* 12(14), 5707–5717.
11. Gorman, C. M. and Howard, B. H. (1983) Expression of recombinant plasmids in mammalian cells is enhanced by sodium butyrate. *Nucleic Acids Res.* 11(21), 7631–7648.
12. Luthman, H. and Magnusson, G. (1983) High efficiency polyoma DNA transfection of chloroquine treated cells. *Nucleic Acids Res.* 11(5), 1295–1308.

CHAPTER 4

Polybrene/DMSO-Assisted Gene Transfer

Rémy Aubin, Michael Weinfeld,
and Malcolm C. Paterson

1. Introduction

Efforts to expand the current repertory of cell types amenable to transfection have often been thwarted by a common obstacle—namely, the low tolerance displayed by the recipient cells toward the gene-transfer regimen itself. As a result, several laboratories have turned to the use of synthetic polycations for delivering copious amounts of exogenous DNA to target cells without compromising their viability or clonogenicity. One of these compounds, polybrene, is mostly known for its ability to enhance the infectivity of retroviruses in culture by serving as an electrostatic bridge between the negatively charged viral particles and the anionic components residing on the surface of recipient cell membranes. Recently we, as well as others (*1–4*), have demonstrated that introduction of naked foreign DNA can be accomplished with high efficiency in a variety of mammalian cell types by exploiting a two-stage gene-transfer schedule in which polybrene is used first to promote the binding of DNA molecules to the target cell population, and dimethyl sulfoxide (DMSO) is then employed to permeabilize the DNA-coated cells. The method is simple to perform and has proven very effective, producing stable transfection frequencies on the order of 0.01–0.1% with only

From: *Methods in Molecular Biology, Vol. 7: Gene Transfer and Expression Protocols*
Edited by: E. J. Murray © 1991 The Humana Press Inc., Clifton, NJ

nanogram quantities of input DNA. In a typical experiment, the process is initiated by bathing the recipient cell population in growth medium supplemented with polybrene and the transfecting DNA. Following a period of incubation during which polybrene–DNA complexes are allowed to form and attach to the cell surface, the cells are permeabilized by a brief exposure to growth medium containing DMSO in order to facilitate the uptake of the adsorbed complexes. The cells are then rinsed to remove the DMSO, and the transfected cell population is allowed to recover in fresh growth medium before being submitted to a dominant selection schedule or assayed for the "transient" expression of the transfected gene.

In the first part of this chapter, a description of the basic protocol is provided, using the mouse fibroblast line NIH 3T3 as an example. In the second part, conditions deemed optimal for the transfection of several human fibroblast cultures are summarized.

2. Materials

1. Polybrene: Dissolve polybrene (1,5-dimethyl-1,5-undecamethylene polymethobromide; Aldrich Chemical Co., Milwaukee, WI) to 1 mg/mL in Ca^{2+}/Mg^{2+} -free Hanks balanced salt solution (HBSS). Sterilize by filtration (0.22 μm) and store 0.25-mL vols at –20°C in sterile microcentrifuge tubes. Once thawed, a tube of polybrene solution should not be refrozen for future use.

2. G418: G418 sulfate (Geneticin®) is usually supplied at potencies ranging between 450 and 600 μg of active product/mg of powder. Prepare a 10 mg/mL stock solution at full potency by dissolving the necessary amount of powder in HBSS. Sterilize by filtration (0.22 μm) and store 5–10 mL vols at –20°C. The G418 solution will resist repeated freeze-thawing.

3. Dimethyl sulfoxide (DMSO): Although, in principle, any lot of DMSO suitable for cell culture may be used, we have found that the product available from Fisher Scientific Co. (Spectranalyzed DMSO, UV cutoff at 262 nm; Cat. No. D-136) offers the most consistent performance.

4. Growth media: Murine NIH 3T3 fibroblasts are cultivated in Dulbecco's Modified Eagle's Medium (DMEM; 1× liquid, 4500 mg/L D-glucose, with L-glutamine, without sodium pyruvate). Human fibroblasts are grown in Ham's F12 Nutrient Mixture (1× liquid, with L-glutamine). Growth media are supplemented with 10 or 15% (v/v) fetal calf serum , 1mM L-glutamine, 100 U/mL penicillin, and 100 μg/mL streptomycin sulfate prior to use and stored at 4°C. Complete medium should be used within 14 d.

5. Trypsin (10× stock; 2.5% trypsin in 0.8 g/L NaCl): Prepare a 1× working solution by diluting the stock in sterile phosphate-buffered saline. Working solutions should be stored at –20°C. Repeated cycles of freezing and thawing will reduce the potency of the solution considerably.

6. Crystal violet staining solution: The working solution consists of 0.5% (w/v) crystal violet in 40% (v/v) methanol.

3. Methods

3.1. Basic Protocol

1. NIH 3T3 fibroblasts are propagated in monolayer culture using DMEM (4500 mg/mL glucose) supplemented with 10% fetal calf serum (FCS), 1 mM L-glutamine, 100 U/mL penicillin, and 100 µg/mL streptomycin sulfate (henceforth referred to as complete medium). The cells are maintained in a 37°C incubator providing a humidified (75–85%) atmosphere of 5% CO_2 in 95% air and are fed complete medium twice weekly. Cells destined for gene transfer should be routinely passaged in late log phase and never be allowed to remain in a confluent state for more than 24 h prior to seeding.

2. On the day preceding transfection, harvest log to late-log cultures by brief exposure to dilute (0.25%) trypsin, and seed NIH 3T3 cells at a density of 5×10^5 cells/60-mm dish. Place the dishes in the incubator and allow the cells to attach and resume growth overnight.

3. The next day, initiate the process of DNA adsorption by replacing the growth medium in each dish with 2.0 mL of an "adsorption cocktail" consisting of 5.0 µg/mL polybrene and between 5 and 25 ng/mL form I pSV2*neo* plasmid DNA in prewarmed (37°C) complete medium. Prepare the cocktail immediately before use in a sterile culture tube by adding the medium first, the plasmid DNA second, and the polybrene last. Vortex the solution after the addition of plasmid DNA and polybrene. (NOTE: Never add polybrene directly to DNA, since this will cause irreversible precipitation to occur.) Distribute the solution evenly over the cell monolayer, and return the dishes to the incubator. Allow DNA–polybrene complexes to attach to the cells overnight (*see* Notes 1 and 2).

4. Following adsorption, proceed to permeabilize the cells with DMSO. The permeabilization solution consists of complete medium augmented to 15% (v/v) DMSO. Prepare the solution immediately before use in a glass bottle and place in a water bath equilibrated to 37°C. Remove the adsorption cocktail by aspiration, and cover each monolayer with 4.0 mL of the permeabilization medium. Distribute the solution evenly across

the cells by swirling each dish gently for 10–15 s. Transfer the dishes to the incubator, and allow cell permeabilization to proceed for 4.5 min. Ensure adequate heat exchange by placing each dish in contact with the incubator shelf (i.e., do not stack the dishes). (NOTE: Keep the permeabilization medium at 37°C throughout the procedure.) In addition, to minimize the toxicity of the treatment, the permeabilization solution should be added from the side of each dish, rather than directly over the monolayer (*see* Notes 3 and 4).

5. Remove the DMSO solution by aspiration and rinse the cells twice with 5 mL of prewarmed complete medium. To do this, add the medium from the side of each dish at a moderate rate and swirl the dish slowly for 10–15 s to remove excess DMSO. It is very important at this stage to begin the rinsing schedule promptly after exposure to the permeabilization solution and to maintain the rinse medium at 37°C.

6. Cover the cells with another 5 mL of growth medium following the last rinse and allow the "transfectants" to recover for 24 h in the incubator.

7. Following recovery, reseed the transfectants at a density of $2.0–2.5 \times 10^5$ cells in 100-mm dishes containing 10 mL of warm complete medium supplemented with 500 mg/mL active G418. Replenish the selection medium every fourth day over a 14–18-d period.

8. Determine the number of drug-resistant colonies by staining the dishes with crystal violet. To do this, decant the medium into a designated receptacle, and rinse the dishes briefly under a gentle stream of tap water. Drain the dishes and pour approx 5 mL of crystal violet staining solution into each dish. Allow colonies to be fixed and stained for 5 min. Decant the staining solution (which can be reused), and rinse the dishes thoroughly but gently under tap water. Allow the dishes to dry in an inclined position. Score the colonies by visual inspection. The protocol will yield transfection frequencies varying between 0.02 and 0.1% over a dose range of 10–50 ng input form I pSV2*neo* plasmid DNA (*see* Note 5).

A schematic representation of the basic polybrene/DMSO-assisted gene-transfer protocol is provided in Fig. 1.

3.2. Optimized Parameters for Polybrene/DMSO-Assisted Gene Transfer of Cultured Human Fibroblasts

A description of the human fibroblast cultures considered in this section is presented in Table 1. All are available from the NIGMS Human Genetic Mutant Cell Repository (Camden, NJ). Conditions deemed optimal for these fibroblast types are summarized in Table 2. Using this table as a guide,

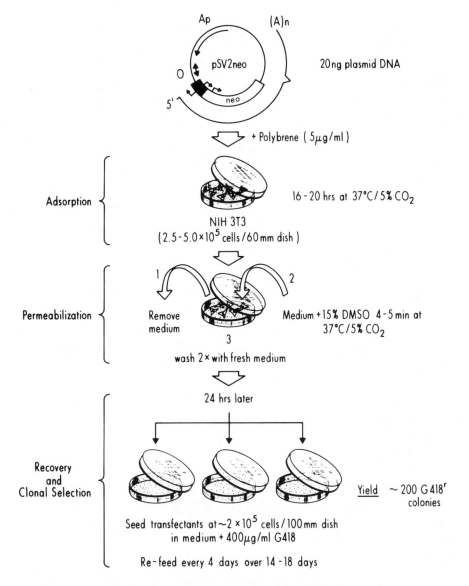

Fig. 1. Schematic outline of polybrene/DMSO-assisted gene transfer as optimized for NIH 3T3 fibroblasts.

polybrene/DMSO-assisted gene transfer can be performed by simply incorporating the appropriate set of conditions into the basic transfection schedule outlined in the preceding section. Parameters for the transfection of individual fibroblast cultures were optimized using 100 ng/mL form I pSV2*neo* plasmid DNA, a concentration that effectively saturates all available DNA binding sites on the cell surfaces. The protocols routinely provide transfec-

Table 1
Description of Human Fibroblast Cultures[a]

Designation	Age	Sex	Race	Comments
GM10	12 FW	M	Bl	Normal fetal strain
GM11	8 FW	M	Bl	Normal fetal strain
GM38	9	F	Bl	Normal nonfetal strain
GM43	32	F	Bl	Normal adult strain
GM730	45	F	Wh	Normal adult strain
GM969	2	F	Wh	Normal nonfetal strain
GM4312A	7	F	Or	SV40-transformed XP20S; xeroderma pigmentosum group A; UV sensitive
GM5849	18	M		SV40-transformed GM5823A (AT5BIVA); ataxia telangiectasia; radiosensitive
GM637A	18	F	Wh	SV40-transformed; normal

[a]Abbreviations: Bl, black; F, female; FW, fetal weeks; M, male; Or, oriental; Wh, white.

tion frequencies in the range of 0.01–0.04 for the nonimmortalized fibroblast strains, and in the range of 0.05–0.08% for the SV40-transformed lines (*see* Notes 6–8).

4. Notes

1. During the adsorption phase, complete and uniform DNA binding to recipient cell monolayers can be assured by swirling the dishes periodically.
2. Large volumes (i.e., 100 mL) of adsorption cocktail can be prepared to accommodate experiments involving many dishes.
3. The most critical determinant of success is the DMSO permeabilization schedule. To ensure reproducibility between experiments and maximize cell survival and clonogenicity, the following points should be kept in mind:
   a. The permeabilization solution should be prepared in a glass bottle. If polystyrene or polypropylene culture tubes are used, the solution must be utilized within 1 h following preparation. This is particularly important for solutions containing more than 15% (v/v) DMSO, because the solvent properties of this com-

Table 2
Summary of Optimized Parameters for Polybrene/DMSO-Assisted Gene Transfer of Human Fibroblast Cultures

Designation	Growth medium[a]	Seeding density[b]	Polybrene, μg/mL	DMSO, %	Shock, min	G418, μg/mL
GM10	Ham's F12/10% FCS	3.5×10^5	6.25	30	5	65
GM11	Ham's F12/10% FCS	3.5×10^5	6.25	30	5	65
GM38	Ham's F12/10% FCS	3.5×10^5	2.5	30 or 25	5 / 18	50
GM43	Ham's F12/10% FCS	3.5×10^5	2.5	30	5	50
GM730	Ham's F12/10% FCS	3.5×10^5	2.5	30 or 25	5 / 18	50
GM969	Ham's F12/10% FCS	3.5×10^5	2.5	30 or 25	5 / 18	75
GM4312A	Ham's F12/15% FCS	5×10^5	7.5	15	5	75
GM5849	Ham's F12/15% FCS	5×10^5	5.0	15	5	50
GM0637A	Ham's F12/15% FCS	5×10^5	7.5	15	5	50

[a]Growth medium also contains 1mM L-glutamine, 100 U/mL penicillin, and 100 μg/mL streptomycin sulfate.
[b]Expressed as the number of viable cells/60-mm-diam-diameter culture dish.

pound will promote the release of toxic plastisizers into the mixture.

b. The addition of DMSO to complete medium is exothermic. Therefore, ensure that the permeabilization solution is equilibrated to 37°C before use.

c. Maintain the permeabilization solution and the rinse medium at 37°C throughout the procedure. Dishes can be insulated from the cold metal surface of the biological safety cabinet by being placed on a thick paper towel.

d. Under optimal conditions, the permeabilization schedule should produce no more than 15% cell killing, as determined by colony-forming ability.

4. Whereas polybrene can be applied to many cell types over a wide range of concentrations and exposure times without adverse effects, the DMSO permeabilization schedule must be configured independently for each cell strain. Unfortunately, we have not found the CAT assay to be a reliable predictor of optimal DMSO treatment. This is mainly because elevated concentrations of DMSO favor the influx of the reporter gene at the expense of long-term cell viability and cloning efficiency. The assay therefore measures high levels of CAT activity in an essentially moribund cell population. The labor and tedium involved in determining the best regimen for stable transfection can be reduced, however, by performing the following preliminary experiment: Using 60-mm dishes, seed the cells at a density estimated to produce a monolayer occupying approx 70% of the dish surface area. Using a fixed pSV2*neo* concentration of 100 ng/mL and a DMSO exposure time of 5 min at 37°C, transfect single dishes in which only the polybrene and DMSO concentrations are varied. Select the cells without reseeding, using a concentration of G418 previously determined to be fully toxic within the first 7 d of exposure to the cell type under evaluation.

5. Linearizing the donor DNA before gene transfer will boost stable transfection frequencies by a factor of 2 or 3. Chloroquine or sodium butyrate were observed to be without effect.

6. Cell surface sites available for the binding of polybrene–DNA complexes are saturable at relatively low DNA concentrations (i.e., 200 ng of pSV2*neo* DNA/5×10^5 fibroblasts). This should be taken into account in cotransfection experiments in which a nonselectable gene will compete against a vector bearing the selectable marker for binding sites on the recipient cell membrane.

7. We have adapted the SV40-transformed human fibroblast lines to the Ham's F12/15% FCS medium formulation in order to obtain uniform growth kinetics, high plating efficiency (>85%; defined as the proportion of cells in the innoculum capable of attaching to the dish), and high cloning efficiency (typically between 40 and 50%; defined on the basis of colony-forming ability in the absence of feeder cells). In our hands, cultures propagated in DMEM/10% FCS handled poorly, providing plating efficiencies of 40% and cloning efficiencies below 0.01%.

8. For transfection experiments performed in 100-mm dishes, SV40-transformed and nonimmortalized human fibroblasts should be seeded to obtain 10^6 and 8.5×10^5 cells/dish, respectively. In addition, 4.5 mL of adsorption cocktail, 6 mL of permeabilization solution, and two rinses of 10 mL each should be used.

References

1. Kawai, S. and Nishizawa, M. (1984) New procedure for DNA transfection with polycation and dimethyl sulfoxide. *Mol. Cell. Biol.* **4,** 1172–1174.
2. Morgan, T. L., Maher, V. M., and McCormick, J. J. (1986) Optimal parameters for the polybrene-induced DNA transfection of diploid human fibroblasts. *In Vitro Cell. Dev. Biol.* **22,** 317–319.
3. Chaney, W. G., Howard, D. R., Pollard, J. W., Sallustio, S., and Stanley, P. (1986) High-frequency transfection of CHO cells using polybrene. *Somatic Cell Mol. Genet.* **12,** 237–244.
4. Aubin, R. J., Weinfeld, M., and Paterson, M. C. (1988) Factors influencing the efficiency and reproducibility of polybrene-assisted gene transfer. *Somatic Cell Mol. Genet.* **14,** 155–167.

CHAPTER 5

Electroporation Technique of DNA Transfection

Sarah C. Spencer

1. Introduction

Electroporation is a simple and rapid procedure by which DNA may be transferred into cells. Essentially, a high voltage pulse is applied to a suspension of cells and DNA placed between electrodes in a suitable cuvet. It is thought that this pulse induces local areas of cell-membrane breakdown, or pores, through which the DNA then enters the cell. Once these pores have resealed, normal cell functions can continue. Since this transfection method involves a physical effect of the delivered pulse on the cell membrane, it can potentially be used for most cells, independent of their phagocytic capacity as required for transfection by the calcium phosphate coprecipitation technique (*see* Chapter 2, this vol.).

The following range of cells have all been successfully electroporated: Mouse fibroblasts (L, NIH 3T3), pre-B cells (Abelson virus transformed), thymomas (RlA), T-cell clones (Dl0.G4.1); human lymphoblastoid cells (Epstein-Barr virus transformed), hematopoietic stem cells, peripheral blood T-cells, T-cell lines (HSB-2, TALL-l), a monocytic cell line (U937), an erythroleukemia line (K562), and Chinese Hamster Ovary cells (CHO), as described in refs. *1–6.*

From: *Methods in Molecular Biology, Vol. 7: Gene Transfer and Expression Protocols*
Edited by: E. J. Murray © 1991 The Humana Press Inc., Clifton, NJ

Electroporation can be used to obtain both short-term (transient) or long-term (stable) transfectants. For some cells, the efficiency of transfection is at least as good as that obtained by calcium phosphate *(2)*; in other cells, efficiencies may be greater or less. Transfection by electroporation offers certain advantages over other methods. Insertion by electroporation can result in gene copy numbers ranging from one to 20, differing from the large tandem arrays frequently seen following calcium phosphate *(7)*. Achieving such low gene copy numbers is useful when the transfected cells are to be used for gene expression studies. In addition, following electroporation, nuclear uptake and incorporation of DNA takes place without rearrangement or extensive modification of the termini *(7)*. Although plasmid DNA is generally transfected, genomic DNA (>65 kb) can also be used *(8)*.

Although many parameters should be considered when attempting to electroporate a cell or cell line for the first time, published conditions that work for a similar cell type are a useful starting point. Two examples (a fibroblast line and a thymoma line) will be described in the Methods Section below. To achieve optimal transfection efficiencies, these variables would need to be finely adjusted for each cell line. These variable aspects will be briefly described here.

Several electroporation machines that are safe and easy to use are currently available, offering different types of pulses. Firstly, capacitor discharge devices (e.g., Bio-Rad Gene Pulser) can be used to deliver pulses that then decay exponentially. A range of capacitance settings can be selected, as can the applied voltage; the machine will then indicate the actual time of the discharge. Both high-voltage low-capacitance (hence short-time) and low-voltage high-capacitance (hence long-time) conditions may be selected. Special disposable cuvets (with covers to maintain sterility) are needed, although the volume of cell suspension to be pulsed can be varied. Other electroporation devices can deliver square wave pulses (e.g., Hoefer Pro-Genetor pulse controller). In this particular device, the pulse voltage and duration can be selected. Cuvets are not needed, since the electrode fits directly into the wells of a tissue-culture plate. Other square-wave-type machines offer the facility for accurately delivering more than one pulse, possibly multiple pulses separated by a predetermined time interval (e.g., Baekon 2000). It is not yet clear whether one of these machine types is best for electroporation of a particular type of cell. Whichever machine is available or selected, successful transfection may be possible only within a narrow voltage range.

The choice of electroporation buffer is critical for this technique, since the composition and electrical resistance of the electroporation medium will greatly affect the time of pulse that can be delivered. Cells in high-ionic-strength media (e.g., phosphate-buffered saline) manifest shorter time constants than those in HEPES-buffered isotonic sucrose media, if all other parameters are fixed. In addition, the salt conditions around the cells influence cell survival. An ideal medium would lead to minimal detrimental effects during the critical period when the pores are induced. Such a medium would reassemble the cytosol and would also facilitate rapid resealing to restore cell function. (For a detailed assessment, *see* ref. *9*.)

Electroporation may be carried out either at room temperature or, more usually, with incubations on ice. Prechilling avoids cell damage through local heating during pulsing, whereas resting on ice after pulsing prolongs the period when the pores are open so that DNA may enter over an extended time span. However, raising the temperature after pulse delivery reseals the pores and enables the cells to survive unfavorable media. The latter can also be achieved by addition of a large volume of culture medium.

The form of DNA used for transfection is important. Unlike the use of circular plasmid DNA for the calcium phosphate technique, in order to obtain stable transfectants by electroporation, it is usually necessary to linearize plasmids at a site outside the transcriptional unit by digestion with a suitable restriction enzyme. For transient expression this is not desirable, since it results in decreased transient transfection efficiency *(1)*. In either case, DNA concentrations in the range 1–80 µg/mL are effective. For at least some cells it is possible to cotransfect two linearized plasmids, provided a suitable DNA ratio is used to achieve stable selection of both genes. Thus, it is not essential to link genes covalently to selectable markers, although for cells with low transfection efficiencies, this step would be advisable. For some cells, the use of carrier DNA can increase transfection efficiency. Again, the amount used should be titrated; sonicated salmonsperm DNA can be effective at 300 µg/mL, but is toxic at high concentrations *(2)*.

The best results are obtained with electroporation if the cells to be transfected are actively growing and dividing, rather than from confluent cultures. In the case of resting cells that do not normally divide, using a stimulus to induce proliferation (e.g., phytohemagglutinin for human T-cells) could be one way to make them transfectable *(4)*. The density of cells in the cuvet is also important and should be in the range 10^6–10^7/mL, since at lower concentrations, poor cell recovery occurs, and at higher concentrations, undesirable cell fusion starts to take place.

A method will be described for electroporation leading to stable transfection of two genes (a murine Major Histocompatibility Complex class I gene and neomycin selectable gene) in mouse L-cells (fibroblast) and mouse

RlA cells (thymoma). For the L-cells, a low capacitance condition is needed, but a harsher, higher capacitance is applied for the smaller R1A cells (the latter cannot be transfected by calcium phosphate).

2. Materials

1. Plasmids containing the bacterial neomycin phosphotransferase gene (pSV2*neo*) and the murine MHC class I D^d gene purified by cesium chloride gradient ultracentrifugation.
2. Restriction enzymes and appropriate digestion buffers as recommended by the manufacturer.
3. Phenol: Equilibrated with 0.1*M* Tris, pH 8.0, and 0.2% 2-mercaptoethanol; containing 8-hydroxyquinoline (Sigma).
4. 3*M* sodium acetate, pH 5.2, and 100% ethanol for DNA precipitations.
5. TE buffer: 10 m*M* Tris-HCl, 1 m*M* EDTA, pH 7.4; sterilized by passage through a 0.22 µm filter.
6. Carrier DNA: Salmon-sperm DNA (Sigma D-1626) at 10 mg/mL in TE buffer (dissolved overnight at 37°C) sonicated to less than 2 kb.
7. Phosphate-buffered saline: Dulbecco's "A," containing 8 g NaCl, 0.2 g KCl, 0.2 g KH_2PO_4, 1.15 g Na_2HPO_4/L, sterilized by autoclaving.
8. Complete culture medium: Dulbecco's Modified Eagle's Medium supplemented with glutamine, penicillin, streptomycin, bicarbonate, HEPES, 2-mercaptoethanol, and 10% heat-inactivated fetal calf serum.
9. Trypsin/EDTA for harvesting adherent cells.
10. Geneticin sulfate (G418) stock solution, 2 mg/mL in complete medium (sterilized by passage through a 0.22-µm filter). The minimum concentration found to kill untransfected L-cells is 0.8 mg/mL (for R1A cells, 1.8 mg/mL), although the concentration required must be determined for each batch of G418 (*see* Chapter 19).
11. Actively dividing cell cultures: L-cells should be approaching confluence ($1–1.5 \times 10^7$ from a 75 cm^2 culture flask), R1A cells at $1–2 \times 10^7$/mL culture. For each transfection, 2×10^6 cells are needed.
12. Bio-Rad Gene Pulser (with Capacitance Extender fitted) and cuvets (these can be reused up to five times if thoroughly washed with dH$_2$O, sterilized with 70% alcohol, and rinsed five times with PBS before use).

3. Methods

3.1. Electroporation of L-Cells

1. In separate Eppendorf tubes, linearize 5 µg pSV2*neo* and 20 µg D^d in the appropriate digestion buffer in a vol of 100 µL with appropriate restric-

tion enymes. (It is a good idea to check that linearization is completed by analysis on a mini-gel; *see* Note 1.)

2. To remove the restriction enzymes (and hence avoid further DNA digestion when both DNAs are later mixed), add 100 μL of phenol to each digest. Mix until an emulsion forms and then centrifuge each for 10 min in an Eppendorf centrifuge at 4°C.

3. Pipet the upper (aqueous) layers to fresh tubes with caps. To concentrate and sterilize each, add one-tenth of the 3*M* sodium acetate, mix, and then add 2 vol ice-cold ethanol. Store for a minimum of 1 h at –70°C to allow the DNAs to precipitate. Centrifuge as before.

4. In a laminar flow hood, carefully remove the supernatants with a needle and syringe and discard. Allow the pellets to air-dry for 30 min, then thoroughly dissolve them in sterile TE buffer to 2 μg/μL (*see* Note 2).

5. Similarly sterilize 250 μg (25 μL of 10 mg/mL) sonicated salmon-sperm DNA by addition of 75 μL distilled H_2O, 10 μL 3*M* sodium acetate, and 200 μL ethanol. Precipitate and resuspend in 25 μL sterile TE buffer.

6. Under sterile conditions, harvest the L-cells with trypsin/EDTA, add complete medium, and spin down. Wash the cell pellet thoroughly with PBS (4 washes, 5 mL each) and resuspend the pellet to 2.5×10^6 viable cells/mL in PBS. Cell viability should be 90–95%.

7. Transfer 0.8 mL of cell suspension to a cuvet. Add the sonicated salmon-sperm DNA (250 μg in 25 μL), pSV2*neo* (5 μg in 2.5 μL) and D^d (20 μg in 10 μL), mixing thoroughly after each addition. Cap the cuvet and place on ice for 10 min.

8. Meanwhile, place 15 mL of complete medium at room temperature into a 75-cm² flask.

9. Mix the cuvet contents briefly with a graduated 1-mL plastic pipet to ensure that the cells have not settled out. Place in the cuvet holder and deliver a pulse of 1000 V at 25 μF. A release of gas may be seen on the electrodes (*see* Note 3).

10. One minute after pulsing, gently transfer the cuvet contents to the medium in the flask, and then incubate for 48 h (37°C, 5% CO_2).

11. Discard the medium and give fresh medium containing 0.8 mg/mL G418.

12. After 10–14 d, G418-resistant colonies should be visible by eye (20–200/flask). These can be harvested separately as clones or collectively (bulk) and analyzed with the fluorescence-activated cell sorter after staining with a suitable monoclonal antibody reactive with surface D^d antigen. In one experiment, all G418-resistant cells were also expressing the D^d antigen (*see* Notes 4–6).

3.2. Electroporation of RlA Cells

1. The plasmid DNAs are linearized and sterilized as described above. Optimal transfection requires 12 μg pSV2*neo* and 50 μg D^d, and these should be redissolved in TE buffer to 5 μg/μL.

2. The required number of cells is washed free of FCS and resuspended to 2.5×10^6/mL in PBS. Following DNA addition and prechilling on ice, the electroporation machine should be set at 350 V, 960 μF for pulsing. This will give considerable frothing!

3. After 1 min, gently transfer the cell suspension (but not the froth) to 4 mL of complete medium in one well of a 12-well culture plate and incubate for 48 h at 37°C, 5% CO_2.

4. Harvest the cells, pellet them, and resuspend in 24 mL complete medium containing 1.8 mg/mL G418. Plate six wells (4 mL each).

5. By day 10, colonies of G418-resistant cells are visible by eye. These cells divide more frequently than many other lines and can soon be analyzed for surface D^d antigen expression, as indicated above. In one experiment, 50% G418-resistant RlA cells were expressing the D^d antigen. In a separate transfection of a $K^d K^k$ hybrid gene, 100% G418-resistant cells were also expressing surface K^d antigen.

4. Notes

1. It is usually more convenient to linearize and sterilize a larger amount of pSV2*neo* (for example, 100 μL at μg/mL), and sonicated salmon-sperm DNA (for instance, 200 μL at 10 mg/mL). These can be stored at –20°C and thawed as required, refreezing after use.

2. It is most convenient and easiest to resuspend the pelleted DNA in TE buffer as described, but it should be remembered that this is not isotonic. The above volumes recommended for resuspending the DNAs are tolerated by these cells, but should not be exceeded, especially for osmotically fragile cells. It is possible that the slightly hyposmotic conditions that result contribute to successful electroporation *(2)*.

3. The conditions described above, with the pulse delivered from a capacitor discharge device, result in only 40–80% cell recovery when assessed at 24 h by dye exclusion (*see* Note 6). Conditions causing some cell death are generally needed for successful transfection of the remaining cells with this type of device.

4. When attempting electroporation for the first time, confirm these conditions for transfection of L-cells with linearized selector plasmid alone. When other cells are considered, the initial conditions to be tested (e.g.,

capacitance setting) could be based on those published for a similar cell type, provided that the type of electroporation machine to be used is similar. Unfortunately, the effective voltage intensity may be so cell-dependent that transfection occurs only if the exact voltage from a narrow range is selected. Suitably small voltage increments would be needed to locate this. Cell death being observed only after a certain voltage is exceeded would help to narrow down the possibilities.

5. As mentioned in the Introduction Section, several other parameters can also be altered, including the electroporation buffer, temperature and timing, and cell and DNA concentration.

6. Once colonies of stable transfectants can be obtained, it is comparatively straightforward to determine whether the transfection efficiency can be increased. If no transfection at all is occurring, it might be useful to monitor the induction of a state of permeability to dyes in the electroporated cells. For example, permeabilized cells take up the fluorescent dye Lucifer yellow (M_r 457 dalton) *(10)*. Since not all permeabilized cells fully recover, it is important to also record cell survival after resealing or at 24 h. Both aims may be achieved in one approach if access to a fluorescence-activated cell sorter is possible *(11)*. Propidium iodide (PI) is added to the cell suspension immediately after pulsing and the cells held on ice for 10 min. After a period of resealing in complete medium at 37°C, fluorescein diacetate (FDA) is added. Permeabilized viable cells fluoresce both red (following uptake of PI) and green (since live cells hydrolyze the FDA to fluorescein). Permeabilized cells that have failed to reseal are red only. Achieving doubly stained cells is a fast way to monitor early electroporation attempts with a new cell line.

If these dyes affect the ionic strength of the buffer, they are best added during a postpulsing incubation on ice. It should be remembered that dye uptake will differ from DNA uptake—it has been suggested that DNA enters the permeabilized cells electrophoretically during the pulse itself, rather than by simple diffusion *(12)*.

References

1. Potter, H. (1988) Electroporation in biology: Methods, applications and instrumentation. *Anal. Biochem.* **174,** 361–373.
2. Chu, G., Hayakawa, H., and Berg, P. (1987) Electroporation for the efficient transfection of mammalian cells with DNA. *Nucleic Acids Res.* **15,** 1311–1326.
3. Ohtani, K., Nakamura, M., Saito, S., Nagata, K., Sugamura, K., and Hinuma, Y. (1989) Electroporation: Application to human lymphoid cell lines for stable introduction of a transactivator gene of human T-cell leukemia virus type I. *Nucleic Acids Res.* **17,** 1589–1604.

4. Cheynier, R., Soulha, M., Laure, F., Vol, J. C., Reveil, B., Gallo, R. C., Sarin, P. S., and Zagoury, D. (1988) HIV-l expression by T8 lymphocytes after transfection. *AIDS Res. Human Retroviruses* **4,** 43–50.

5. Toneguzzo, F. and Keating, A. (1986) Stable expression of selectable genes introduced into human hematopoietic stem cells by electric field-mediated DNA transfer. *Proc. Natl. Acad. Sci. USA* **83,** 3496–3499.

6. Kaye, J. and Hedrick, S. M. (1988) Analysis of specificity for antigen, Mls, and allogeneic MHC by transfer of T-cell receptor α- and β-chain genes. *Nature* **336,** 580–583.

7. Toneguzzo, F., Keating, A., Glynn, S., and McDonald, K. (1988) Electric field-mediated gene transfer: Characterization of DNA transfer and patterns of integration in lymphoid cells. *Nucleic Acids Res.* **16,** 5515–5532.

8. Jastreboff, M. M., Ito, E., Bertino, J. R., and Narayanan, R. (1987) Use of electroporation for high-molecular-weight DNA-mediated gene transfer. *Exp. Cell Res.* **171,** 513–517.

9. Michel, M. R., Elgizoli, M., Koblet, H. and Kempf, C. (1988) Diffusion loading conditions determine recovery of protein synthesis in electroporated P3X63Ag8 cells. *Experientia* **44,** 199–203.

10. Mir, L. M., Banoun, H., and Paoletti, C. (1988) Introduction of definite amounts of nonpermeant molecules into living cells after electropermeabilization: Direct access to the cytosol. *Exp. Cell Res.* **175,** 15–25.

11. O'Hare, M. J., Asche, W., Williams, L., and Ormerod, M. G. (1988) Optimization of transfection of breast epithelial cells by electroporation. *DNA* (in press).

12. Winterbourne, D. J., Thomas, S., Hermon-Taylor, J., Hussain, I., and Johnstone, A. P. (1988) Electric shock-mediated transfection of cells. Characterization and optimization of electrical parameters. *Biochem. J.* **251,** 427–434.

CHAPTER 6

Irradiation and Fusion Gene Transfer

Peter N. Goodfellow

1. Introduction

The fusion of human and rodent somatic cells is usually followed by the spontaneous loss of human chromosomes from the hybrid cells *(1)*. The correlation between the presence of a human chromosome retained in the hybrid cell and the presence of a human phenotypic trait is the basis of human gene mapping by somatic cell genetics *(2)*. This method for constructing physical maps has been central to human genetics and has resulted in the chromosomal assignment of several hundred genes *(see* ref. *3)*. Unfortunately, subchromosomal gene localization by this approach is limited by the paucity of suitable translocation and deletion chromosomes.

Molecular methods for constructing physical maps of the human genome have improved dramatically with the introduction of pulsed-field gel electrophoresis *(4,5)*, and yeast artificial chromosomes (YACs) *(6)*. Nevertheless, routine analysis and cloning of DNA fragments in the megabase range are still difficult.

In an attempt to span the gap left by the resolution of somatic-cell genetics and molecular methods, we have explored two techniques that combine chromosome fragmentation with somatic cell genetics. The first method, chromosome-mediated gene transfer (CMGT), exploits calcium phosphate to promote uptake of purified human chromosomes by recipient rodent cells

From: *Methods in Molecular Biology, Vol. 7: Gene Transfer and Expression Protocols*
Edited by: E. J. Murray © 1991 The Humana Press Inc., Clifton, NJ

(*7*; *see also* Chapter 10, this vol). At some point during the preparation or uptake of the donor chromosomes, they break and only fragments are incorporated into the recipient cell genome. The second method, irradiation and fusion gene transfer (IFGT), was originally described by Goss and Harris *(8)*, and was based on an idea proposed by Pontecorvo *(9)*. Human donor cells are irradiated with γ-rays, and the chromosome fragments generated are rescued by fusion with a rodent cell.

CMGT has several drawbacks, including the major disadvantages of the selective retention of sequences from centromeric regions as well as the rearrangement of DNA within transferred fragments *(10)*. Because of the drawbacks of CMGT, we have sought to develop IFGT; this review describes our recent experiences and is designed to provide a starting protocol for others interested in exploring this approach. It should be stressed that IFGT is a technique under development, and many of the opinions expressed herein will require modification with time.

1.1. Principles of IFGT

The initial experiments performed by Goss and Harris were limited by two problems:

1. The donor cell was a human cell containing the whole human genome.
2. The human genetic region of interest had to be retrieved by selecting for hybrid cells retaining this region.

The requirement for selection limited the regions of the genome available for study, and the human donor cell frequently contributed chromosome fragments from regions other than those required. A major advance was made when D. Cox (personal communication) made the discovery that it was possible to avoid direct selection for human material. Figure 1 describes the basic experiment as performed by Cox and colleagues. A hamster cell containing a single human chromosome is lethally irradiated and then fused with a second hamster cell.

Although selection is applied to isolate hybrids, no selection is applied for retention of human material. The human material is retained in the hybrid cells by association with hamster chromosomes or, occasionally, as reduced human chromosomes (*see* Fig. 1 in ref. *11*).

There are two basic applications for this technique: The first is the isolation of hybrids containing small defined fragments of specific human chromosomes that can be used for the isolation of human DNA sequences. In this application, IFGT can play a central role in reverse-genetics strategies designed to isolate genes important in human genetic disease *(12,13)*. The

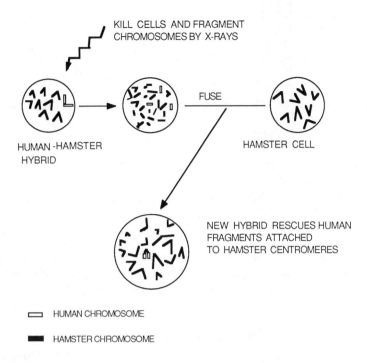

Fig. 1. A strategy for producing hybrids containing nonselected fragments of human chromosomes.

second application is in the construction of whole chromosome genetic maps. After low-dose irradiation of the donor hybrid (<10,000 rads), about 50% of the subsequent hybrid clones are positive for any single marker. If it is assumed that the chance of any two markers being present will depend on the distance between them as well as the average size of retained chromosome fragments, then it is possible to construct chromosome maps based on IFGT data. Preliminary maps of this kind show promise for genetic analysis (D. Cox, personal communication; P. Goodfellow and T. Bishop, unpublished observation).

1.2. A Comparison Between IFGT and CMGT

IFGT and CMGT both produce hybrid clones containing multiple subchromosomal fragments. It has not been possible to deliberately isolate clones with single human fragments in either technique; such clones arise by chance. The size of the fragments produced by IFGT may be controllable by irradiation dose; the size of the fragments in the CMGT hybrids cannot be controlled. CMGT requires a selection for the human genetic material, IFGT does not.

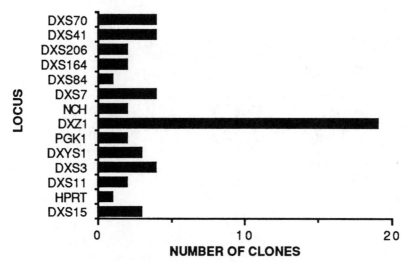

Fig. 2. Marker retention in IFGT clones containing fragments of the human X chromosomes. The data is taken from Benham et al. *(11),* and represents clones obtained after 20,000- and 50,000-rad irradiations of the donor cells.

In both methods, alphoid sequences derived from the human centromeric region are overrepresented (Fig. 2). The alphoid sequences are rearranged, and their retention may have implications for their function. The sequences present in CMGT hybrids are usually, but not always, extensively rearranged. Apart from the alphoid sequences, the sequences present in IFGT show less evidence of within-fragment rearrangement than CMGT (unpublished observation; D. Cox, personal communication). This question requires further investigation. In our experience, IFGT and CMGT clones are usually unstable.

In summary, IFGT can be used to generate hybrids that contain subfragments of donor chromosomes. These hybrids may find a use in reverse genetics strategies and in genome mapping.

2. Materials

IFGT is a technique that requires the culture and cloning of somatic cells. Good cell husbandry and a well-equipped tissue-culture laboratory are essential.

2.1. Irradiation of Donor Cells

1. Tissue-culture medium: The specific medium is not important; we use Dulbecco's Modified Eagle's Medium supplemented with 10% fetal bovine serum.

2. Donor cells: Hamster–human hybrid containing a single human chromosome (*see* Note 1).
3. X-ray source: Pantak HF30 industrial X-ray unit.

2.2. Fusion and Growth of Hybrid Cells

1. Recipient cells: Hamster cell line (*see* Notes 1 and 2).
2. Selection medium: Selection agent added to growth medium (*see* Note 2).
3. PBSA: Phosphate-buffered saline without calcium or magnesium.
4. PEG, 50% v/v: 5.5 g of PEG4000 (Baker) and 5 mL of serum-free growth medium, mixed and autoclaved. The final pH should be adjusted, if necessary, to 8.2. The solution can be stored for at least 1 wk at 4°C, but the pH should be rechecked before use.

3. Methods

In our experiments, we have concentrated on high-dose irradiation in an attempt to generate small fragments for use in reverse-genetics experiments. The experiment can be broken into three stages: irradiation of the donor cell, fusion and growth of hybrids, and analysis of hybrid clones.

3.1. Irradiation of the Donor Cell

1. Before confluence, harvest 5×10^6 donor cells (a hamster–human hybrid containing a single human chromosome) and suspend in 10 mL of serum containing medium in a plastic universal.
2. Expose the cells at room temperature to irradiation produced by an industrial X-ray unit on maximum setting (320 KV; 10.0 mA). This results in an irradiation rate of about 1000 rads/min; however, because of cooling problems with the machine, a total dose of 40,000–50,000 rads takes about $1^1/2$ h (*see* Note 3).

3.2. Fusion

The donor cell is killed by the irradiation, and a selection is used to kill the recipient cell to permit the outgrowth of the hybrid cells (*see* Note 2).

1. Harvest recipient cells (A23) and resuspend in medium to obtain single cell suspension.
2. Combine the irradiated donor cells with 5×10^6 recipient cells and spin to a common pellet in a conical-base centrifuge tube (1500*g* for 15 min at room temperature).
3. Wash once in PBSA and spin again as above.

4. Remove the supernatant and loosen the pellet by tapping the side of the tube. Add, drop by drop, 1mL of PEG solution, prewarmed to 37°C (*see* Note 4).
5. Incubate for 1 min at 37°C.
6. Add 5 mL of PBSA over a period of 1–2 min. Mix the contents of the tube by gently stirring with the pipet.
7. Add 5 mL of PBSA supplemented with 10% fetal bovine serum.
8. Pellet the cells as in step 2. Remove the supernatant and plate the cells in growth medium (for fast-growing cells, plate at 2×10^5 cells/90-mm tissue-culture plates).
9. Add selective media after 24 h (*see* Note 2). Change the medium every 3–4 d.
10. Colonies should appear in 14–21 d (*see* Note 5).

3.3. Analysis of Hybrid Clones

Only 10–20% of the clones produced from high-dose irradiation experiments have maintained the human DNA after either prolonged culture or freezing and thawing. We have addressed this problem of instability by growing clones to about 5×10^8 cells and making a large batch of DNA at a single time-point (*see* Chapter 9). Although this limits the usefulness of IFGT, the production of a large stock of DNA enables the construction of λ genomic libraries that can be used indefinitely.

If the investigator is interested in only one region on the donor chromosome, it should be possible to screen the clones in an early stage, using PCR methods (*see* Chapter 31) if suitable primers can be designed for the locus of interest.

Figures 2 and 3 summarize an IFGT experiment designed to produce hybrids containing fragments of the X chromosome *(11)*. From Fig. 2, it is clear that there is a more frequent retention of alphoid sequences (locus name *DXZ1*) than other human X-located sequences. The probability of retention of the other X-located sequences is approx the same for all loci tested, including the telomeric sequences *DXYS14*. The generated hybrids contain discrete fragments of the X chromosome; further investigation of these clones has demonstrated that markers known to be closely located in the genome are often transferred together (Table 4 in ref. *11*).

4. Notes

1. Not all combinations of donor and recipient cells appear to work in IFGT. Hamster–human hybrids have been used successfully as donors

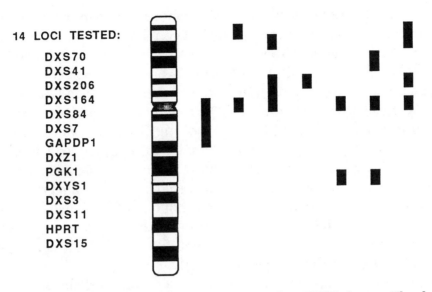

14 LOCI TESTED:

DXS70
DXS41
DXS206
DXS164
DXS84
DXS7
GAPDP1
DXZ1
PGK1
DXYS1
DXS3
DXS11
HPRT
DXS15

Fig. 3. Human chromosome fragments retained in IFGT clones. The data are taken from Benham et al. *(11)*, and represent clones obtained after 50,000-rad irradiation of the donor cells. Each set of vertical bars represents a separate clone.

to transmit human chromosome fragments to hamster recipient cells. Hybrids containing fragments of human chromosomes 4, 9, 10, 21, and X have been created with a hamster background (*11,12;* D. Cox, personal communication; P. Goodfellow et al., unpublished observations). Combinations of cells that have not worked include: (a) mouse–human hybrid donors transferring human fragments to mouse or hamster recipients, and (b) human–mouse hybrid donors transferring mouse fragments to human or hamster cells. Why these combinations have failed is not obvious. Recent experiments by D. Housman and colleagues suggest that the mouse cell line 3T3 can be successfully used as a recipient (personal communication).

2. One of the most convenient selection systems is the hypoxanthine, aminopterin, thymidine (HAT) method of Szybalski et al. *(14)*; a protocol for making HAT medium is presented in Chapter 20, this volume. If no selection is to be applied to the human DNA, then the recipient hamster cell should lack the enzyme for which the original hamster parent of the hybrid is positive. The two hamster cell lines that we have used are A23 *(15)*, which is thymidine kinase negative, and W3GH *(8)*, which is hypoxanthine phosphoribosyl transferase negative.

3. Although the rate of irradiation is likely to be as important as the total

dose, we have not investigated this parameter. In an initial set of experiments using a hamster–human hybrid containing a human X chromosome, three irradiation doses were investigated: 6000, 20,000, and 50,000 rads (*11*). At 6000 rads, two classes of hybrids were obtained; one class had undetectable human DNA and the second class had large amounts of X-chromosome material. At 20,000 and 50,000 rads, the majority of hybrid clones had small fragments of the X chromosome. Low-dose irradiation may be the method of choice for map construction, where high marker frequency produces more information per clone. It is also possible that low-dose irradiation may result in less rearrangement within fragments. Other variables that have not been tested include the temperature at which cells are irradiated and recovery time after irradiation.

4. A discussion of the effect on fusion of different PEG batches and grades can be found in Goodfellow et al. (*16*).

5. Using this method for cell fusion, the frequency is usually better than 1 hybrid/10^5 parental cells.

Acknowledgments

The work described in this article has been performed in collaboration with a large number of colleagues. I thank all of them for their contributions. Editorial assistance in preparing this manuscript was provided by C. Middlemiss and B. Martin.

References

1. Weiss, M. A. and Green, H. (1967) Human–mouse hybrid cell lines containing partial complements of human chromosomes and functioning human genes. *Proc. Natl. Acad. Sci. USA* **58,** 1104–1111.

2. Ruddle, F. H. (1972) Linkage analysis using somatic cell hybrids. *Adv. Hum. Genet.* **3,** 173–235.

3. Human gene mapping 9. (1987) *Cytogenet. Cell Genet.* **46,** 1–762.

4. Carle, G. F. and Olson, M. V. (1984) Separation of chromosomal DNA molecules from yeast by orthogonal-field-alteration gel electrophoresis. *Nucleic Acids Res.* **12,** 5647–5664.

5. Schwartz, D. C. and Cantor, C. R. (1984) Separation of yeast chromosome-sized DNAs by pulsed field gradient gel electrphoresis. *Cell* **37,** 67–75.

6. Brownstein, B. H., Silverman, G. A., Little, R. D., Burke, D. T., Korsmeyer, S. J., Schlessinger, D., and Olson, M. J. (1989) Isolation of single-copy human genes from a library of yeast artificial chromosome clones. *Science* **244,** 1348–1351.

7. McBride, O. W. and Ozer, H. L. (1973) Transfer of genetic information by purified metaphase chromosomes. *Proc. Natl. Acad. Sci USA* **70,** 1258–1262.

8. Goss, S. J. and Harris, H. (1975) New method for mapping genes in human chromosomes. *Nature* **255,** 680–683.

9. Pontecorvo, G. (1971) Induction of directional chromosome elimination in somatic cell hybrids. *Nature* **230,** 367–369.

10. Goodfellow, P. N. and Pritchard, C. A. (1988) Chromosome fragmentation by chromosome mediated gene transfer. *Cancer Surv.* **7,** 251–265.

11. Benham, F., Hart, K., Crolla, J., Bobrow, M., Francavilla, M., and Goodfellow, P. N. (1989) A method for generating hybrids containing nonselected fragments of human chromosomes. *Genomics* **4,** 509–517.

12. Cox, D. R., Pritchard, C. A., Uglum, E., Casher, D., Kobom, J., and Myers, R. M. (1989) Segregation of the Huntington disease region of human chromosome 4 in a somatic cell hybrid. *Genomics* **4,** 397–407.

13. Pritchard, C. A., Casher, D., Uglum, E., Cox, D. R., and Myers, R. M. (1989) Isolation and field inversion gel electrophoresis analysis of DNA markers located close to the Huntington disease gene. *Genomics* **4,** 408–418.

14. Szybalski, W., Szybalska, E. H., and Ragni, G. (1962) Genetic studies with human cell lines. *Natl. Cancer Inst. Monogr.* **7,** 75–79.

15. Westerveld, A., Visser, R. P. L. S., Khan, P. M., and Bootsma, D. (1971) Loss of human genetics markers in man–Chinese hamster somatic cell hybrids. *Nature* **234,** 20–24.

16. Goodfellow, P. N., Pritchard, C. A., and Banting, G. S. (1988) Techniques for mammalian genome transfer, in *Genome Analysis: A Practical Approach* (Davies, K., ed.) IRL, Oxford, pp. 1–18.

CHAPTER 7

Direct Use of λ Phage Particles for DNA Transfection

Masahiro Ishiura

1. Introduction

Recent progress in techniques for the transfer of genes into cultured mammalian cells has made possible the isolation of various interesting genes from other mammalian cells, and also the study of the function and the regulation of gene expression of mammalian genes in vivo. Various transfection techniques have been developed: incubation of recipient cells with genes in the presence of diethylaminoethyldextran (*see* Chapter 3, this vol.; ref. *1*); incubation of the cells with metaphase chromosomes and poly-L-ornithine *(2)*; and incubation of the cells with coprecipitates of calcium phosphate and genetic material, such as DNA (Chapter 2; refs. *3,4*), metaphase chromosomes (Chapter 10; ref. *5*), and λ phage particles *(6,7)*. Other methods for gene transfer have also been developed: direct injection of DNA into the nuclei of recipient cells *(8,9)*; use of viral vectors (Chapters 11–15; for review, *see also* ref. *10*); fusion of the recipient cells with bacterial spheroplasts *(11)* or liposomes *(10–14)*; and fusion of cells, mediated by HVJ (Sendai virus), with liposomes *(15–17)* or reconstituted erythrocyte membrane vesicles *(18)*. The cell membranes of recipient cells have also been rendered permeable to genetic material by electric pulses (Chapter 5; ref. *19*).

From: *Methods in Molecular Biology, Vol. 7: Gene Transfer and Expression Protocols*
Edited by: E. J. Murray © 1991 The Humana Press Inc., Clifton, NJ

We describe here an efficient procedure for transferring mammalian genes that have been cloned in a λ phage vector or in a cosmid vector (*see* Note 1; ref. *6*). In this procedure, λ phage particles that contain recombinant phage DNA or recombinant cosmid DNA, in place of either DNA or chromosome, are coprecipitated with calcium phosphate and applied to recipient cells. It is not necessary to extract and purify DNA from recombinant phages. Once isolated, phage particles that harbor a specific gene are directly transferred into the cells. The efficiency of gene transfer (namely, the number of transformant colonies/λ phage particle/10^6 recipient cells) by this procedure is very high (10^{-5}), using small amounts of phage particles without additional carrier DNA. Furthermore, once established, the transformed cells obtained by the procedure are extremely stable in the absence of selective drugs *(6,7)*. Therefore, this procedure is particularly attractive in obtaining stably transformed cells that carry low copy numbers of a transferred gene with long flanking sequences without additional carrier DNA sequences. This method has been successfully applied to the isolation of a specific gene. Okayama and Berg *(20)* have developed a phage vector for transferring a cDNA library into cultured mammalian cells by the phage transfer method described here. They have attained a frequency of gene transfer of 10^{-2} and successfully isolated cDNA clones for the human hypoxanthine-guanine phosphoribosyltransferase.

The phage transfer method is mediated by coprecipitation of calcium phosphate (Table 1), and several parameters govern the efficiency of gene transfer (*see* Figs. 1–5). They include the cell density of preculture, culture media, the buffer used for coprecipitation of phage particles with calcium phosphate and its pH, the period of coprecipitation, the vol of calcium phosphate suspension added, the time of absorption of phage particles, and the expression time required for the thymidine kinase *(tk)* gene of herpes simplex virus type 1 (HSV-1). The most important parameter is the pH of the buffer used for coprecipitation of phage particles with calcium phosphate.

Recombinant phages are grown in liquid cultures using *E. coli* K12 Dp50SupF as a host, according to the protocol of Blattner et al. *(21)*, and purified from the cultures by polyethylene glycol mediated phage precipitation and two subsequent CsCl centrifugations *(22)*. Dialysis membranes used for the preparation of phages are pretreated by the procedure described previously *(23)*. Preparation and titration of phage λ have also been described in detail in a previous vol. of this series of publications *(24)*, and in a standard manual for molecular cloning *(25)*.

Table 1
Effect of Calcium Phosphate on Gene Transfer

Experiment	Condition[a]	Tk[+] colonies/dish			
1	Complete	163,	210,	253,	(209)[b]
	– CaCl$_2$	0,	0,	0	(0)
	– Phosphate	0,	0,	0	(0)
2	Complete	167,	268,	367,	(267)
	– CaCl$_2$	0,	1,	1	(1)
	– Phosphate	0,	1,	2	(1)

[a]Experiments were carried out under the standard conditions, except that phage particles (3×10^{10} PFU/dish) with calcium phosphate (Complete) or without either CaCl$_2$ (– CaCl$_2$) or inorganic phosphate (– Phosphate) were applied to Ltk$^-$ cells.
[b]Average for three dishes.

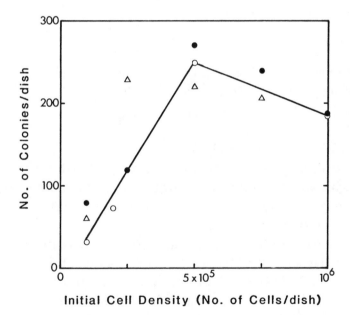

Fig. 1. Effect of the initial cell density of preculture on gene transfer (after ref. 6). Phage dosage, 3×10^{10} PFU/dish. Experiments were carried out under the standard conditions described in the text, except the initial cell density of preculture was different. The results of three separate experiments are shown.

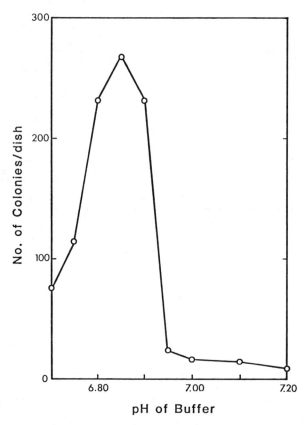

Fig. 2. Effect of pH of the buffer for coprecipitation of phage particles with calcium phosphate on gene transfer (after ref. 6). Phage dosage, 3×10^{10} PFU/dish.

2. Materials

1. Water: Water referred to here is ultrapure water that is prepared by a Milli-Ro, Milli-Q system (Millipore Corp., Bedford, MA).
2. Chemicals and solutions: Unless otherwise stated, all reagents are biochemical grade and all solutions are sterilized by autoclaving and stored at room temperature.
3. Tris: Trizma base (Sigma Chemical Co., St. Louis, MO).
4. NZYDT: 5 g NaCl; 2 g $MgSO_4 \cdot 7H_2O$; 5 g yeast extract (Difco Laboratories, Detroit, MI); 10 g NZ amine type A (Humko Scheffield Chemical, Norwich, NY); 0.04 g thymidine; 0.1 g diaminopimelic acid (Sigma). Dissolve in 1 L of water.
5. NZYDT agar: 11 g Bactoagar (Difco). Dissolve in 1 L of NZYDT.
6. Top agar: 7.5 g Bactoagar. Dissolve in 1 L of NZYDT.
7. Ca–Mg solution: 10 mM $CaCl_2$; 10 mM $MgCl_2$.
8. Chloroform: Use without sterilization. Chloroform is volatile and toxic; therefore, handle it in a well-ventilated place.

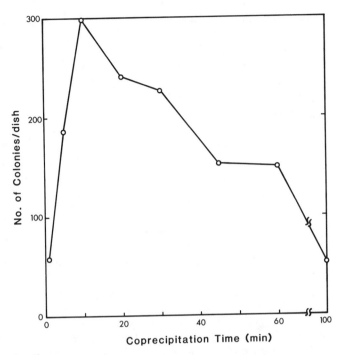

Fig. 3. Effect of the incubation period for coprecipitation of phage particles with calcium phosphate on gene transfer (after ref. *6*). Phage dosage, 3×10^{10} PFU/dish. Experiments were carried out under the standard conditions described in the text, except the incubation period for coprecipitation of phage particles with calcium phosphate was different.

9. PEG: polyethylene glycol 6000.
10. CsCl: Sterilize by heating at 180°C for 3 h.
11. CsCl solution with a density of 1.5: Dissolve 6.4587 g of CsCl in 8 mL of SM (*see* step 15). Prepare the required vol of solution just before use.
12. 50% ethanol.
13. 10 m*M* NaHCO$_3$, 1 m*M* EDTA.
14. Visking dialysis membrane (Union Carbide Corp., Chicago, IL, #8/32): Immerse for 2 h in 2 L of 50% ethanol with one change of the solution. The immersion is repeated sequentially for periods of 1 h in two changes of solution containing 10 m*M* NaHCO$_3$ and 1 m*M* EDTA, and in two changes of water.
15. SM: 100 m*M* NaCl, 50 m*M* Tris-HCl (pH 7.5), 10 m*M* MgSO$_4$, 0.01% gelatin. Adjust the pH to 7.5 at room temperature. Sterilize by autoclaving.
16. 1% gelatin (Difco).
17. 2.5 *M* CaCl$_2$.

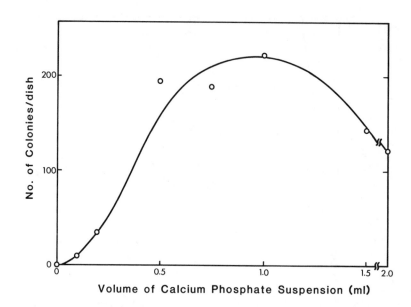

Fig. 4. Effect of the vol of the suspension of calcium phosphate on gene transfer. Phage dosage, 3×10^{10} PFU/dish. Experiments were carried out under the standard conditions described in the text, except the vol of the suspension of calcium phosphate was different.

18. 1 mM Tris-HCl (pH 7.9); adjust the pH to 7.9 at room temperature.
19. Buffered Ca²⁺: 250 mM CaCl$_2$, 0.9 mM Tris-HCl (pH 7.9). Prepare just before use, by mixing aseptically 1 vol of 2.5 M CaCl$_2$ and 9 vol of 1 mM Tris-HCl (pH 7.9). Store at 25°C in a water bath until used.
20. BES saline (×2): 100 mM N,N-bis (2-hydroxyethyl)-2-aminoethane sulfonic acid (BES), 560 mM NaCl, 3 mM Na$_2$HPO$_4$.
21. BES saline: Prepare just before use, by mixing equal vols of BES saline (×2) and water. In order to equilibrate the temperature of the saline to 25°C, stand a glass bottle containing 1 vol of BES saline (×2) and $^1/_2$ vol of water in a water bath at 25°C for 15 min; then adjust the pH to 6.87 with 1 N NaOH. Sterilize by filtration through a Millex-GS 0.22-μm filter (Millipore). Store at 25°C in a water bath until used.
22. HEPES saline: 20 mM N-2-hydroxyethylpiperazine-N'-2-ethanesulfonic acid (HEPES) (Dojin), 137 mM NaCl, 3 mM KCl. Adjust the pH to 7.1 at room temperature.
23. PBS(−): 137 mM NaCl, 3 mM KCl, 8 mM Na$_2$HPO$_4$, 1 mM KH$_2$PO$_4$.
24. 10% formalin: Prepare by mixing 1 vol of formalin (37% formaldehyde aqueous solution) and 9 vol of PBS (−). Use without sterilization. For-

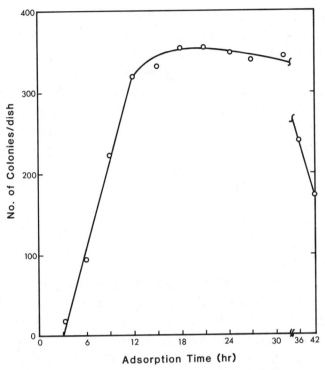

Fig. 5. Effect of the incubation period for adsorption of phage particles to Ltk⁻ cells on gene transfer (after ref. *6*). Phage dosage, 3×10^{10} PFU/dish. Experiments were carried out under the standard conditions described in the text, except the incubation period for adsorption of phage particles to Ltk⁻ cells was different.

malin is volatile and toxic; therefore, handle it in a well-ventilated place or in a fume hood.

25. 0.1% crystal violet: Dissolve 1 g crystal violet in 1 L of water and filter through a filter paper. Use without sterilization.

26. α-MEM: Alpha modification of Eagle's Minimum Essential Medium (MEM) with Earles's salts, but without ribosides, or deoxyribosides. According to the manufacturer's instruction, prepare by dissolving the desired amount of a blended medium powder (Flow Laboratories, McLean, VA, No. 10–311 [α-MEM with glutamine and without NaHCO₃]) and NaHCO₃ in water. Sterilize by filtration through a 0.22-μm filter. Store at 4°C and use within 20 d of preparation.

27. Calf serum: Check the ability of several test lots of sera to support cell growth and colony formation, and select a lot with high ability (*see* Note 2). Be careful not to use sera contaminated with mycoplasma (*see* Note 3.) Store at –80°C. Thaw just before use and store at 4°C.

28. Culture medium: α-MEM supplemented with 10% calf serum. Prepare by mixing aseptically 1 vol of calf serum and 9 vol of α-MEM.
29. EDTA: 0.2 g EDTA-Na$_2$. Dissolve in 1 L of PBS(–).
30. 0.25% Trypsin (*see* Note 4): 2.5 g trypsin. Dissolve in 1 L of PBS(–) with stirring at 4°C (for several h), and remove insoluble materials by centrifugation at 10,000 rpm for 10 min at 2°C, using a J2-21 centrifuge and a JA-10 rotor (Beckman Instruments Inc., Palo Alto, CA). Sterilize by filtration through a 0.45-µm filter and then through a 0.22-µm filter (*see above*). Handling of trypsin should be carried out in a cold room. Use for preparation of EDTA-trypsin as soon as possible. Store on ice until used.
31. EDTA-trypsin: Prepare by mixing aseptically equal vols of EDTA and trypsin. Store in 50- or 100-mL aliquots at –20°C. Thaw just before use and store at 4°C.
32. 200 mL HAT mixture (250×) (*see* Note 4): 750 mg hypoxanthine; 10 mg aminopterin; 250 mg thymidine; 1.5 g glycine. Dissolve in 150 mL of warm water (37°C) by adding about 10 mL of 1 *N* NaOH. Adjust the vol to 200 mL with water and sterilize by filtration through a Millex–GS filter (*see above*). Store at –20°C in small aliquots until used. Thaw just before use by incubating in a water bath at 37°C.
33. HAT medium: Prepare by mixing aseptically 1 vol of culture medium and 0.004 vol of HAT mixture. Store at 4°C.
34. Dimethylsulfoxide (Nakarai, UVS35 No. 134–35 for spectrometry); store in small aliquots at –20°C. Thaw an aliquot just before use and discard the aliquot after use.
35. Glycerol; store at room temperature.
36. A recombinant Charon 4A phage that carries the HSV–1 *tk* gene. Store the suspension of the phage (or cleared phage lysates of *Escherichia coli* host bacteria) at 4°C under sterile conditions for short-term storage (<1 mo) and at –80°C in the presence of 15% glycerol or 5% dimethylsulfoxide for long-term storage.
37. *E. coli* K 12 strain Dp50SupF *(21)*: Store at 4°C on a NZYDT agar plate for short-term storage (<2 wk) and at –80°C in the presence of 15% glycerol for long-term storage.
38. Ltk⁻ cells: L-cells deficient in *tk* activity *(6)*. Maintain in 10-cm Falcon dishes (Becton Dickinson and Co., Oxnard, CA, No. 3003) that contain 10 mL of culture medium. Unless otherwise stated, cells are incubated at 37°C under 5% CO_2 in air in a CO_2 incubator, and cell handling is carried out aseptically in a clean bench. Cells for preculture (*see below*) should be in the logarithmic phase of growth (*see* Notes 3 and 5).

3. Methods

3.1. Preparation of Phage Particles for Gene Transfer

1. Recombinant Charon 4A phage is grown in liquid cultures using *E. coli* K12 Dp50SupF as a host. First, thaw Dp50SupF bacteria stored at −80°C and streak them on a NZYDT agar plate, and then incubate the plate at 37°C overnight.

2. The next day, isolate a single colony from the plate and inoculate it into 5 mL of NZYDT in a long test tube (total, 10 mL in two tubes). Incubate the test tube at 37°C with shaking at 175 rpm overnight.

3. The next morning, use 10 mL of the culture to inoculate 200 mL of NZYDT in a 500-mL flask and incubate the flask at 37°C with shaking at 130 rpm. Monitor cell growth by measuring the optical density at 600 nm (OD_{600}). The doubling time of cells is about 90 min. Use the cells for the infection of phages when the OD_{600} of culture reaches about 0.5–0.8 and cells are growing in the midlogarithmic phase of growth (*see* Note 6).

4. Determine the required number of flasks (usually three flasks) for the growth of phage (*see below*, step 9). Calculate the required vol of bacterial culture. Twenty OD_{600} units of bacteria (*see* Note 7) are used for each liter of culture for the growth of phage.

5. For absorption of phage, mix each 10 mL of bacterial culture and Ca–Mg solution in a 100-mL flask, and then add 10^7 plaque-forming units (PFU) of recombinant phage to the mixture. Mix the contents gently and incubate the flask at 37°C in a water bath for 20 min without agitation.

6. Inoculate the mixture into 1 L of NZYDT in a 3-L flask and incubate the flask at 37°C with shaking at 130 rpm until a sign of cell lysis appears. Incubation time is usually 10 h (*see* Note 8).

7. To lyse the cells, add 5 mL of chloroform to each flask containing 1 L of culture. Mix the contents in the flask and stand the flask at room temperature for 20 min.

8. To remove cell debris, centrifuge the culture at 10,000 rpm for 25 min at 2°C in a Beckman JA-10 rotor (*see* Note 9).

9. Collect the supernatant, which contains phages. Store a 1-mL aliquot at 4°C for the titration of phages in the cleared lysates. Titrate the phage as described below (*see* Section 3.2.). The titer of phage should be about 10^{10} PFU/mL of lysate or higher.

10. Phages are precipitated from the cleared lysates with polyethylene glycol. First, to remove materials that become insoluble in the presence of

NaCl, add 60 g NaCl to each liter of supernatant. Gently stir the mixture at 4°C, using a magnetic stirrer, until the NaCl is dissolved.

11. To remove the insoluble materials, centrifuge the mixture at 10,000 rpm for 25 min at 2°C in a JA-10 rotor.

12. Collect the supernatant. Gently add 70 g PEG to each liter of supernatant. Gently stir the mixture at 4°C until the PEG is dissolved. Then stand the mixture in a cold room overnight without stirring (*see* Note 10).

13. The next morning, to collect precipitated phages, centrifuge the mixture at 10,000 rpm for 30 min at 2°C in a JA-10 rotor.

14. Remove the supernatant completely, and add 10 mL of SM for each liter of initial culture to pellets. Resuspend the pellets by gentle pipeting, and transfer the suspension into a Dounce homogenizer. Homogenize the suspension with 10 strokes of a loose pestle in the homogenizer.

15. Phages are purified by two subsequent CsCl centrifugations. First, transfer the suspension into a 50-mL measuring cylinder and make up the vol of the suspension to 40 mL with SM.

16. Transfer the suspension into a 200-mL flask, add 32.290 g CsCl, and gently stir the mixture at room temperature with a magnetic stirrer until the CsCl is dissolved.

17. To evaporate residual chloroform, gently rotate the flask, uncapped, at 37°C for 30 min (*see* Note 11).

18. For the banding of phages, centrifuge the sample at 25,000 rpm for 14 h at 4°C in Beckman angle titanium rotor 50.2Ti (*see* Note 12). After centrifugation a phage band should be visible.

19. Collect a phage band from the top of centrifuge tubes using a 50-µL glass micropipet connected to a peristatic pump.

20. Make up the vol of the collected fractions to about 10 mL with CsCl solution with a density of 1.5.

21. For the rebanding of phages, centrifuge the sample at 30,000 rpm for 20 h at 4°C in a Beckman angle titanium rotor 50Ti (*see* Note 12).

22. Collect a phage band from the final CsCl density gradient, as described above, and transfer into a Visking dialysis membrane.

23. To remove CsCl, dialyse the suspension of purified phage (<1 mL) against 1 L of SM at 4°C with three changes of SM at intervals of 6 h.

24. Transfer the suspension of phage into a 5-mL graduated glass centrifuge tube with a screw cap.

25. Measure the vol of the suspension. To stabilize phages, add 0.01 vol of 1% gelatin to the suspension.

26. To sterilize the suspension of phage, add 0.01 vol of chloroform to the suspension and mix the contents well.

27. Incubate the mixture at room temperature for 20 min with occasional stirring.
28. To remove the chloroform, centrifuge the mixture at 5000 rpm for 20 min.
29. Transfer the upper aqueous layer, which contains the phages, to a 50-mL glass centrifuge bottle with a round bottom and a screw cap. To evaporate residual chloroform, open the cap of the bottle and incubate the suspension of phage at 37°C for 1 h with gentle rotation.
30. Transfer the suspension of phage into a 2-mL stock vial and store it at 4°C until used.

3.2. Titration of Phages

1. Prepare a series of tenfold dilutions of the preparations of purified phages or the cleared lysates, using SM as a diluent.
2. Melt the top agar using an autoclave or a microwave, and store the melted agar at 50°C in a water bath until used.
3. For absorption of phages, gently mix each 100 μL of the overnight culture of Dp50SupF, Ca–Mg solution, and diluted phage suspension in small test tubes, and incubate the mixture at 37°C in a water bath for 15 min.
4. Add 2.5 mL of the melted top agar into each test tube, gently mix the contents, and pour them each onto a 10-cm NZYDT agar plate. Stand the plates at room temperature until the agar solidifies.
5. Incubate the plates upside down at 37°C overnight without agitation.
6. In the next morning or afternoon, count the number of plaques on plates (at least three plates for each preparation of phage) and, from the average number of plaques/plate, calculate the PFU/mL of the preparation of phages.

3.3. Preculture of Recipient Cells

1. Cell monolayers on stock dishes are dissociated with treatment of the cells with trypsin and EDTA. First, remove culture medium from stock dishes that contain Ltk⁻ cells in the logarithmic phase of growth (*see* Notes 2, 3, and 5).
2. To wash the cells, add 10 mL of PBS(–) to each dish, gently rotate the dish on a culture tray, and then remove PBS(–).
3. To dissociate the cells, add 5 mL of EDTA-trypsin to each dish and incubate the dish at 37°C for 10–15 min.
4. Gently swirl the dish and confirm dissociation of cells by microscopic observation.

5. Add 10 mL of culture medium to each dish and dissociate cells completely by gentle pipeting, using a Pasteur pipet.
6. Transfer the suspension of cells into a sterile 50-mL centrifuge tube and collect cells by low-speed centrifugation at 1500 rpm for 5 min at 2°C.
7. Remove the supernatant completely, add 20 mL of culture medium/ dish into the tube, and resuspend the cells by gentle pipeting with a Pasteur pipet.
8. Store cells on ice until used.
9. Determine cell density by counting the cell number, using a hemocytometer.
10. Determine the required number of dishes for experiments and calculate the required vol of cell suspension for inoculation from the cell density. Each 10-cm dish is inoculated with 10 mL of culture medium that contain 5×10^5 cells (Fig. 1; *see also* Note 13).
11. Prepare the cell suspension in culture medium for inoculation by mixing the calculated vols of the medium and the stock cell suspension in a 500-mL glass bottle (*see* Note 14).
12. Add 10 mL of cell suspension to each dish using a 10-mL pipet.
13. To allow the cells to distribute homogeneously on the dish, shake the dishes on a culture tray, gently and reciprocally. Turn the tray 90° and then shake them again.
14. Incubate the cells in a CO_2 incubator for 24 h.
15. Confirm good plating of cells by microscopic observation (*see* Note 5).

3.4. Dilution of Phage and Coprecipitation of Phage Particles with Calcium Phosphate

1. For experiments of gene transfer, prepare a suspension of phage of a desired concentration and of a desired vol by diluting with SM (*see* Note 15).
2. Transfer the required vol of the suspension of phage into a polycarbonate (Beckman, bottles for a J2-21 centrifuge, such as No. 870177 [50 mL], No. 334843 [250 mL], and No. 3411236 [500 mL]) or polypropylene (No. 870178 [50 mL], No. 341237 [250 mL], and No. 339996 [500-mL]) bottle with a round bottom and a screw cap (*see* Note 16).
3. The suspension of phage that contains buffered Ca is prepared just before use. Slowly add an equal vol of freshly prepared buffered Ca^{2+} (25°C) to the bottle that contains the suspension of phage while gently swirling the bottle. Stand the bottle at room temperature until used.
4. Phage particles are coprecipitated with calcium phosphate. Slowly add 1 vol of BES saline (25°C) dropwise down the side of the bottle that

contains the suspension of phage while gently swirling the bottle (Fig. 2; *see also* Note 14).

5. To develop a fine precipitate of calcium phosphate, incubate the mixture in a water bath at 25°C for 10 min. Confirm that a fine precipitate develops (Fig. 3).

6. Gently add 1 mL of the preparation to the medium on recipient cells of each dish, using a 5-mL plastic pipet (Fig. 4). To allow the preparation to distribute homogeneously on the cells, gently swirl the dishes on a culture tray.

7. Incubate the cells in a CO_2 incubator for 24 h (Fig. 5). During this incubation, cells are allowed to incorporate phage particles. Confirm that the fine precipitates of calcium phosphate covers the surface of the cells.

3.5. Culture for Expression and HAT Selection

1. Remove the medium from the dishes by aspiration.

2. To wash the cells, gently add 10 mL of HEPES saline (room temperature) dropwise down the side of each dish (*see* Note 17). Gently swirl the dishes on a culture tray and remove the saline by aspiration. Throughout this step, be careful not to disturb the cells.

3. Add 10 mL of fresh culture medium (room temperature) to each dish as gently as possible, as described in step 2, and incubate the cells in a CO_2 incubator (*see* Note 18).

4. The next day, change the medium and then further incubate the cells overnight as above. Total incubation time is 40 h. During this incubation, cells are allowed to express the transferred gene.

5. Transformant cells that carry and express the HSV-1 *tk* gene are selected in HAT medium. Remove the medium from the dishes. Add 10 mL of HAT medium (room temperature) to each dish. Incubate the cells for 10 d with four changes of HAT medium, as above. Renew the medium every day for the first 3 d, and then once every 3 d.

3.6. Colony Count

1. Remove the medium from the dishes by aspiration.

2. To wash the cells, add 10 mL of PBS(–) (room temperature) to each dish, swirl the dishes on a culture tray, and remove PBS(–) by aspiration.

3. Add 5 mL of 10% formalin to each dish and fix the cells at room temperature for 30 min.

4. Remove formalin from the dishes by decantation.

5. Add 5 mL of 0.1% crystal violet into each dish and stain the cells at room temperature for 30 min.

6. Remove the dye solution from the dishes by decantation. Wash the dishes in running tap water for 1 min and dry the dishes in air.

7. Count the number of colonies on the dishes (at least three dishes for each point) by microscopic observation using a binocular.

8. Calculate the efficiency of gene transfer from the average number of colonies per dish.

4. Notes

1. Recombinant cosmid DNA also can be transferred into cultured mammalian cells by the procedure described here, after packaging the DNA into phage particles in a lysogenized *E. coli* host. Recently, we have developed a cosmid vector and a procedure that enabled us to package recombinant cosmid DNA efficiently into λ phage particles and have succeeded in transferring recombinant cosmid DNA into the cells by the phage transfer method described here *(26)*.

2. Good healthy growth of recipient cells apparently correlates with a high efficiency of gene transfer. In this connection, fetal calf serum is superior to calf serum and newborn calf serum as a supplement of medium for gene transfer.

3. Cells contaminated with mycoplasma show retarded unhealthy growth, and use of such cells as a recipient completely spoil gene-transfer experiments. Discard cells that are suspected of contamination, and decontaminate the CO_2 incubator used for culture of the cells. The sources of the contamination are serum and culture cells that have already been contaminated with mycoplasma.

4. Currently, concentrated solutions of a HAT mixture and trypsin are commercially available.

5. For preculture, do not use cells just after their recovery from storage at $-80°C$. Use the cells after several passages of culture. Discard cells if the cells used for preculture do not show good growth or if they are poorly dissociated by trypsinization. Also discard cells if the precultured cells do not show a high efficiency of plating (usually, floating cells should not be evident).

6. *E. coli* cells for phage infection should be in the midlogarithmic phase of growth. Otherwise, a poor yield of phage results.

7. One OD_{600} unit of bacteria corresponds to about 4×10^8 cells.

8. The yield of phage is maximum just before cell lysis. The optimal incubation time is 9–15 h and differs from culture to culture. The signs of cell lysis can be monitored by treatment of cells with chloroform. Re-

move 1-mL aliquots of culture at intervals during incubation, and add a few drops of chloroform to the aliquot. Incubate at room temperature for 20 min. If cell lysis begins in the culture, the culture treated with chloroform will show a clear appearance.

9. Never use polycarbonate centrifuge tubes, because chloroform destroys polycarbonate.

10. If necessary, you can move to the next step after standing the mixture in a cold room for 1 h.

11. Usually, step 17, Section 3.1., can be omitted.

12. A vertical rotor can be used for the banding of phage.

13. The procedure described here can be applied to different kinds of cells and different selection-maker genes with a slight modification. With a rat fibroblast cell line, F2408tk^- *(6)*, we can obtain essentially the same efficiency of gene transfer. The initial cell density of preculture should be increased to 1.0×10^6 cells/dish, because this cell line is more sensitive to the application of phage particles.

14. When the competence of α-MEM to sustain gene transfer is defined as 100%, those of F-12, Eagle's MEM, and Dulbecco's Modified MEM (with 2 g NaHCO$_3$/L) are 21, 89, and 94%, respectively. In most cases, various kinds of cells grow well in α-MEM or Dulbecco's Modified MEM. When the competence of BES buffer to sustain gene transfer is defined as 100%, those of piperazine-*N,N'-bis*(2-ethanesulfonic acid) (PIPES), 3-(*N*-morpholino) propane sulfonic acid (MOPES), and HEPES buffers are 100, 94, and 70%, respectively.

15. Application of over 10^{10} PFU of phage particles/dish is toxic to cultured mammalian cells, resulting in a greatly reduced efficiency of gene transfer (Table 2). It is uncertain what causes this toxic effect. Bacterial DNA *(27)* and protein *(28)* have been reported to be toxic to cultured mammalian cells in gene transfer. It is also possible that, if large amounts of phage particles are applied to the cells, either the DNA sequences of vector arms or the coat proteins of phage *per se* (or both) might be toxic to the cells.

16. The procedure described here can also be applied to DNA. The efficiency of gene transfer is comparable to or higher than those obtained by various procedures of the calcium phosphate coprecipitation method. Chen and Okayama *(28)* have reported the very high frequency gene transfer of plasmid DNA into various cultured mammalian cells, including an SV40-transformed human fibroblast cell line (frequencies, 10–50%), by the procedure described here with slight modifications. If a

Table 2
Effect of Carrier Phage Dosage on Gene Transfer[a]

Dosage of carrier phage, PFU/dish	tk^+ Colonies/dish			
0	258	410	—[b]	(334)[c]
10^8	288	324	332	(315)
10^9	344	344	396	(361)
10^{10}	126	132	152	(137)
10^{11}	0	4	14	(4)

[a]Experiments were carried out under the standard conditions, except that phage particles (3×10^{10} PFU/dish) were coprecipitated with calcium phosphate in the presence of various titers of Charon 4A library phage for human DNA and applied to Ltk⁻ cells (after ref. 6).
[b]Contaminated.
[c]Average for three dishes.

recombinant phage does not carry a mammalian selective marker gene, we can isolate transformant cells that carry the transferred recombinant phage DNA by the procedure of contransformation *(29)*.

17. Use of PBS(–) in place of HBS for washing cells that have been treated with the suspension of precipitates of calcium phosphate reduces the efficiency of gene transfer. Use of cold HBS also reduces the efficiency.

18. In contrast to the DNA and chromosome transfer described previously, treatment of recipient cells with dimethyl sulfoxide, glycerol, or sucrose at the end of the absorption period does not significantly affect the efficiency of gene transfer.

19. λ Phage particles containing recombinant DNA also may be efficiently introduced into recipient cells by other methods, such as the microinjection method, the HVJ-aided fusion method, using either liposomes *(15–17)* or reconstituted erythrocyte membrane vesicles *(18)*, and the electroporation method *(19)*.

References

1. Pagano, J. S., McCutchan, J. H., and Vaheri, A. (1967) Factors influencing the enhancement of the infectivity of poliovirus RNA by diethylaminoethyl-dextran. *J. Virol.* **1**, 891–897.

2. McBride, O. W. and Ozer, H. L. (1973) Transfer of genetic information by purified metaphase chromosomes. *Proc. Natl. Acad. Sci. USA* **70**, 1258–1262.

3. Graham, F. L. and van der Eb, A. J. (1973) A new technique for the assay of infectivity of human adenovirus 5 DNA. *Virology* **52,** 456–461.
4. Wigler, M., Pellicer, A., Siverstein, S., and Axel, R. (1978) Biochemical transfer of single-copy eucaryotic genes using total cellular DNA as donor. *Cell* **14,** 725–731.
5. Spandidos, D. and Siminovitch, L. (1977) Transfer of codominant markers by isolated metaphase chromosomes in Chinese hamster ovary cells. *Proc. Natl. Acad. Sci. USA* **74,** 3480–3484.
6. Ishiura, M., Hirose, S., Uchida, T., Hamada, Y., Suzuki, Y., and Okada, Y. (1982) Phage particle-mediated gene transfer to cultured mammalian cells. *Mol. Cell. Biol.* **2,** 607–616.
7. Ishiura, M., Uchida, T., and Okada, Y. (1989) Stability of the transformants obtained by phage particle-mediated gene transfer. *Cell Struct. Funct.* **14,** 495–499.
8. Capecchi, M. R. (1980) High efficiency transformation by direct microinjection of DNA into cultured mammalian cells. *Cell* **22,** 479–488.
9. Anderson, F. W., Killos, L., Sanders-Haigh, L., Kretschmer, P. J., and Diacumakos, E. G. (1980) Replication and expression of thymidine kinase and human globin genes microinjected into mouse fibroblasts. *Proc. Natl. Acad. Sci. USA* **77,** 5399–5403.
10. Gulzman, Y., ed. (1982) *Eukaryotic Viral Vectors* (Cold Spring Harbor Laboratory, Cold Spring Harbor, NY).
11. Shaffner, W. (1980) Direct transfer of cloned genes from bacteria to mammalian cells. *Proc. Natl. Acad. Sci. USA* **81,** 2163–2167.
12. Fraley, R., Subramani, S., Berg, P., and Papahadjopoulos, D. (1980) Introduction of liposome-encapsulated SV40 DNA into cells. *J. Biol. Chem.* **255,** 10431–10435.
13. Mukherjee, A. B., Orloff, S., Butler, J. Deb., Triche, T., Lalley, P., and Schlman, J. D. (1978) Entrapment of metaphase chromosomes into phospholipid vesicles (lipochromosomes): Carrier potential in gene transfer. *Proc. Natl. Acad. Sci. USA* **75,** 1361–1365.
14. Wong, T.–K., Nicolau, C., and Hofsneider, P. H. (1980) Appearance of β-lactamase activity in animal cells upon liposome-mediated gene transfer. *Gene* **10,** 87–94.
15. Volsky, D. J., Gross, T., Sinangil, F., Kuszynski, C., Bartzatt, R., Dambaugh, T., and Kieff, E. (1984) Expression of Epstein-Barr virus (EBV) DNA and cloned DNA fragments in human lymphocytes following Sendai virus envelope-mediated gene transfer. *Proc. Natl. Acad. Sci. USA* **81,** 5926–5930.
16. Nakanishi, M., Uchida, T., Sugawa, H., Ishiura, M., and Okada, Y. (1985) Efficient introduction of contents of liposomes into cells using HVJ (Sendai virus). *Exp. Cell Res.* **159,** 399–409.
17. Kaneda, Y., Uchida, T., Kim, J., Ishiura, M., and Okada, Y. (1987) The improved efficient method for introducing macromolecules into cells using HVJ (Sendai virus) liposomes with gangliosides. *Exp. Cell Res.* **173,** 56–69.
18. Sugawa, H., Uchida, T., Yoneda, Y., Ishiura, M., and Okada, Y. (1985) Large macromolecules can be introduced into cultured mammalian cells using erythrocyte membrane vesicles. *Exp. Cell Res.* **159,** 410–418.
19. Neumann, E., Schaffer–Ridder, M., Wang, Y., and Hofschneider, P. H. (1982) Gene transfer into mouse myeloma cells by electroporation in high electric fields. *EMBO J.* **1,** 841–843.
20. Okayama, H. and Berg, P. (1983) Bacteriophage lambda vector for transducing a cDNA clone library into mammalian cells. *Mol. Cell. Biol.* **5,** 1136–1142.

21. Blattner, F. R., Williams, B. G., Blechl, A. E., Thompson, K. D., Faber, H. E., Furlong, L. A., Grunwald, D. J., Kiefer, D. O., Moore, D. D., Schumm, J. W., Sheldon, E. L., and Smithies, O. (1977) Charon phages: Safer derivatives of bacteriophage lambda for DNA cloning. *Science* **196**, 161–169.

22. Yamamoto, K. R., Alberts, B. M., Benzinger, R., Lawhorne, L., and Treiber, C. (1970) Rapid bacteriophage sedimentation in the presence of polyethylene glycol and its application to large scale virus purification. *Virology* **40**, 734–744.

23. McPhie, P. (1971) Dialysis, in *Methods in Enzymology*, vol. 22 (William, B. J., ed.), Academic, NY, pp. 23–32.

24. Dale, J. W. and Greenaway, P. J. (1985) Preparation and assay of phage lambda, in *Methods in Molecular Biology*, vol. 2 (Walker, J., ed.), Humana Press, Clifton, NJ, pp. 201–209.

25. Maniatis, T., Fritsch, E. F., and Sambrook, J. (1982) *Molecular Cloning: A Laboratory Manual* (Cold Spring Harbor Laboratory, Cold Spring Harbor, NY).

26. Ishiura, M., Ohashi, H., Uchida, T., and Okada, Y. (1989) Phage particle-mediated gene transfer of recombinant cosmids to cultured mammalian cells. *Gene* **82**, 281–289.

27. Yoder, J. I. and Ganesan, A. T. (1983) Procaryotic genomic DNA inhibits mammalian cell transformation. *Mol. Cell. Biol.* **3**, 956–959.

28. Chen, C. and Okayama, H. (1987) High-efficiency transformation of mammalian cells by plasmid DNA. *Mol. Cell. Biol.* **7**, 2745–2752.

29. Wigler, M., Sweet, R., Sim, G. K., Wold, B., Pellicer, A., Lacy, E., Maniatis, T., Silverstein, S., and Axel, R. (1979) Transformation of mammalian cells with genes from procaryotes and eucaryotes. *Cell* **16**, 777–785.

CHAPTER 8

Cationic Liposome-Mediated Transfection with Lipofectin™ Reagent

Philip L. Felgner

1. Introduction

Since their original description, liposomes have been discussed as vehicles that could be used as carriers of pharmaceutically active agents (*1*), and their potential for use as carriers of genetic information has been examined (*2,3*). Some encouraging DNA-delivery results have been obtained; however, the methodology has had some fundamental difficulties (*4–8*). Chief among these is that liposomes do not generally fuse with the target cell surface, but are taken up phagocytically, and the polynucleotides are subsequently subjected to the action of digestive enzymes in the lysosomal compartment. Another practical problem with conventional liposome technology results because the internal dimensions of typical liposomes may be too small to accommodate large macromolecules, such as DNA or RNA, resulting in low capturing efficiency. In addition, conventional liposomal methodology involves a relatively inconvenient multistep preparation procedure.

The Lipofectin™ reagent is a preparation of cationic liposomes composed of a novel positively charged lipid, DOTMA (*N*[1-(2,3-dioleyloxy) propyl]-*N,N,N*-trimethylammonium), and DOPE (dioleoyl phosphatidyl

From: *Methods in Molecular Biology, Vol. 7: Gene Transfer and Expression Protocols*
Edited by: E. J. Murray © 1991 The Humana Press Inc., Clifton, NJ

ethanolamine), that overcomes some of these difficulties *(9)*. DOTMA was designed by applying physical chemical principles pertaining to molecular shape and hydrophobicity *(10)* to form stable cationic bilayers. Cationic vesicles containing DOTMA interact spontaneously and rapidly with polyanions such as DNA and RNA, resulting in liposome/polynucleotide complexes that capture 100% of the polynucleotide *(9,11)*. The resulting polycationic complexes are taken up by the anionic surfaces of tissue culture cells with an efficiency 10–100 times greater than negatively charged or neutral liposomes (S. Foung and P. Felgner, unpublished results). The fusogenic behavior of DOTMA results in functional intracellular delivery of polynucleotide *(12)* in a manner that bypasses degradative enzymes present in the lysosomal compartment *(13)*. All of these attributes result in a transfection methodology that is convenient, reproducible, and efficient, and is effective in a wide variety of tissue culture cell types and for different classes of polynucleotides, including DNA, messenger RNA *(14)*, and double-stranded RNA *(15)*.

The Lipofectin™ methodology is particularly notable for its simplicity. An aliquot of the sterile aqueous reagent is simply introduced into a DNA or RNA solution, and the mixture is added on tissue culture cells. The efficiency of the method is essentially unaffected by pH between 6.0–8.0 (P. Felgner, unpublished). This factor, among others, contributes to its convenience and reproducibility. For instance, a pH difference of as little as 0.1 pH unit in a calcium phosphate transfection experiment can make the difference between a positive and a negative result *(16)*. Other factors, such as precise mixing protocols, careful attention to the level of DNA in the experiment, and the presence of low levels of contaminants, are less important to the outcome of a Lipofectin™ experiment. In addition, large DNA molecules, such as baculovirus DNA (130 kb), have been successfully transfected into tissue culture cells (J. Barnett, personal communication).

Another attractive feature of the method is that relatively crude preparations of plasmid DNA, such as those made in "mini-preps," are efficiently introduced into cells. This allows for screening of large numbers of different DNAs. For example, the products of site-directed mutagenesis can be conveniently transfected without the need for the time consuming purification required by other methods (P. Felgner, unpublished).

Particularly exciting, Lipofectin™ has recently been found to be broadly applicable for the delivery and expression of messenger RNA in a wide variety of both adherent and suspension culture cell lines *(14)*. This has opened a new experimental approach to characterization of mRNA structure and function, which was not previously amenable to study using more conventional transfection procedures. For example, expression efficiency of mRNA synthesized in vitro has been shown to be strongly dependent on the presence of specific untranslated elements in the RNA construction (14). In addition, Lipofectin™ was also exploited successfully to deliver Sinbus virion RNA or infectious RNA transcribed in vitro, resulting in active virus particles (17).

Slightly different protocols have emerged. Each protocol avoids the aggregation of the DNA and liposomes that can reduce the efficiency of the method. Each protocol may be used interchangeably; however, for fine-tuning and optimization, they should be compared. The procedures work similarly for DNA and RNA transfections, although particular 5' and 3' untranslated elements must be present in the mRNA transcript in order to obtain expression in intact cells. These mRNA structural requirements are related to the biology of handling mRNA in intact cells rather than being requirements of the delivery system.

2. Materials

1. Tissue culture medium: Tissue culture conditions may vary, depending on the requirements of the cell line. Typically, Eagle's (EMEM) or Dulbecco's Minimum Essential Medium (DMEM), 10% fetal calf serum (FCS) or fetal bovine serum (FBS), and an antibiotic solution (Fungi Bact Solution, Irvine Scientific, Irvine, CA, which contains penicillin, streptomycin, and fungizone) are used to maintain cell lines. However, we recommend the use of Opti-MEM I (GIBCO) medium during the transfection step with this procedure. Opti-MEM I provides good cell viability under the reduced serum conditions that are required for optimal transfection activity with Lipofectin™ (*see* Notes 2 and 3). Opti-MEM may be used with or without β-mercaptoethanol.
2. Lipofectin™ (GIBCO/BRL).
3. Polystyrene tubes (Falcon): 17 × 100 mm (#2059) or 12 × 175 mm (#2058).
4. Tissue culture dishes: Either 60 mm or 100 mm.
5. Sterile water.
6. DNA samples: These may be CsCl-purified (*see* Chapter 1) or relatively impure minipreparations.
7. Phosphate-buffered saline (PBS): Optional.

3. Methods

3.1. Cationic Liposome-Mediated Transfection Protocol
3.1.1. Using Plasmid DNA

1. Seed 0.5×10^6 cells onto 60-mm plates and incubate overnight at 37°C. Any standard medium may be used, for example, 5 mL EMEM with 10% (v/v) FCS (*see* Note 1). Cells are typically about 80% confluent prior to transfection for transient assays because lower cell densities, for some cell lines, may result in increased toxicity during the transfection step.
2. Immediately prior to transfection, wash the cells three times with serum-free medium (*see* Notes 2 and 3). PBS is acceptable for this procedure, although any medium without serum may be used.
3. Dilute the Lipofectin™ reagent by adding to 1 vol of Opti-MEM I, and dilute the DNA with 1 vol of Opti-MEM I. For example, with 1×10^6 cells on a 60-mm dish, add 30 µg Lipofectin™ Reagent to 1.5 mL of Opti-MEM I, and 5 µg DNA into 1.5 mL of Opti-MEM I (*see* Note 4). The quantity of DNA and Lipofectin™ reagent required to produce an optimal signal varies with the cell type (*9*).
4. Combine the diluted reagents from the previous step (*see* Note 5) and add the mixture onto the washed tissue culture cells (*see* Note 6).
5. Incubate the cells at 37°C in a humidified environment with 5–10% CO_2 for 6 h (*see* Note 7).
6. Add 3 mL of medium with 20% (v/v) FCS. Other sources of serum may be used instead of fetal calf, depending on the viability of the cell type.
7. Incubate the cells for 24–48 h at 37°C in a humidified environment with 5–10% CO_2.
8. Harvest and assay for gene activity (*see* Chapters 3, 16, 17, and 18, this vol). The conditions required for optimum transfection efficiency may now be determined (*see* Notes 8 and 9).

3.1.2. Performing Bulk Transfections Using Plasmid DNA

For some experiments, it may be more convenient to prepare enough complex for several transfections in a concentrated stock. The important aspect of this procedure is that the stock solution should be prepared in water, rather than in saline solution or medium. This avoids an ionic strength mediated aggregation effect (*12,19*).

1. For each 60-mm dish, dilute 5 µg of DNA to 50 µL in water and 30 µg of Lipofectin™ reagent to 50 µL in water. Saline solutions cannot be used when the DNA and Lipofectin™ reagent are relatively concentrated.

2. Combine the solutions in a polystyrene tube and mix gently. Do not vortex. The solution may be slightly cloudy and still be effective. If a thick, thread-like precipitate forms, the transfection efficiency will be greatly reduced. Complexes stored at 4°C for 1 wk have been tested and are as active as freshly prepared complexes. Avoid polypropylene tubes, since the complexes tend to adhere to them (*see* Note 4).

3. Immediately prior to transfection, wash the cells three times with serum-free medium.

4. Add 3.0 mL Opti-MEM I to each well.

5. Add 100 μL of the DNA/liposome complex to each 60-mm well. The complex must be added dropwise, as uniformly as possible, across the entire plate. Addition of the complex to an isolated area of the plate will result in cell death in that area.

6. Proceed as described in Section 3.1.1., step 5.

3.2. Transfection Using RNA

The procedures required for RNA transfection are identical with the DNA methodology, except that the optimum quantity of Lipofectin™ required per unit mass of RNA may differ. In addition, it is important to recognize that messages that can be translated in in vitro reticulocyte lysate systems may not be active on intact cells. Intracellular activity requires a message that is flanked by untranslated elements. B. Malone et al. *(14)* describes an exemplary luciferase message that contains the 5' and 3' untranslated regions present in the Xenopus β-globin mRNA, in addition to a 3' poly A tail and a 5' Me-G cap. All of these untranslated elements are shown to be necessary for significant expression in intact cells (*see* Notes 10 and 11).

Cationic lipid delivery technology is emerging as a field of study *(19)*, suggesting that alternative cationic lipid molecules, improved formulations, and methodology enhancements may continue to be identified. Procedures for obtaining activity in the presence of serum, which would be expected to lower the toxicity of the treatment, would be particularly welcomed. Other enhancements leading to delivery of antisense molecules and ribozymes may be expected. Further improvements may result in a reagent for intracellular protein delivery and in vivo gene expression.

4. Notes

1. The small (30 nm in diameter) cationic lipid vesicles in the reagent can fuse to form large (>1 μm in diameter) multilamellar structures in the presence of polyvalent anions, such as EDTA, citrate, or phosphate *(12)*.

Preparations of these large fused vesicles are less efficacious than the small vesicles. Therefore, tissue culture media containing high concentrations of polyanionic buffers should be avoided. For example, transfections of 3T3 cells carried out in the presence of EMEM, which contains 1 mM phosphate, results in much higher levels of transient expression than similar transfections using RPMI, which contains 10 mM phosphate (Gary Rhodes, personal communication).

2. There are components present in serum that can inhibit Lipofectin™-mediated transfection. Since it can be shown that several purified chondroitin and heparin sulfates are inhibitory *(11)*, similar polyanionic factors present in serum may be responsible for this inhibitory effect. These polyanionic factors would be expected to compete with polynucleotides for binding to the cationic lipid vesicles. Alternatively (or simultaneously), they could bind to and neutralize the charge on the cationic lipid/ polynucleotide complexes, rendering them less subject to uptake by the anionic target cell surface. Although a wide variety of serum-free media give good results with lipofection, in a number of cell lines, Opti-MEM 1 (GIBCO/BRL) gives the best results with respect to both viability in the presence of Lipofectin™ and the level of expression obtained.

3. The toxicity of the treatment varies among different cell types, and elimination of serum from the transfection media further reduces viability. Screening of serum-free media has identified Opti-MEM as an acceptable serum-free medium, which results in improved viability, relative to EMEM or DMEM, in a number of different cell types.

4. Large nonfunctional polynucleotide/lipid aggregates can form when the polynucleotide concentration during formation of the Lipofectin™/ polynucleotide complexes is too high (approx 100 μg/mL or greater). Formation of these large aggregates is exacerbated by increased ionic strength; if it is desirable to prepare a concentrated stock solution of premixed Lipofectin™/polynucleotide complexes, they should be prepared at low ionic strength. In an effort to maintain both the polynucleotide and Lipofectin™ concentrations at the lowest possible concentration, prior to complex formation, the polynucleotide and Lipofectin™ should be separately diluted into equal vols of media and then mixed.

5. The concentration-dependent, ionic species and ionic strength-dependent aggregates that can form under different conditions are sticky, and they can be seen to adhere to glassware and to plastic. Polypropylene and glass attract these aggregates more than polystyrene. For this reason, polystyrene mixing containers are preferred.

6. It is not necessary to mix the lipid and the DNA prior to adding them to

the culture dish; the two components can be added sequentially. Either the lipid or the DNA can be added first, incubated for up to 1 h, and then the second component added. If, however, the DNA or the lipid is washed off the cells before addition of the second component, expression is prevented. These results indicate that the polynucleotide delivery occurs after formation of a complex among the cationic liposomes, the DNA, and the cell surface, rather than through leaky cells caused by damage to the cell surface by the Lipofectin™ reagent.

7. Optimum transfection activity occurs under conditions in which the net negative charge on the polynucleotide is substantially reduced. Quantitation of uptake of fluorescent complexes in the fluorescent-activated cell sorter indicates that complexes with an excess of positive charge are taken up by hybridoma cells 10–100-fold more effectively than neutral or negatively charged complexes (S. Foung and P. Felgner, unpublished). The optimum transfection activity for DNA and double-stranded RNA occurs when the ratio of positively charged molar equivalents (contributed by DOTMA) exceeds by 1.1–2.5 the number of molar equivalents of negative charge contributed by the polynucleotide. The molarity of DOTMA (mol wt, 669.5) in a 1 mg/mL Lipofectin™ solution that contains 50/50 (w/w) of DOPE (neutral lipid) is 0.75 mM; the molar equivalents of negative charge in a 1 mg/mL polynucleotide solution (average mol wt of the nucleotide monomer = 330) is 3 mM. Based on this estimate, the optimum activity occurs when the total mass of lipid (DOTMA + DOPE) exceeds the mass of polynucleotide by four- to tenfold. The amount of lipid required for optimum mRNA expression is less by a factor of about two; the optimum range for mRNA expression occurs when the mass of lipid exceeds the mRNA by two- to fivefold.

8. Although these protocols appear to be broadly applicable to many cell lines, careful optimization may be desirable for some applications. A general optimization procedure can be performed in two stages. The first step involves determining the toxic level of Lipofectin™ reagent for the cell line being tested. Toxicity varies among different cell types, but for 1×10^6 cells in 3 mL of medium, 60–80 µg of Lipofectin™ reagent usually causes cell death. Toxicity is indicated when cells round up and lift off the tissue culture dish. The reagent can be used successfully at about 50% below its toxic level. At this dose, the DNA level can be increased on separate culture dishes to give the maximum signal *(9)*. This signal usually occurs when the Lipofectin™ reagent/DNA ratio is in the range of 2:1–10:1 (w/w). The theoretical basis for an optimum 4:1 weight ratio has been previously discussed *(18)*.

9. An abbreviated optimization procedure that is particularly useful when quantities of plasmid are limited involves applying an acceptable quantity of plasmid to several tissue culture dishes and varying the quantity of Lipofectin™ reagent added.

10. RNasin may be included in the mRNA stock solution at 1–20 U/µg of mRNA without reducing RNA expression (J. Wolff, personal communication).

11. Carrier RNA at a ratio of 20:1–3:1 (carrier:message) can be used together with the message. Ribosomal RNA results in somewhat better activity than yeast transfer RNA (B. Malone, personal communication). ,

References

1. Bangham, A. D. (1981) Introduction, in *Liposomes from Physical Structure to Therapeutic Application* (Knight, G., ed.) Elsevier North-Holland, New York.

2. Straubinger, R. M. and Papahadjopoulos, D. (1983) Liposomes as carriers for intracellular delivery of nucleic acids. *Methods Enzymol.* **101,** 512–527.

3. Cudd, A. and Nicolau, C. (1984) Entrapment of recombinant DNA in liposomes and its transfer and expression of eukaryotic cells, *Liposome Technology* vol. II, CRC, Boca Raton, FL, pp. 207–221.

4. Mannino, R. J. and Fould-Fogerite, S. (1988) Liposome mediated gene transfer. *Biotechniques* **6,** 682–690.

5. Itani, T., Ariga, H., Yamaguchi, N., Tadakuma, T., and Yasuda, T. (1987) A simple and efficient liposome method for transfection of DNA into mammalian cells grown in suspension. *Gene* **56,** 267–276.

6. Nicolau, C., Legrand, A., and Grosse, G. E. (1987) Liposomes as carriers for in vivo gene transfer and expression. *Meth. Enzymol.* **149,** 157–176.

7. Wang, C. Y. and Huang, L. (1987) Ph-sensitive immunoliposomes mediate target cell-specific delivery and controlled expression of a foreign gene in mouse. *Proc. Natl. Acad.Sci. USA* **84,** 7851–7855.

8. Kaneda Y., Iwai, K., and Ucheda, T. (1989) Increased expression of DNA cointroduced with nuclear protein in adult rat liver. *Science* **243,** 375–378.

9. Felgner, P. L., Gadek, T. R., Holm, M., Roman, R., Chan, H. W., Wenze, M., Northrop, J. P., Ringold, G. M., and Danielsen, M. (1987) Lipofection: A highly efficient, lipid-mediated DNA- transfection procedure. *Proc. Natl. Acad. Sci. USA* **84,** 7413–7417.

10. Israelachvili, J. N., Mitchell, D. J., and Ninham, B. W. (1977) Theory of self-assembly of lipid bilayers and vesicles. *Biochim. Biophys. Acta* **470,** 185–201.

11. Felgner, P. L. and Holm, M. (1989) Cationic liposome-mediated transfection. *Focus* **11:2,** 21–25.

12. Düzgünes, N., Goldstein, J. A., Friend, D. S., and Felgner, P. L. (1989) Fusion of liposomes containing a novel cationic lipid N[1-(2,3-Dioleyloxy)Propyl]-N,N,N-Trimethylammonium: Induction by multivalent anions and asymmetric fusions with acidic phospholipid vesicles. *Biochemistry* **28,** 9179–9184.

13. Felgner, P. L. and Ringold, G. M. (1989) Cationic liposome-mediated transfection. *Nature* **337,** 387,388.

14. Malone, R., Felgner, P. L., and Verma, I. (1989) Lipofectin-mediated RNA transfection. *Proc. Natl. Acad. Sci. USA* **86,** 6077–6081.
15. Reid, T. R., Felgner, P. L., and Ringold, G. M. High efficiency RNA transfection using lipofectin: Poly IC mediated cytotoxicity in interferon treated cells (submitted to *J. Biol. Chem.*).
16. Chen, C. A. and Okayama, H. (1988) High-efficiency transformation of mammalian cells by plasmid DNA. *Biotechniques* **6,** 632–638.
17. Weiss, B., Nitschko, H., Ghattas, I., Wright, R., and Shlesinger, S. (1989) Evidence for specificity in the encapsidation of sindbis RNAs. *J. Virol.* **63,** 5310–5318.
18. Chang, A. C. Y. and Brenner, D. G. (1988) Cationic liposome-mediated transfection: A new for the introduction of DNA into mammalian cells. *Focus* **10,** 66–69.
19. Stamatatos, L., Leventis, R., Zuckermann, M. J., and Silvius, J. R. (1988) Interactions of cationic lipid vesicles with negatively charged phospholipid vesicles and biological membranes. *Biochemistry* **27,** 3917–3925.

CHAPTER 9

Preparation of High-Molecular-Weight DNA for Use in DNA Transfection

Secondary Transfections for Cloning Active Genes by Direct Phenotypic Selection

Michael A. Tainsky

1. Introduction

1.1. Applications of Transfections of Genomic DNA Samples

Calcium phosphate mediated transfection of genomic DNA samples into mammalian recipient cells can be used to isolate specific genes of interest. In theory, for any phenotype for which there is a suitable selection in cell culture, a gene sequence encoding that phenotype can be transferred and will complement the selection. If the donor sequences are derived from a different species of origin, the presence of the donor DNA in the recipient cell can be confirmed by Southern blotting, using a repeat DNA sequence probe from the donor species. Wigler and coworkers *(1)* found that in each cycle of transfection, the donor sequences represent approx 0.1% of the recipient cell's DNA. Therefore, after a second cycle of transfection using DNA from the first-cycle transfectant, the selected recipient cell will contain essentially a single gene and adjacent sequences.

From: *Methods in Molecular Biology, Vol. 7: Gene Transfer and Expression Protocols*
Edited by: E. J. Murray © 1991 The Humana Press Inc., Clifton, NJ

The genes of interest in the donor DNA can be cloned from libraries of DNA prepared from a secondary or tertiary transfectant, using a repeat sequence probe to screen that library. Alternatively, marker sequences can be ligated to the donor DNA *(2)*; if the marker survives two cycles of transfection remaining adjacent to the gene of interest, then its presence can be used to clone the gene of interest from the selected recipient cell. In the latter situation, the donor DNA and recipient cell can be from the same species and the marker sequence can be used to isolate clones of the gene of interest.

1.2. Development of Suitable Selections for Assaying a Biological Activity

The success of transfection experiments for the isolation of a specific gene by direct phenotypic selection is dependent on both techniques for the experiment and a systematic design for the transfection and selection of phenotypically transformed recipient cells. Although this chapter will provide the experimental methods and techniques, the design of the selection is at least as important and is dependent on the investigator's specific requirements. The simplest selections involve biochemical transformation of cells to be able to grow in metabolically restrictive media, such as HAT medium (hypoxanthine, aminopterin, thymidine; *see* Chapter 20, this vol) *(3)*, or in the presence of a cytotoxic antibiotic, such as G418 or hygromycin (*see* Chapter 19, this vol) *(4)*. In each case, genes that confer resistance to such cell culture media selections can be transfected into mammalian cells. Other selections that are commonly employed utilize formation of morphologically transformed foci in monolayers of normal cells *(5)* or tumorigenic transformation of such cells *(6)* by transfection of oncogene-containing DNA samples. Bassin and coworkers *(7)* have developed conditions to isolate genes that confer reversion of the transformed phenotype. Using such assays, Noda and coworkers *(8)*, as well as Schaefer and coworkers *(9)*, have isolated genes that can revert *ras*-transformed cells from a cDNA library and human genomic DNA, respectively. The key to such selective cell systems is to have a low spontaneous frequency of appearance of the selected phenotype, to have a transfection frequency high enough to obtain multiple primary transformants, and to have a method of confirming that each primary transformant contains donor DNA.

1.3. Limitations of Transfection Technology

The presence of a gene of interest in a donor DNA is not sufficient to ensure the transfer, selection, and isolation of that gene. There are several limitations of transfection technology for isolating eukaryotic genes.

1. The size of the gene must be sufficiently small for the gene to survive DNA preparation intact and pure enough to minimize toxicity to recipient cells at maximum transfection efficiency. In practice, genes as large as 100 kb have been successfully transfected. The details of preparing high-mol-wt DNA will be described in the Methods Section.
2. The gene should be expressed in the cell or tissue of origin, because features of gene structure that reduce expression, such as DNA methylation, will be retained during DNA preparation.
3. If the phenotype for which the selection is designed is contained in more than one unlinked gene, it is statistically unlikely (10^{-3}/gene) that the function can be isolated using transfection and direct phenotypic selection.

Assuming that these criteria are not problematic, isolation of the gene of interest can be facilitated by a systematic design of the transfection experiment.

2. Materials

Molecular biological grade phenol, SDS, and other salt and buffers can be purchased from many companies. A high grade of chloroform should be used. All reagents are prepared in nanopure water. Glass cloning cylinders were purchased from Belco Glass Co., Vineland, NJ.

2.1. Extraction of DNA from Cell Cultures

1. Tris-buffered saline (TBS): 20 mM Tris-HCl, pH 8.0, and 140 mM NaCl. Autoclave prior to using.
2. Ethylenediamine tetraacetic acid (EDTA): 0.5M EDTA is prepared by neutralizing to pH 8.0 with 4N NaOH. Autoclave prior to using.
3. Lysis buffer: TBS with 50 mM EDTA, 100 μg/mL proteinase K, 0.5% SDS.
4. Phenol/chloroform 1:1, v/v.
5. Chloroform.
6. Dialysis tubing (6000 M_r lower exclusion) is hydrated and boiled for 20 min in 0.5M EDTA, and a second time in nanopure H_2O. It is stored in the H_2O in which it was boiled at 4°C for up to 1 mo.
7. Tris/EDTA (TE): 10 mM Tris-HCl, pH 8.0, and 1 mM EDTA. Autoclave prior to using.
8. DNase-free RNase: Prepared by boiling RNase A for 15 min at 2 mg/mL solution in H_2O.
9. Ligated bacteriophage l DNA as mol wt markers.
10. Disposable cell scrapers.

2.2. Extraction of DNA from Tissue Samples

1. Liquid nitrogen.
2. Motorized blender with metal chamber.
3. 150 mM NaCl in TE.
4. Remaining reagents as described in Section 2.1.

3. Methods

3.1. Preparation of Donor DNA

3.1.1. From Cell Cultures

1. Grow the cells just to confluence in either tissue culture flasks or roller bottles. Wash the cells with cold TBS until no further red color from the tissue culture medium is detectable in the washes, and then one additional time. This generally requires three washes.
2. Cover the cells in lysis buffer, 3 mL/150-cm² culture flask, and leave for 10 min at room temperature.
3. The cell lysate is then transferred with the help of disposable scrapers to disposable 50-mL screw-cap centrifuge tubes (up to 20 mL of lysate/tube) and the mixture incubated at 50°C for 3h.
4. DNase-free RNase is added to the lysate, to a final concentration of 10 μg/mL, for 2 h at 37°C to allow the cellular RNA to be degraded.
5. The mixture is then rocked very gently with an equal vol of phenol/chloroform for 10–20 min. Care must be taken to rock the solution gently to avoid reducing the size of the DNA.
6. The mixture is then centrifuged for 30 min at 5000 rpm. This will generate an upper aqueous phase; a thick, opaque interphase; and a lower phase of phenol/chloroform. The upper phase contains the DNA and is removed with a large-bore plastic disposable pipet.
7. Repeat the phenol/chloroform extraction once. If the resulting solution is clear, it is then extracted with chloroform. If the solution contains any opacity, then the phenol/chloroform extraction is repeated.
8. After extraction with chloroform, the upper aqueous phase is dialyzed against three changes of 100 vol of TE in the cold (24 h for each change). The extent of residual protein in the DNA preparation is determined by reading the UV absorbance at 260 and 280 nm. The A_{260}/A_{280} ratio should be >1.8 for use in transfection.
9. The integrity of the DNA preparation can be established by electrophoresis on 0.4% agarose gels at 4°C at low voltage, using ligated

bacteriophage λ DNA ladder as standards. The cellular DNA should migrate as a smear between 100 and 200 kbp in length (*see* Note 1).

3.1.2. From Tissue Samples

DNA from tissues is prepared by a modification of the above method:

1. The tissue, either fresh or previously frozen in liquid nitrogen, is placed with liquid nitrogen in a stainless steel motorized blender until a powder has formed.
2. The resulting fine powder is suspended in 10 vol of lysis buffer and incubated for 3 h and for 2 h at 37°C with RNase, as described above for cellular DNA preparation. DNA prepared from tissues tends to contain more protein; when the above procedure is applied to tissue samples, it is very difficult to remove all of the opacity from the aqueous phase after phenol/chloroform extraction. If this occurs, after three phenol/chloroform extractions, continue to step 3.
3. Proceed with chloroform extraction and dialyze overnight against 100 vol of TE with NaCl added to 150 mM.
4. The resulting solution after dialysis is then reextracted twice with phenol/chloroform, then chloroform-extracted as above for cell cultures, and dialyzed against three changes of 100 vol of TE in the cold (24 h for each change).
5. The resulting preparation is generally free of protein, as judged by A_{260}/A_{280} ratio.

3.2. Establishing a Significant Biological Assay

There are two general approaches for transfecting and isolating a particular gene. One method involves transfection and subsequent direct phenotypic selection, such as growth in selective media *(1)*; morphological phenotype, such as muscle cell differentiation *(11)*, biological markers *(12)*, focus formation *(5)*; or using an immunological selection (*see* Chapters 26 and 27, this vol). Alternatively, the genomic DNA is cotransfected with a drug-selectable plasmid DNA, such as pSV2*neo (10)*. If a sufficient number (>3000) of selected cells are obtained, then the population will contain all donor-cell sequences represented in at least one cell. This population can then be tested further for the phenotype being sought in a second selection, as described above. This second approach has the disadvantage of every cell containing the genomic sequences; detection of repeated DNA sequences by Southern blotting of the recipient cells as a confirmation of the transfer of donor-cell genomic DNA sequences must await a second cycle of transfection.

3.3. Analysis of Transfected Sequences

Because the goal of transfection experiments is to isolate the gene coding for the phenotype to be studied, it is important to set up the primary transfections in a fashion that will facilitate this end. We generally maintain independent primary transfection plates of cells. During subculture and subsequent selection, the cells from individual plates are never pooled. The number of plates used depends on the transfection efficiency, so that >3000 colonies can be tested for phenotypic conversion. Therefore, one can obtain truly independent primary transfectants from which independent secondary selectants can be acquired. If foci or colonies of selected cells are obtained, then they are isolated with glass cloning cylinders and transferred by trypsinization to 35-mm tissue culture dishes. These cultures are expanded for DNA preparation. Analysis of transfected sequences in successfully selected secondary transfectants by Southern blotting with repeat sequence or marker probes will reveal whether consistent restriction enzyme fragments are present (*see* Notes 3 and 4). If so, molecular cloning of such consistent restriction enzyme fragments will provide the first pieces of the gene (*see* Vol 2, this series).

Once candidate cell selectants have been isolated, they are cryopreserved to avoid loss resulting from accidents or contamination. Sufficient DNA is prepared to screen for the transfected sequences by Southern blotting. If this can be achieved quickly, the cells are maintained in culture for that period. If not, then the cells are disposed of and, when blot analysis is complete, cryopreserved cells are revived and used for larger-scale DNA preparation for subsequent transfections and cloning.

If repeat sequence probes will be used for the subsequent cloning, we have found that cloning gel-purified consistent restriction enzyme fragments and then using them as probes to screen a representative genomic library from a secondary transfectant yields the biologically active gene more quickly than trying to sort out clones derived from screening the representative genomic library with the repeat sequence probe. This is because of cross hybridization of the repeats from different species, which is less of a problem when cloning from specifically enriched gel-purified fragments.

4. Notes

1. The DNA preparations are not precipitated and spooled out on a glass wand if DNA with a very high mol wt is desired.
2. Southern blotting of primary transfectants with a repeat sequence probe

tends to give strong hybridization to numerous bands. Sometimes, though rarely, it is difficult to resolve individual bands.

3. Avoid the temptation to place control donor DNA on the same Southern blot when probing for repeat sequences, since this can soak up a lot of probe. It is better to place the positive control lanes in a separate bag for hybridization using the same amout of probe.

4. The source of repeat sequence probe can be either a cloned repeat sequence DNA fragment or total genomic DNA from the donor species. In either case, the hybridization and washing conditions need to be set up such that DNA from an untransfected recipient cell on the Southern blot is not hybridizing and a positive control has a strong signal. We have found that when total genomic DNA is labeled for a probe, the hybridization and washing conditions need to be stringent, whereas the cloned repeat sequence probes require less stringency to retain a strong signal.

References

1. Wigler, M., Sweet, R., Sim, G. K., Wold, B., Pellicer, A., Lacy, E., Maniatis, T., Silverstein, S., and Axel, R. (1977) Transformation of mammalian cells with genes from procaryotes and eucaryotes. *Cell* 16, 777–785.
2. Westerveld, A., Hjoeijamakers, J. H. J., Duin, M., de Wit, J., Odijk, H., Pasternik, A., and Bootsma, D. (1984) Molecular cloning of a human DNA repair gene. *Nature* 310, 425–429.
3. Szybalski, W., Szybalska, E. H., and Ragni, G. (1962) Genetic studies with human cell lines. *Natl. Cancer Monogr.* 7, 75–79.
4. Southern, P. J. and Berg, P. (1982) Transformation of mammalian cells to antibiotic resistance with a bacterial gene under control of the SV40 early region promotor. *Mol. Appl. Genet.* 1, 327–341.
5. Shih, C., Shilo, B. Z., Goldfarb, M. P., Dannenberg, A., and Weinberg, R. A. (1979) Passage of phenotypes of chemically transformed cells via transfection of DNA and chromatin. *Proc. Natl. Acad. Sci. USA* 76, 5714–5718.
6. Blair, D. G., Cooper, C. S., Oskarsson, M. K., Eader, L. A., and Vande Woude, G. F. (1982) New method for detecting cellular transforming genes. *Science* 218, 1122–1125.
7. Benade, L. E., Talbot, N., Tagliaferri, P., Hardy, C., Card, J., Noda, M., Najam, N., and Bassin, R. H. (1986) Ouabain sensitivity is linked to *ras* transformation in human HOS cells. *Biochem. Biophys. Res. Commun.* 136, 807–814.
8. Noda, M., Kitayama, H., Matsuzaki, T., Sugimoto, Y., Okayama, H., Bassin, R. H., and Ikawa, Y. (1989) Detection of genes with a potential for suppressing the transformed phenotype associated with activated *ras* genes. *Proc. Natl. Acad. Sci. USA* 86, 162–166.
9. Schafer, R., Iyer, J., Iten, E., and Nirkko, A. C. (1988) Partial reversion of the transformed phenotype in Hras-transfected tumorigenic cells by transfer of a human gene. *Proc. Natl. Acad. Sci. USA* 85, 1590–1594.

10. Southern, P. J. and Berg, P. (1982) Transformation of mammalian cells to antibiotic resistance with a bacterial gene under control of the SV40 early region promoter. *J. Mol. Appl. Genet.* **1,** 327–341.

11. Pinney, D. E., Pearson White, S. H., Konieczny, S. F., Latham, K. E., and Emerson, C. P., Jr. (1988) Myogenic lineage determination and differentiation: Evidence for a regulatory gene pathway. *Cell* **53,** 781–793.

12. Littman, D. R., Thomas, Y., Maddon, P. J., Chess, L., and Axel, R. (1985) The isolation and sequence of the gene encoding T8: A molecule defining functional classes of T lymphocytes. *Cell* **40,** 237–246.

CHAPTER 10

Chromosome-Mediated Gene Transfer

Janet M. Shipley and Denise Sheer

1. Introduction

McBride and Ozer *(1)* were the first to show that purified metaphase chromosomes could act as vectors in transferring genetic information into mammalian cells. This technique, termed chromosome-mediated gene transfer (CMGT), involves the transfer of subchromosomal fragments from the cells of one species (the donor, usually human) to those of another (the recipient, usually a rodent) that have the ability to maintain them. CMGT thus fills a gap between the isolation of whole chromosomes, produced by cell fusion and microcell-mediated gene transfer, and the isolation of relatively short stretches of DNA by cloning or transfection methods.

CMGT is an important technique that has made a significant contribution to two main areas of research. First, it has been used as a strategy for enrichment cloning and for mapping genetic markers along the length of a chromosome. Second, it has been used as an assay for transforming genes, and has potential for the study of functional aspects of large and complex loci. CMGT will probably continue to play a role in the definition of disease loci.

CMGT is a technique very similar to the more familiar DNA-mediated gene transfer or DNA transfection. The main difference is that the donor DNA in CMGT is present in the form of complete chromosomes rather than

From: *Methods in Molecular Biology, Vol. 7: Gene Transfer and Expression Protocols*
Edited by: E. J. Murray © 1991 The Humana Press Inc., Clifton, NJ

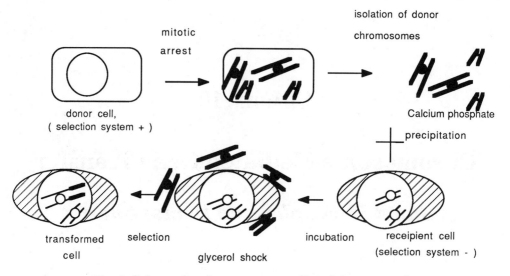

Fig. 1. Scheme for chromosome-mediated gene transfer.

as pure DNA. The method to be described for producing CMGT hybrids is outlined in Fig. 1. Donor cells are treated with a metaphase block, such as colchicine, in order to obtain a maximum number of cells containing chromosomes at metaphase. The plasma membrane is disrupted and the chromosomes separated from whole nuclei by differential centrifugation *(2)*. Coprecipitates form when the chromosomes in phosphate buffer are mixed with calcium chloride and the resulting preparation is added to the recipient cells, which are typically grown in a monolayer *(3)*. Subsequent glycerol or dimethyl sulfoxide (DMSO) treatment can increase the efficiency of transfection *(4)*. The recipient cells are then returned to their usual growing conditions for a short time before selection.

Due consideration to a strategy for rescuing or identifying tranfectants is crucial to the success of the technique. Some of these are outlined below.

A variety of phenotypic selection criteria for oncogenic transforming activity may be possible. These include focus formation with loss of contact inhibition, anchorage-independent growth, and direct selection for tumorigenicity *(5)*. This is an extension of tumor-DNA-mediated transfection *(6)* and means that by definition, the isolated CMGT transfectants contain DNA that may be implicated in neoplasia. Transforming activity has also been used to isolate specific regions containing disease loci; for example, the activated oncogenes c-Harvey-*ras* (HRAS 1) and MET have been used as dominant selectable markers *(5,7)* in the cotransfer of the aniridia–Wilms' tumor region *(8)* and the cystic fibrosis locus *(7)*, respectively.

Alternatively, one can rescue hybrids that express an endogenous biochemical marker from the donor on the background of a deficient recipient cell line. The best known examples are the human phosphoribosyl transferase (*hprt*) gene on the long arm of human chromosome X *(9)* and the thymidine kinase *(tk)* gene on the long arm of human chromosome 17 *(10)*. As an example, *tk* selection was used to produce a panel of CMGT hybrids containing fragments of chromosome 17 *(11)*. These allowed markers to be ordered along the length of the chromosome when used in conjunction with *in situ* hybridization and the analysis of somatic cell hybrids containing well-defined breaks on chromosome 17 *(11)*. Using the defined CMGT panel, new probes could easily be assigned a provisional location. Some of the hybrids containing small regions of chromosome 17 are particularly relevant to the study of the acute promyelocytic leukemia translocation breakpoint region and the gene for von Recklinghausen's neurofibromatosis *(11)*. They may be an appropriate source for constructing gene libraries enriched for these regions, as has been done for the distal region of chromosome X *(12)*.

Biochemical markers, such as HPRT and TK, limit selection to a few specific areas of the genome. One way of selecting alternative regions is to use species-specific monoclonal antibodies that recognize cell-surface antigens *(13,14)*. There are at least 30 such antibodies available for humans *(15)*. Porteous *(16)* has suggested direct visualization of the expressing clones in a rosseting assay with the monoclonal antibodies coupled to red blood cells.

A fluorescence-activated cell sorter (FACS) can be used sequentially to clone cells expressing a particular antigen *(14)*. However, disadvantages are a tendency to select for the most highly expressing clones, and a possible association with secondary amplification. Pritchard and Goodfellow *(17,18)* avoided the need for sequential rounds of enrichment by preselecting for cells that were more likely to be expressing the cell-surface marker before turning to the FACS. Plasmid DNA containing an antibiotic-resistant marker (pSV*neo*), was cotransfected with chromosomes from a somatic cell hybrid containing chromosome Y as its only human content. The uptake and maintenance of pSV*neo*, which allowed only those cells resistant to G418 to grow, indicated a positive transfection event by CMGT. This enriched population was then sorted for transfectants expressing the 12E7 surface antigen and thus containing fragments of the Y chromosome. The procaryotic vector was in some cases shown to have integrated into the Y chromosome *(17)*.

Integration of pSV*neo* into the Y chromosome illustrates an alternative selective strategy in which the procaryotic vector containing the selectable marker integrates into, or near, the region of interest. This has the advantage over cell sorting of maintaining continual selective pressure. Integration into a particular region can be achieved by a random or a nonrandom approach.

After random insertion of a vector carrying a selectable gene into the donor's genome, a chromosome of interest can be isolated by microcell- mediated gene transfer. This hybrid can then act as the donor for CMGT with selection for the different regions of the chromosome where the marker has integrated *(19)*. A method of mass screening colonies by molecular hybridization with donor DNA has been used in conjunction with this method *(19)*. This may have potential for screening transfectants when the donor cell line is a hybrid containing a single chromosome or subchromosomal fragment from the species of interest and there is no other obvious selective strategy.

Nonrandom insertion or gene-targeting of a marker can be accomplished by splicing the marker to be integrated with a DNA probe from a gene in the region of interest. This DNA may then be integrated into the site of the gene by homologous recombination *(20,21)*.

Stable hybrids produced by CMGT usually contain a subchromosomal fragment or fragments attached to one or more of the recipient's chromosomes. Alternatively, a fragment may include its own centromere, and there seems to be a preferential retention of alphoid sequences associated with human centromeres and the regions adjacent to them *(18)*. The amount of donor DNA maintained is usually in the region of 1–50 Mbp but ranges from 100 kb to 100 Mbp *(5)*. The DNA donor of most transfectants appear to suffer from multiple interstitial deletions *(5,22)*, and other rearrangements, such as translocations and amplification, are also possible. Evaluation of the extent of deletions or rearrangements is usually appropriate before using transfectants; some of the ways of doing this are outlined in the Notes Section.

2. Materials

1. Sterile phosphate-buffered saline (PBSA).
2. $1.25 M$ $CaCl_2$: Autoclave and store at 4°C.
3. Solution 1 (lysis buffer): 10 mM HEPES, pH 7.1; 3 mM $CaCl_2$. Autoclave and store at 4°C.
4. Solution 2: 25 mM HEPES, pH 7.1; 134 mM NaCl; 5 mM KCl; 5 mM glucose; 0.7 mM Na_2HPO_4. Filter-sterilize and store at –20°C.
5. Solution 3 (washing buffer): Same as solution 2, but without glucose. Autoclave and store at –20°C.

6. Colcemid® solution (GIBCO/BRL): 10-µg/mL sterile stock solution in Hanks' balanced salt solution. Store at 4°C.

3. Method

1. The donor cells are blocked in metaphase for 16–24 h using 0.1 µg/mL Colcemid®. Approximately 2×10^8 rapidly dividing cells are required to give sufficient chromosomes.
2. The cells are removed, by trypsin treatment or scraping, pelleted, and washed in 10 mL of cold PBSA in a plastic conical-based centrifuge tube.
3. The cells are then resuspended in cold solution 1 (lysis buffer) and mixed gently by drawing the suspension up and down a plastic pipet. The solution and all the plasticware should be at 4°C.
4. After standing on ice for 30 min, the suspension is passed through a 21-gage needle 10 times.
5. Differential centrifugation then separates the chromosomes from the rest of the cellular material *(2)*. This is done by spinning at 150*g* for 7 min and collecting the supernatant, which is then spun at 1500*g* for 25 min. The pellet is resuspended in more cold lysis buffer and spun again at 150*g* for 7 min and then the supernatant spun at 1500*g* for 25 min. All centrifugation should be carried out at 4°C. The chromosomes in the final pellet are then resuspended in 9 mL of cold solution 2.
6. Calcium chloride (1.25*M*, 1 mL) is slowly added dropwise while the suspension is being bubbled with air from a Pasteur pipet. This is left at 4°C for 20–30 min to allow a coprecipitate of calcium phosphate and chromosomes to form.
7. Then 1 mL of the coprecipitate is added to each of ten 10-cm-diameter Petri dishes containing 5×10^5 recipient cells that were plated out the previous day. The dishes are then incubated at 37°C for 4 h.
8. The cells are washed using warm solution 3, and 1 mL of 15% glycerol (in solution 3) is added and left for 4 min. Excessive treatment can remove cells from the surface of the dish.
9. The glycerol solution is quickly but carefully washed off using solution 3 at 37°C, rinsing two or three times before returning the cells to normal media. Selection would normally be applied about 24 h later.
10. It usually takes 2–3 wk before colonies consisting of around 50 cells become visible. It is best not to pick too many colonies from a single plate, since it is possible that they may actually be derived from a single transfected cell. Clones can be expanded and grown up for DNA, chromosome, or expression studies.

4. Notes

1. There are many factors that contribute to the efficiency of transfection. One can expect a transfection frequency in the range of one in 10^5 to one in 5×10^5 cells with donor chromosomes carrying a selectable marker. If this is not achieved, an important consideration (beyond care at the various stages pointed out in the method) is the choice and condition of the cells. Rapidly dividing cells will yield more chromosomes, so optimal culturing conditions are important; growing many more cells may be necessary to obtain sufficient chromosomes. An aliquot can be taken before adding $CaCl_2$, pelleted, and resuspended in fixative consisting of 1:3 glacial acetic acid:methanol. This can be dropped onto a slide, stained with Giemsa's stain, and examined under the microscope to give an idea of the quality of the harvest. Applying 10 chromosomes/recipient cell is recommended *(17)*. The recipient cells must have the ability to grow from single cells into colonies.

2. As with all tissue culture on a large scale (particularly when cells are grown in dishes for any length of time), great care should be taken to avoid infections. It is advisable to make stocks of transfected cells at the earliest possible stage.

3. Some evaluation of stability may be appropriate. One way to assess this is by determining the number of colonies surviving with and without selection for a given transfectant *(17)*.

4. A detailed analysis of the transfectant's donor DNA content may be appropriate, and, since further rearrangements are always possible during culturing, checking after expansion is advised. There are many ways for assessing the donor DNA, including the following:

   a. Estimating the total amount of DNA from dot blots *(17; see also* Chapter 28*)*.

   b. Defining transfectants by the presence or absence of DNA sequences and expressed markers (isoenzymes and cell-surface markers).

   c. Cytogenetic analysis after *in situ* hybridization with total donor DNA or probes that flank a region of interest.

   d. Pulsed-field gel electrophoresis analysis for long-range mapping *(23)*.

   e. L1 "fingerprinting," which augments conventional mapping information *(24)*, can be used with CMGT DNA *(5)*. Members of the L1 (formerly Kpn1) family of human repeat sequences produce a distinct hybridization pattern (or "fingerprint") with an appropriate restriction enzyme, usually Kpnl, since many of the L1 sequences have lost one or more of their internal consensus sites. Some transformants have banding patterns that appear to be subsets of each other and of whole chromosomes, and others do not, which suggests rearrangements of the donor DNA. The human DNA content can be estimated from the overall intensity of hybridization to the bands recognized by the L1 probe. It is also possible to estimate the distances between linked markers by comparing the L1 "fingerprint" with single-copy cotransfer data (5).

5. An alternative technique for isolating subchromosomal fragments in somatic cells is termed irradiation and fusion gene transfer (IFGT). This involves X-irradiating the donor hybrid to cause breaks prior to fusion, followed by selective pressure, if applicable (25, Chapter 6). IFGT appears to have fewer problems with deletions, particularly if the fragments are $<10^7$ bp, so it may be the method of choice for producing libraries from small regions of the genome (26).

References

1. McBride, O. W. and Ozer, H. L. (1973) Transfer of genetic information by purified metaphase chromosomes. *Proc. Natl. Acad. Sci. USA* **70**, 1258–1262.
2. Weiss, J. H., Nelson, D. L., Pryborski, M. J., Chaplin, D. D., Mulligan R. C., Housman, D. E., and Seidman, J. G. (1984) Eukaryotic chromosome transfer. Linkage of the murine major histocompatability complex to an inserted selectable marker. *Proc. Natl. Acad. Sci. USA* **81**, 4879–4883.
3. Spandidos, D. A. and Siminovitch, L. (1977) Transfer of codominant markers by isolated metaphase chromosomes in Chinese hamster ovary cells. *Proc. Natl. Acad. Sci. USA* **74**, 3480–3484.
4. Gross, T. A., Squires, S., Martin, P., and Baker, and R. M. (1979) Chromosome-mediated gene transfer in an intraspecific human cell system. *J. Cell Biol.* **83**, 453.
5. Porteous, D. J., Morten J. E. N., Cranston, G., Fletcher, J. M., Mitchell, A., van Heyningen, V., Fantes, J. A., Boyd, P. A., and Hastie, N. D. (1986) Molecular and physical arrangements of human DNA in HRAS-1 selected chromosome mediated transfectants. *Mol. Cell. Biol.* **6**, 2223–2232.
6. Morten, J. E. N., Hirst, M. C., and Porteous, D. J. (1987) The c-H-*ras*-1 oncogene in chromosome mediated gene transfer. *Anticancer Res.* **7**, 573–588.
7. Scambler, P. J., Law, H. Y., Williamson, R., and Cooper, C. S. (1987) Chromosome mediated gene transfer of six DNA markers linked to the cystic fibrosis locus on human chromosome seven. *Nucleic Acid Res.* **14**, 7159–7174.
8. van Heyningen, V. and Porteous, D. J. (1986) Mapping a chromosome to find a gene. *Trends Genet.* **2**, 4,5.
9. Murphy, P. D., Miller, C. L., and Ruddle, F. H. (1985) Quantitation of the transgenome size in chromosome-mediated gene transfer lines. *Cytogenet. Cell Genet.* **39**, 125–133.

10. Klobutcher, L. A. and Ruddle, F. H. (1979) Phenotype stabilization and integration of transferred material in chromosome-mediated gene transfer. *Nature* **280,** 657–660.

11. Xu, W., Gorman, P. A., Rider, S. H., Hedge, P. J., Moore, G, Pritchard, C., Sheer, D., and Solomon, E. (1988) Construction of a genetic map of the human chromosome 17 by use of chromosome mediated gene transfer. *Proc. Natl. Acad. Sci. USA* **85,** 8563–8567.

12. Murphy, P. D. and Ruddle, F. H. (1985) Isolation and regional mapping of random X sequences from distal human X chromosome. *Somat. Cell Mol. Genet.* **11,** 433–444.

13. Goodfellow, P. N., Banting, G.,Wiles, M. V., Tunnacliffe, A., Parkar, M., Solomon, E., Dalchau, R., and Fabre, J. W. (1982) The gene, MIC4, which controls expression of the antigen defined by monoclonal antibody F10.44.2, is on human chromosome 11. *Eur. J. Immunol.* **12,** 659–663.

14. Kuhn, L. C., McClelland, A., and Ruddle, F. H. (1984) Gene transfer, expression, and molecular cloning of the human transferrin gene. *Cell* **37,** 95–103.

15. McAlpine, P. J., Shows, T. B., Miller, R. L., Boucheix, C., Stranc, L. C., Berent, T. G., Pakstis, A. J., and Douté, R. C. (1989) The 1989 catalog of mapped genes and report of the nomenclature committee. *Cytogenet. Cell Genet.* **51,** 13–66.

16. Porteous, D. J. (1987) Chromosome mediated gene transfer: A functional assay for complex loci and an aid to human genome mapping. *Trends Genet.* **3,** 171–182.

17. Pritchard, C. and Goodfellow, P. (1986) Development of new methods in human genome mapping: Selection for fragments of the human Y chromosome after chromosome mediated gene transfer. *EMBO J.* **5,** 979–985.

18. Pritchard, C. and Goodfellow, P. N. (1987) Investigation of chromosome-mediated gene transfer using the HPRT region of the human X chromosome as a model. *Genes Dev.* **1,** 172–178.

19. Siden, T. S., Hoglund, M., and Rohme, D. (1989) Construction of microcell hybrid panel containing different *neo* gene insertions in mouse chromosome 17 used for chromosome mediated gene transfer. *Somat. Cell Mol. Genet.* **15,** 245.

20. Capecchi, M. R. (1989) The new mouse genetics: Altering genome by gene targeting. *Trends Genet.* **5,** 70–76.

21. Dorin, J. R., Inglis, J. D., and Porteous, D. J. (1989) Selection for precise chromosomal targeting of a dominant marker by homologous recombination. *Science* **243,** 1357–1360.

22. Goodfellow, P. N. and Pritchard, C. A. (1988) Chromosome fragmentation by chromosome mediated gene transfer. *Cancer Surv.* **7,** 251–265.

23. Brickmore,W. A., Maule, J. C., van Heyningen, V., and Porteous, D. J. (1989) Long-range structure of H-*ras* 1-selected transgenomes. *Somat. Cell Mol. Genet.* **15,** 229–235.

24. Gusella, J. F., Jones, C., Kao, F., Housman, D., and Puck, T. T. (1982) Genetic fine-structure in human chromosome 11 by use of repetitive DNA sequences. *Proc. Natl. Acad. Sci. USA* **79,** 7804–7808.

25. Goss, S. J. and Harris, H. (1975) New method for mapping genes in human chromosomes. *Nature* **255,** 680–683.

26. Benham, F., Hart, K., Crolla, J., Bobrow, M., Francavilla, M., and Goodfellow, P. N. (1989) A method for generating hybrids containing nonselected fragments of human chromosomes. *Genomics* **4,** 509–517.

CHAPTER 11

Manipulation of Adenovirus Vectors

Frank L. Graham and Ludvik Prevec

1. Introduction

Adenoviruses are intermediate-sized DNA viruses with genomes, consisting of linear double-stranded DNA molecules of approx 36,000 bp. The virion is an icosahedron about 70 nm in diameter, consisting exclusively of protein and DNA. Adenoviruses have been isolated from a large number of different species (mammalian and fowl) and over 100 different serotypes have been reported, some 43 of them human. The human adenoviruses, particularly types 2, 5, and 12, have been the most extensively characterized, and these viruses have served as valuable tools in the study of the molecular biology of DNA replication, transcription, RNA processing, and protein synthesis in mammalian cells. *See* ref. *1* for a general review.

For a number of reasons, adenoviruses are attracting increasing attention as potential mammalian cell expression vectors and recombinant vaccines (for an excellent recent review of adenovirus vectors, *see* ref. *2*). Not only is the viral particle relatively stable, but also, in the case of serotypes commonly used as vectors to date, the viral genome does not undergo rearrangement at a high rate, and insertions of foreign genes are generally maintained without change through successive rounds of viral replication. The adenovirus genome is also relatively easy to manipulate by recombinant DNA techniques, and the virus replicates efficiently in permissive cells. Infected cells

From: *Methods in Molecular Biology, Vol. 7: Gene Transfer and Expression Protocols*
Edited by: E. J. Murray © 1991 The Humana Press Inc., Clifton, NJ

produce 1000–10,000 plaque-forming units (PFU), and the virus remains concentrated within the cell long after yields have reached maximum levels, making collection and concentration of virus extremely easy. Since a large fraction of the infected cell protein and DNA is viral at late stages of infection, adenoviruses are very attractive as vectors for high-level expression of proteins in mammalian cells. Furthermore, because adenoviruses can transform a variety of different cell types, resulting in the integration of viral DNA into the host-cell chromosome, adenoviruses carrying foreign DNA may serve as efficient gene transfer vectors in mammalian cells. Finally, the availability of over 40 different human serotypes, and of many different viruses isolated from other animals, affords considerable versatility in the selection of appropriate viruses for specific purposes.

This chapter outlines the methods for growing, titrating, and purifying adenoviruses; for extracting viral DNA from purified virions, and from infected cells; for rescuing inserts of foreign DNA into the viral genome; and for assessing the expression of inserted genes in adenovirus vectors. The details derive from our work with human adenovirus type 5 (Ad5), but the principles should apply to manipulation of other adenovirus serotypes.

Figure 1 shows a simplified map of the Ad5 genome, with a few key landmarks (for more details, *see* ref. *1*). The replication cycle of the virus can be divided into two phases: early, corresponding to events occurring before the onset of viral DNA replication; and late, corresponding to the period after initiation of DNA replication. During the early phase, four noncontiguous regions of the genome are expressed: early region 1 (E1), which comprises Ela and Elb; E2; E3; and E4. After the onset of DNA replication, the major late promoter (MLP) located at 16 map units (mμ) drives much of the viral transcription. Transcription originating from the MLP terminates near the right end of the genome, and the late transcripts are processed into a complex array of different mRNAs (not shown in Fig. 1) that encode most of the structural virion proteins.

Some of the restriction enzyme sites most frequently used in the manipulation of Ad5 DNA are shown in Fig. 1. ClaI cuts only once near the left end (2.5 mμ) in wild-type Ad5 DNA; Bam HI cleaves wild-type DNA once at 59.5 mμ and EcoRI cuts twice, at 76.0 and 83.5 mμ. XbaI makes four cuts in wild-type DNA, but a useful mutant, *dl*309 *(3),* has retained only the XbaI site at 3.7 mμ in E1—*dl*309 DNA and the enzymes ClaI and XbaI are widely used in the construction of Ad5 mutants and vectors containing altered E1 sequences.

There are at least three regions of the viral genome that can accept insertions or substitutions of DNA to generate a helper independent virus. These are in E1, in E3, and in a short region between E4 and the end of the genome

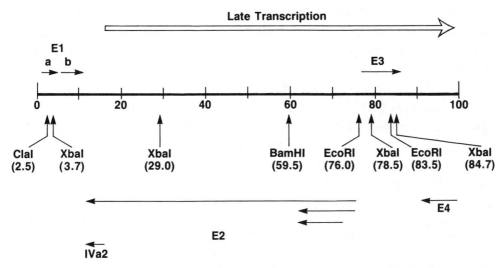

Fig. 1. Structure of the Ad5 genome. Locations of a few restriction enzyme sites are indicated in map units (mμ) (100 mμ = 100% = 36 kb). Arrows indicate transcriptional units.

(*see* ref. 2 and studies cited therein). Our work has involved insertions or substitutions, principally in E3 and to some extent in E1, and the methods outlined in the following sections deal specifically with construction of vectors having inserts of foreign genes in either of those two regions. However, with minor modifications, the techniques we describe should be applicable to insertion of DNA into any nonessential region of the genome.

E1 is not required for viral replication in human 293 cells (a line that is transformed by Ad5 DNA and contains and expresses the left end of the genome) (4), and E3 is nonessential for replication of adenovirus in cultured human cells. The most DNA that can be packaged in virions is approx 105% of the wild-type genome (5), for a capacity of about 2 kb of extra DNA. To incorporate larger DNA segments, it is necessary to compensate by deleting appropriate amounts of viral DNA. One of the most useful deletions is made by collapsing the two naturally occurring XbaI sites within E3 (Fig. 1) to remove 1.9 kb of viral DNA (6,7). This results in vectors having a capacity for approx 4 kb of foreign DNA and having the ability to replicate in any of the cell lines commonly used for adenovirus propagation, such as HeLa or KB cells. Approximately 3 kb can be deleted from E1 to generate vectors restricted to growth in 293 cells and able to accept inserts of 5 kb. Combining E1 and E3 deletions in a single vector should result in a capacity of approx 7 kb. It is important to point out, however, that the E1 deletion must not extend into the E1 region containing the coding sequences for protein IX (from 10 to 11 mμ), since protein IX is a virion structural component that is necessary for packaging full length viral genomes, and deleting this gene results in a net decrease in capacity *(5)*. If the generation of helper/dependent vectors is a suitable option, then, except for the extreme terminal sequences (which must be retained to allow DNA replication) and sequences near the left end (which are needed in *cis* for packaging), theoretically, almost the entire genome (approx 35 kb) can be substituted with foreign DNA.

Most of the nondefective vectors constructed by us and others have the 1.9 kb deletion in the E3 region and use the XbaI site at this position as a cloning site. Inserts in E3 can have either the E3 parallel or the E3 antiparallel orientation; this is an important distinction, because expression of E3 inserts in the parallel (left to right) orientation seems to be primarily a result of transcripts originating from somewhere to the left in the viral genome, either from the E3 promoter or from the MLP (cf. *8–10*).

There are certain basic steps that are followed prior to rescuing genes into the viral genome. These involve relatively straightforward recombinant DNA manipulations in which the gene to be cloned in viral DNA is first inserted into a subsegment of the viral genome, itself cloned in a bacterial plasmid. The resulting chimeric construct is then cotransfected into mammalian cells, along with appropriately prepared viral DNA, by conventional DNA transfer techniques. Usually, rescue is achieved by in vivo recombination in the transfected cells, but prior in vitro ligation is also an option. Figure 2 illustrates the procedure for rescue of either E1 insertions (shown below the Ad5 map) or E3 insertions (above map) into the viral genome by cotransfection with appropriately restricted viral DNA (cleavage of viral DNA reduces the infectivity of the parental viral DNA and enhances the efficiency of isolation of recombinant vectors resulting from in vivo recombination).

For E1 inserts, the first requirement is a bacterial plasmid containing the left end of the genome and having an appropriate deleting E1 sequences and a restriction site into which to clone a foreign gene. In the example shown in the lower part of Fig. 2, the requisite plasmid is pXCX2 *(11)*. This is a plasmid containing the left 16% of the Ad5 genome cloned in pBR322, minus a deletion in E1 from 1.3 to 9.3 mμ, and having a unique XbaI cloning site for insertion of foreign DNA. The resulting construct is cotransfected into 293 cells along with virion DNA, usually derived from *dl*309 virus, that has been cleaved at the left end to eliminate or at least reduce infectivity of the parental viral DNA. In vivo recombination results in rescue of the cloned viral sequences into the left end of the genome. Rescue into E3 is a similar process. In this case, one starts with a plasmid such as pFGdX1 *(7)*, which con-

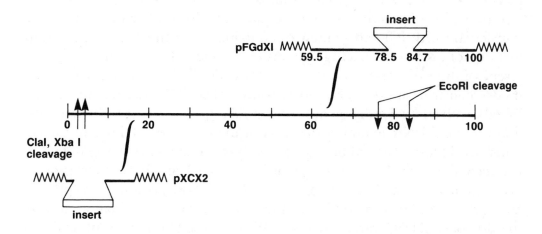

Fig. 2. Strategy for rescue of foreign DNA into the Ad5 genome. Rescue by in vivo recombination is shown schematically for inserts in region E1 (below genome map) or in region E3 (above map). Ad5 sequences are indicated by solid lines, insertions by open bars, and bacterial plasmid sequences, which are linked to viral DNA in plasmids pFGdX1 and pXCX2, by jagged lines. Relevant restriction enzyme digestion sites are indicated for rescue of E3 insertions (EcoRI digestion of wild-type virion DNA) or E1 insertions (ClaI and XbaI digestion of *dl*309 DNA). *See text* for further details.

tains the right 40% of the genome from 59.5 to 100 mμ with a deletion in E3 and, again, a unique XbaI restriction enzyme site for cloning. Wild-type virion DNA is cut with EcoRI as shown and cotransfected with plasmid DNA, again resulting in recombination in vivo. Resulting plaques are isolated, expanded, and screened by restriction analysis to identify the desired recombinant. These methods are usually satisfactory, but there is often a background of infectious parental DNA, which can be a serious problem if the desired vector replicates significantly slower than wild-type virus.

To circumvent potential problems posed by infectious parental virion DNA, we have developed alternative methods that became feasible following the discovery that adenovirus DNA can circularize in infected cells *(12)*, and that circular forms of the genome can be cloned as infectious plasmids *(13,14)*. One such plasmid, pFG140, has been described previously *(13)* and consists of a circular *dl*309 genome with an insert at 3.7 mμ of a small 2.2 kb DNA segment carrying ampicillin resistance and a bacterial origin of replication that permits propagation in *E. coli*. From pFG140, a series of simple recombinant DNA manipulations was used to substitute the 2.2-kb insert with a 4.4

kb DNA segment, resulting in a plasmid designated pJM17 *(15)*. Because an insertion of 4.4 kb is too large to be packaged into infectious virions, co-transfection with left-end sequences containing substitutions or insertions that do not exceed the packaging constraints selects for recombination and rescue of the E1 inserts into infectious virus. Similar approaches have been used to construct another pFG140 derivative, pFG173 (F. L. Graham, unpublished), with a lethal deletion around the E3 region to select for recombination with viral DNA spanning that part of the genome. Neither of the co-transfected plasmids need be digested with restriction enzymes to obtain in vivo recombination. The advantages of this approach are that the background of infectious parental DNA is zero (when pFG173 is used) or low (using pJM17) and, once the appropriate plasmids have been made, purification and restriction of viral DNA can be avoided. We have used both conventional and these newer techniques to construct over 20 vectors expressing various gene products. The protocols described below are ones that have been used routinely in the course of that work.

2. Materials

2.1. Propagation, Titration, and Purification of Adenovirus

1. Cell lines and media: Wild-type and E3–Ad5 can be propagated in most standard human cell lines, such as HeLa or KB; E1–mutants are propagated in 293 monolayer cells *(4)* or in 293N3S suspension cultures *(16)*. For all DNA transfections and most virus plaque assays, we recommend 293 cells. Any of the standard growth media, such as Minimal Eagle's Medium (MEM), a-MEM, or MEMF 11, supplemented with bovine serum (e.g., 10% fetal bovine serum or newborn calf serum), can be used for cell culture. We generally use MEMF 11 + either 2 or 5% heat-inactivated horse serum (HS) for propagation of virus.

2. Phosphate buffered saline (PBS^{2+}) is prepared as follows:
    Solution A: 80 g NaCl, 2 g KCl, 11.5 g Na_2HPO_4, 2 g KH_2PO_4 /L of distilled H_2O;
    Solution B: 1 g $CaCl_2.2H_2O$/100 mL H_2O; and
    Solution C: 1 g $MgCl_2.6H_2O$/100 mL H_2O.
    Sterilize solutions A, B, and C separately by autoclaving. For 1L of PBS^{2+}, mix 880 mL of sterile H_2O with 100 mL of solution A, and then add 10 mL each of solutions B and C. For 1L of PBS^{2-}, mix 900 mL of H_2O with 100 mL of Solution A.

3. Overlay for plaque assays and transfections: Prepare 400 mL of $2 \times$ MEMF

11 + 100 U/mL penicillin + 100 µg/mL streptomycin + 8 mL of 5% yeast extract. This can be stored for a few weeks at 4°C. To make 200 mL of complete overlay (20 60-mm dishes) prepare 100 mL of 2 × MEMF 11 + 10 mL inactivated HS, and autoclave 100 mL H_2O + 1 g agarose. Bring the agarose and F11 to 44°C before mixing and use within about 1h.

4. Crystal violet for fixing and staining cell monolayers: Dissolve 2 g crystal violet in 20 mL methanol, and add 144 mL PBS^{2-} and 36 mL formaldehyde. Filter through Whatman no. 1 filter paper to remove any particulate matter prior to use.
5. Neutral red is purchased as a sterile stock solution of 0.33g/L neutral red (sodium salt).
6. 10% glycerol in PBS^{2+}. Glycerol can be sterilized by autoclaving prior to mixing with PBS.
7. Tris-HCl buffer, 0.1 M and 0.01 M, pH 8.0.
8. Carnoy's fixative: methanol:glacial acetic acid, 3:1.
9. 1% sodium citrate: 1 g sodium citrate dihydrate dissolved in 100 mL H_2O.
10. Orcein staining solution: 2% orcein in 50% acetic acid. Filter through Whatman No. 1 paper.
11. Sodium deoxycholate: 5 g/100 mL H_2O.
12. Saturated CsCl: At room temperature, add sufficient CsCl to 0.01 M Tris-HCl, pH 8.0; 0.001 M EDTA to saturate the buffer. Store at 4°C, but bring to room temperature prior to use.

2.2. Adenovirus DNA Purification

1. 0.01 M Tris-HCl, pH 8.0.
2. Pronase stock solution: Dissolve pronase at 5 mg/mL in 0.01 M Tris-HCl, pH 7.5; preincubate at 56°C for 15 min, and then incubate at 37°C for 1 h. Aliquot into plastic tubes and store at –20°C. Pronase solution is thawed and diluted in buffer just prior to use for DNA extraction from purified virus (1 mg/mL pronase in 0.01 M Tris-HCl, pH 7.5; 0.01 M EDTA; 1% SDS) and from infected cell monolayers (0.5 mg/mL pronase in 0.01 M Tris-HCl, pH 7.5; 0.01 M EDTA; 0.5% SDS).
3. Phenol: Distilled or nucleic-acid grade phenol is melted and saturated with 0.01 M Tris-HCl, pH 8.0; 0.01 M EDTA. We generally add a few crystals of hydroxyquinoline, which not only inhibits oxidation but also gives a distinctive orange color to the phenol, thus facilitating discrimination between aqueous and phenol phases in DNA extraction procedures.
4. 30% sodium acetate trihydrate.
5. 0.1 × SSC is usually made from 20 × solutions by diluting in H_2O and

autoclaving to sterilize and inactivate nucleases (20 × SSC: 175 g NaCl and 88 g sodium citrate dihydrate/L).

2.3. DNA Transfection and Screening of Plaque Isolates

1. HEPES-buffered saline (HEBS): 5 g/L HEPES (*N*-2-Hydroxyethyl-piperazine-*N*'-2-ethanesulfonic acid) 8 g/L NaCl, 0.37 g/L KCl, 0.125 g/L $Na_2HPO_4.2H_2O$, 1 g/L glucose; final pH 7.1. HEBS is aliquoted into small glass bottles, sterilized by autoclaving, and stored at 4°C with caps tightly closed.
2. Carrier DNA: We use commercially available salmon-sperm DNA. This is dissolved in sterile 0.1 × SSC at approx 1 mg/mL, the exact final concentration determined by OD at 260 nm. This stock solution is stored in small aliquots at –20°C and used at a final concentration of 10 μg/mL HEBS.
3. 2.5 *M* $CaCl_2$: Prepared in distilled H_2O, sterilized by filtration, and stored in small plastic tubes or flasks at 4°C.
4. Restriction enzymes, apparatus for horizontal slab gel electrophoresis, and the like, for analyzing structure of recombinant viruses.

2.4. Detection of Expression

1. Cell-culture media: Complete MEMF 11 supplemented with 5% horse serum; medium lacking methionine (MEMmet⁻) is usually MEM119 with no methionine, supplemented with 2% dialyzed fetal bovine serum.
2. ³⁵S-methionine: Either L-methionine [³⁵S] with a specific activity >800 Ci/mmol or a mixture of predominantly L-methionine [³⁵S] and L-cysteine [³⁵S] can be used.
3. PBS–: Described in Section 2.1.2.
4. RIPA buffer: 0.05 *M* Tris-HCl (pH 7.2), 0.15 *M* NaCl, 0.1% (w/v) SDS, 1% (w/v) sodium deoxycholate, and 1% (v/v) Triton X-100.
5. Protein A Sepharose beads (Pharmacia Inc.) are prepared by swelling 500 mg of beads in 25 mL of RIPA buffer on a roller wheel at 4°C. The beads are washed three times by centrifugation at 1500 rpm for 5 min and resuspended in RIPA buffer. The final pellet is resuspended in 3.5 mL of RIPA buffer and stored at 4°C.
6. Loading buffer: 5% (w/v) SDS, 12.5% (v/v) β-mercaptoethanol, 25% (v/v) glycerol, and 0.1% (w/v) bromophenol blue.
7. Apparatus and materials for SDS polyacrylamide gel electrophoresis of proteins and subsequent detection of radioactive proteins on X-ray film.

3. Methods

3.1. Propagation, Titration, and Purification of Adenovirus

3.1.1. Plaque Assays

1. Set up appropriate cells (HeLa or 293) 1 d prior to use, arranging to have the cells just at confluency when used. The actual split ratio depends on the cell type, but a good rule of thumb is about 6–8 60-mm dishes from each 150-mm dish of 293 cells, and about 20–30 60-mm dishes from each 150-mm dish of HeLa cells.
2. The following day, prepare virus dilutions in PBS^{2+}. Remove the medium and add 0.2 mL virus/dish. Adsorb the virus at room temperature for 30–60 min, occasionally tipping the dishes to spread the suspension over the cell monolayer. To each 60-mm dish, add 10 mL of overlay that has been prepared beforehand and has been equilibrated in a 44°C waterbath.
3. Incubate at 37°C in a CO_2 incubator. On 293 cell monolayers, plaques should be visible within 4–5 d and can be counted at 6–8 d. Plaques on 293 cells can be counted by eye, or the cells can be fixed with formaldehyde, the overlay can be flipped out, and the monolayer stained with crystal violet. Plaques on HeLa cells can be counted after staining with neutral red by overlaying on d 7 or 8 with 5 mL of overlay containing 33 µg/mL neutral red and counting plaques 2–3 days later.

3.1.2. Infection of Cells in Monolayer

1. After determining the number of cells on a dish that is about 80–90% confluent, remove the medium and add appropriately diluted virus in 1 mL PBS^{2+}/150-mm dish, or 0.2 mL/60-mm dish at multiplicity of infection (moi) of 1–10 PFU/cell.
2. Adsorb for 30–60 min, tipping the dishes once or twice to spread the suspension evenly and refeed with MEMF 11 + 2% heat-inactivated horse serum. Incubate the dishes at the appropriate temperature and examine twice daily for signs of cytopathic effect. Virus replication and spread is more rapid in 293 cells, and cytopathic effect is more readily apparent than in infected HeLa or KB cells.
3. When the cytopathic effect is complete (as indicated by rounding up of the cells), harvest by scraping the cells off the plastic and centrifuging infected cells from the medium. For a relatively concentrated stock of virus, resuspend the cell pellet in 2 mL PBS^{2+} + 10% glycerol/dish. Cells

can be broken and virus released by sonication or by freezing and thawing. The medium will also contain substantial amounts of infectious virus at a lower titer than the concentrated cell suspension, and may be useful for some purposes for which a high titer is not needed. Sterile glycerol should be added (to 10%) and the virus stored at −20 to −70°C.

3.1.3. Infection of Cells in Suspension (KB or 293N3S)

1. Grow spinner culture cells to $2–4 \times 10^5$ cells/mL in Joklik's modified MEM + 10% inactivated horse serum. Centrifuge gently to pellet cells, saving 50% of the conditioned medium, and resuspend the cell pellet in 1/10 vol of medium.
2. Add virus at a moi of 10–20 PFU/cell and stir gently at 37°C for 1 h.
3. Bring to the original vol., using 50% fresh medium and 50% conditioned medium, and continue incubating at 37°C. Monitor infection on a twice-daily basis using inclusion body staining (*see* Section 3.1.4.).
4. When inclusion bodies are visible in 80–90% of infected cells (about 11/2–2 d), harvest by centrifugation and resuspend in 10mL PBS^{2+}+10% glycerol/L infected cells for preparation of stocks of crude infectious virus, or resuspend in 0.1*M* Tris-HCl, pH 8.0 (10–20 mL for 1–4 L), for preparation of virus to be used for CsCl banding and DNA extraction.

3.1.4. Inclusion Body Staining

1. Remove a 5-mL aliquot from the infected spinner culture. Centrifuge for 10 min at 1000 rpm and resuspend the cell pellet in 0.5 mL of 1% sodium citrate.
2. Incubate at room temperature for 10 min; then add 0.5 mL Carnoy's fixative and fix for 10 min at room temperature.
3. Add 1 mL of 1% sodium citrate, centrifuge, and resuspend the pellet in a few drops of 1% sodium citrate. Add a drop of fixed cells to a slide and dry for at least 1 h; then add Orcein and a cover-slip and examine in the microscope. Inclusion bodies appear as densely staining nuclear structures resulting from accumulation of large amounts of virus and viral products at late times in infection. A negative control should be included in initial tests.

3.1.5. Purification of Adenovirus: A Rapid, Simple Method

Concentrated crude virus stocks are prepared from infected KB cells or 293N3S cells by pelleting cells infected as described above and resuspending the cell pellet in 5–10 mL of 0.1*M* Tris-HCl, pH 8.0/L of infected cell suspension. This is stored at −70°C until needed.

1. Thaw the frozen crude virus stock and add 1/10 vol 5% sodium deoxycholate. Mix well and incubate on ice for 30 min. This disrupts cells without disrupting virions, and results in a relatively clear, highly viscous suspension.
2. Shear the cellular DNA using a probe-type homogenizer. We have found this step to be necessary to avoid aggregation of virus and cellular material, presumably DNA, during the subsequent CsCl banding step. Viscosity should be reduced so that, when the suspension is pipeted dropwise, there is still some noticeable viscosity, but only slightly more than that of water.
3. Add 1.8 mL saturated CsCl (in 0.01 M Tris-HCl, pH 8.0; 0.001 M EDTA) for each 3.1 mL of virus suspension. Be sure that the saturated CsCl stock is at room temperature prior to use, since this affects the concentration.
4. Distribute virus into Beckman 50Ti quickseal (or similar) tubes and spin in a Beckman 50Ti angle rotor (or a vertical rotor) for 16–20 h at 4°C and 35,000 rpm.
5. Collect the viral bands and pool. (For tubes other than nitrocellulose, one can collect by puncturing the top of the tube with a hot needle, then puncturing the bottom, and controlling the flow of solution out the bottom with a finger over the top hole.)
6. Centrifuge pooled virus in a Beckman SW50.1 rotor at 35,000 rpm, 4°C, for 16–20 h.
7. Collect the virus band. This time, try to collect the virus in a small vol. Banded virus is relatively stable at 4°C in CsCl, though it may eventually fall apart.

3.2. Adenovirus DNA Purification

This is a simple, reliable method for extracting virion DNA from CsCl-purified adenovirus. An alternative, somewhat more involved method is also available, which avoids proteases and phenol, and produces virion DNA with an intact terminal protein (cf. *17,18*). Such DNA–protein complexes are much more infectious than deproteinized virion DNA; however, we do not use this method routinely, since we usually find specific infectivities of pure virion DNA made by the technique outlined below adequate for our purposes.

1. Dialyze the banded virus in boiled dialysis tubing for about 2 h against two changes of approx 100 vol of 0.01 M Tris-HCl, pH 8.0 (keep cold). Often, this causes the virus to precipitate, but for DNA extraction, this is no problem.

2. Prepare the digestion buffer containing 1 mg/mL pronase in 0.01 *M* Tris-HCl, pH 7.5; 0.01 *M* EDTA; 1% SDS.

3. To a Petri dish, add 1 vol of digestion buffer from step 2, and then add the dialyzed virus (1 vol) dropwise, mixing by tipping the dish. The order is important: Always add virus to pronase–SDS digestion buffer, rather than the reverse. Incubate for 2 h at 37°C.

4. Extract once with phenol that has been saturated with 0.01 *M* Tris-HCl, pH 8.0; 0.01 *M* EDTA.

5. Add 1/10 vol of 30% sodium acetate, ethanol-precipitate by adding 2 vol of 96% ethanol, and wash extensively with 96% ethanol. Dry for about 1 h at 37°C and redissolve DNA in 0.1 × SSC. Expect to obtain about 0.5– 1 mg DNA from each liter of original infected cells.

6. Aliquot DNA into several tubes and store at –20°C. Repeated freezing and thawing can degrade viral DNA; otherwise, it should be stable indefinitely.

3.3. Isolation of Expression Vectors by Cotransfection and In Vivo Recombination

This section outlines methods for cotransfecting 293 cells with plasmid and virion DNA, or with two plasmids, for rescue of insertions into the viral genome by recombination in vivo. *See* Fig. 2 for a general outline of the steps involved. If virion DNA is being used, it should be cut with appropriate restriction enzymes, as illustrated in Fig. 2, to reduce the infectivity of parental DNA and enhance the efficiency of recovery of recombinants. If two plasmids containing overlapping viral sequences are used, they should be engineered such that neither, on its own, is capable of generating infectious virus.

3.3.1. DNA Transfection

This is a more-or-less standard protocol for assaying infectivity of adenovirus DNA or for rescue of cloned viral sequences into full length viral genomes by cotransfection. Whether insertions are targeted to E1 or to other regions of the genome, the cell line of choice is always 293, because these cells are good recipients of DNA in DNA-mediated gene-transfer procedures, and generate adenovirus plaques rapidly and efficiently.

We routinely use the procedure outlined below to obtain infectious virus from adenovirus DNA or from plasmids containing the Ad genome. It is essentially unchanged from the original technique for assaying infectious Ad5 DNA (*19*). We have not investigated other methods; the reader is encouraged to evaluate some of the other transfection techniques described in this vol.

The 293 cells should be at low passage (<p50), should be set up the previous day in 60-mm dishes, and should be about 70–80% confluent at the time of use. Do not use growth media with high concentrations of phosphate, such as Joklik's modified MEM, since this interferes with transfections by the calcium phosphate technique.

1. Prepare 1× HEPES-buffered saline (HEBS) + 10 µg/mL salmon-sperm DNA (or other suitable carrier DNA), and mix well by vortexing for 1 min.
2. Aliquot HEBS + carrier DNA into sterile clear plastic tubes (e.g., at 0.5 mL/60-mm dish, four dishes will require 2 mL of HEBS).
3. Add the experimental DNA and mix well. We typically use 5–10 µg plasmid DNA containing the foreign DNA insert, and 2–5 µg restricted virion DNA or 5–10 µg of the second plasmid for each transfected dish.
4. Slowly add 2.5 M CaCl$_2$ (50 µL/mL) for a final concentration of 125 mM.
5. Mix well and incubate at room temperature for 15–30 min. (A fine precipitate should form within a few min.) Add the suspension to the cells without removing the growth medium (0.5 mL/5 mL medium) and incubate at 37°C in a CO$_2$ incubator for 4.5 h. Remove the medium and overlay with MEMF11 + 5% horse serum + 0.5% agarose, prepared as described above, or refeed with MEMF11 + 5% horse serum and incubate at 37°C. Plaques or cytopathic effect should appear after about 5–7 d.

3.3.2. Screening Adenovirus Plaque Isolates

Most screens will utilize 293 cells for expanding plaque isolates because the virus spreads rapidly, and because 293 cells are used for isolating many mutants (e.g., E1 mutants). The protocol below is designed for 293 cells.

1. Set up 60-mm dishes of 293 cells as for plaque assays, i.e., about 80–90% confluent. The denser and older the cell monolayer, the longer it takes for virus cytopathic effect to reach completion. Use dishes the next day.
2. Pick well-isolated plaques from transfected cultures (*see* Section 3.3.1.) by punching out agar plugs using a sterile Pasteur pipet, and transfer mashed agar to 1 mL of PBS^{2+} + 10% glycerol. This can be stored at –70°C until results of the analysis are available.
3. Remove the medium from 293 cell dishes and add 0.2 mL of virus. Distribute over the cell monolayer and adsorb at room temperature for 30 min. Add 5 mL MEMF 11 + 5%HS and incubate at 37°C.
4. Depending on the size of the original plaque and the growth properties of the virus mutant, a cytopathic effect should become visible within 1–2 d. Do not attempt to harvest before the cytopathic effect is absolutely complete, i.e., essentially all cells rounded and many floating (usually 3–4 d).

5. Process the dishes with complete cytopathic effect as follows: Leave dishes undisturbed in the tissue-culture hood for 20–30 min. Gently remove medium with a pipet and save about 4 mL in a sterile glass vial containing 0.5 mL sterile glycerol for storage at –70°C. Remove the residual medium by suction. If all this is done carefully, the majority of loose cells will be left behind in the dish.

6. Add 0.5 mL pronase (0.5 mg/mL pronase + 0.5% SDS prepared as in Section 2.2.) and digest at 37°C for 3–4 h.

7. Transfer the viscous lysate to a 1.5-mL Eppendorf tube (do this by leaving the dishes at an angle so the lysate drains to one edge of dish, and then collecting with a Pasteur pipet) and extract once with 0.5 mL of phenol. Collect the aqueous phase and transfer to a fresh tube.

8. Add 50 µL of 30% sodium acetate and precipitate with 1 mL of 96% ethanol; vortex or mix by tipping the tube. You should get an easily visible fibrous precipitate. Spin and wash twice with 1.5 mL of 96% ethanol to remove phenol.

9. Dry the pellet of crude DNA completely, redissolve in 50 µL of $0.1 \times$ SSC (complete solubilization may take several hours) and digest 5 µL with HindIII (this is the best all-purpose diagnostic enzyme for preliminary analysis of Ad5 DNA) for 3–4 h or, preferably, overnight.

10. Run on a 1% agarose gel with appropriate markers (a HindIII digest of wild-type Ad5 DNA being the best marker) and identify the candidate recombinants. If the cytopathic effect was complete, this procedure should result in a relatively pure preparation of viral DNA, with cellular DNA running as a background smear. There should be very little RNA. Note that in HindIII digests of human DNA, there will be a band of cellular repetitive DNA at around 1.8 kb, not to be confused with viral DNA. Candidates with predicted HindIII restriction patterns should be analyzed with additional enzymes, plaque-purified (using virus from the original agar plug), and reanalyzed.

3.4. Detection of the Expression of Inserts in Adenovirus Vectors

3.4.1. Expression in Virus-Infected Cell Cultures

The most suitable procedure for the detection of a product expressed by adenovirus vectors will, of course, depend on the properties of the protein produced and on the availability and quality of reagents necessary to detect it. For example, products with enzymatic or biological activity may be detected in vector-infected cell extracts or culture fluids using the appropriate assays, whereas foreign-virus glycoproteins with fusion or hemeadsorption activity may be detected on the surface of vector-infected cells using these particular properties. The most generally applicable procedures depend on the ability to detect the expressed protein with conventional antigen–antibody detection procedures, such as ELISA, immunoprecipitation, or Western-blot analysis. The following protocol for immunoprecipitation is one used in our laboratory and, though satisfactory for most purposes, it is far from perfect in view of variable nonspecific precipitation of adenovirus proteins, which may obscure some of expressed products. This procedure of course depends on having a suitable precipitating antibody against the relevant protein, with no contaminating antiadenovirus activity.

1. Infect nearly confluent Hela cell monolayers in 60-mm Petri dishes with the adenovirus vector or with control adenovirus at a moi of 20 PFU/cell, as described in Section 3.1.2. Incubate in MEMF11 + 5% horse serum at 37°C.

2. At 12, 24, and 36 h postinfection, carefully remove medium from the infected cells and wash the cells once with prewarmed MEMmet– medium. Add 1 mL of MEMmet– medium containing 50 µCi of ^{35}S-methionine. Incubate for 2 h at 37°C in CO_2 incubator.

3. Remove the radioactive medium. Rinse the cell monolayer with PBS^{2-}, and scrape the cells into PBS^{2-}, using a rubber policeman. Pellet the cells by centrifugation for 15 min at 1500 rpm, remove the supernatant, and redissolve the cell pellet in 1 mL of RIPA buffer. Reduce the viscosity of the solution by passing the material through a syringe needle or by vigorous vortexing followed by sonication in an immersion bath sonifier. The former procedure is best initiated by drawing the solution up into the syringe barrel prior to attaching the needle, and then putting on the needle and expelling the material carefully through the needle into a tube.

4. Once the viscosity has been reduced to a point at which the solution flows reasonably freely, centrifuge in a microfuge for 15–30 min and collect the supernatant. (During the first few experiments, you may wish to save the pelleted material until you have determined that the protein of interest is not principally in this fraction; however, for most soluble and plasma-membrane-associated proteins, this will not be necessary.)

5. To 500 µL of supernatant add an appropriate vol of antiserum (we generally use 5–10 µL of serum). Then add 100 µL of the suspension of

protein A–Sepharose beads in RIPA buffer. Incubate the final suspension overnight at 4°C in a roller wheel or other suitable mixing device.

6. Pellet the beads by centrifugation for 5–10 min at 1500 rpm and wash the beads by repeated resuspension and pelleting (at least six times). The final pellet is resuspended in 50–100 μL of loading buffer.

7. After 3 min in a boiling water bath, the sample is cooled and centrifuged to pellet the beads. The supernatant is then removed and analyzed by SDS polyacrylamide gel electrophoresis with appropriate controls and size markers, and the radioactivity is detected by autoradiography.

3.4.2. Expression In Vivo Detected
by Antibody Production in Infected Animals

If the inserted protein may induce antibodies that can be readily and selectively detected (for example, if the insert encodes a virus glycoprotein that can induce virus neutralizing antibodies), then an indirect assay for expression of the insert in mice infected with the vector may be useful. We have found, in some cases in which reagents for immunoprecipitation were not available or not suitable, that the following method provided a sensitive test of antigen expression by the adenovirus vector, though this method is not necessarily suited to providing a quantitative measure of levels of expression. *Anyone intending to use this procedure should read carefully the section below relating to biohazards and should consult the relevant governing authorities before proceeding with these experiments.*

1. In general, crude lysates of cells infected with the Ad5 vector, prepared and titered as described above, will be suitable for this procedure, though in some instances, CsCl-purified virus may be required. In this latter case, care must be taken to dialyze extensively against PBS^{2+} + 10% glycerol to remove CsCl from the preparation before it is used. The virus should be titered by plaque assay after dialysis.

2. The vector (crude or purified) in 0.1-mL vol containing 10^8 PFU is injected by the intraperitoneal route into recipient mice. We have routinely used 6- to 8-wk old Balb/C mice, but have no reason to believe that any other strain would not work as well.

3. The mice are bled by tail vein at 2 and 4 wk following immunization and the serum either titered for virus-neutralizing activity or used in an immunoblot or ELISA assay against purified antigen to detect specific antibodies. If a source of labeled antigen not contaminated with adenovirus antigens is available, then immunoprecipitation, PAGE, and autoradiography also can be used to detect the presence of specific antibody.

4. Notes

4.1. Biosafety Considerations in the Production and Use of Infectious Recombinant Vectors

Adenovirus vectors with foreign gene inserts in the E3 region are either directly or potentially infectious in humans or other permissive species. All experimentation with recombinant virus vectors should be carried out in accordance with regulations governing the use of these agents, and with the permission of relevant authorities. No known toxic (or potentially toxic) gene product should be expressed from adenovirus vectors.

Although Ad5 is a ubiquitous human virus infecting many individuals very early in life, there is nonetheless a significant fraction of individuals who do not carry antibodies to this virus. Individuals in this group would be particularly susceptible to infection with Ad5 vectors, and would be subject to seroconversion against any inserted foreign-gene products. This is to be avoided in most cases, especially if the development of antibody may confuse diagnosis or epidemiology of a particular disease. The same consideration should be given to possible animal infection with the vector.

4.2. Potential Pitfalls in the Isolation of Expression Vectors

1. The most common problems likely to be met in the construction of adenovirus expression vectors are, in order of likelihood: a. failure to obtain any plaques following cotransfection; b. failure to obtain recombinants among a large number of plaques screened; and c. failure of the insert to express following rescue.

Inability to obtain plaques can be the result of a number of factors, the most common and easiest to identify being poor transfection efficiencies. A positive control, such as uncut virion DNA, should generate 10–100 plaques/ μg if the Ad DNA has been deproteinized, and 1–2 orders of magnitude more plaques if the terminal protein has been left intact. If the efficiency of plaque production with control DNA is poor, the most likely cause is the condition of the cell monolayer. Assuming 293 cells are being used, it is important that they be at an early passage, not be growing too rapidly, and be slightly less than confluent at the time of use. Suitable cell monolayers should yield visible plaques within 4–5 d following infection with virus or transfection with virion DNA. Other possible explanations for poor transfection efficiencies are incorrect HEBS composition (the pH, in particular, is critical and the phosphate concentration is important as well), and poor-quality DNA, e.g., degraded or sheared viral DNA. If transfection efficiencies are satisfactory with control DNA, but no plaques are obtained with cotransfected cultures, check that the plasmid DNA is "clean." We generally use CsCl-banded plasmid DNA extracted from bacteria treated with chloramphenicol to amplify the plasmid copy number (*see* Chapter 1). Sometimes, linearizing the transfecting plasmid will enhance the recombination efficiencies. PFGdX1, for example, can be cut with BamHI if the insert is lacking BamHI sites. In a "worst-case scenario," transfections seem to be working, but only wild-type parental viruses are found by screening as many as 50–100 candidate plaque isolates obtained from cotransfections of restricted virion DNA and plasmid DNA. Assuming the virion DNA has been completely digested to reduce infectivity, then the unfortunate possibility exists that the insertion being rescued is potentially toxic for the cells or virus. This does not happen often, but it does happen. There is little that can be done if this is the case, but at least it may be possible to determine whether toxicity is the problem by introducing an inactivating mutation into the coding sequences of the insert (e.g., a chain terminator near the start for translation). If the construct now becomes rescuable, then toxicity is in all likelihood preventing replication of the vector carrying the original gene.

2. Our experience has been that vectors containing E3 inserts of foreign genes in the E3 parallel (left to right) orientation almost invariably express the inserted gene as protein, though the levels of expression can vary greatly from one insert to another. Whether the inserted gene has its own promoter or not, expression seems generally to be the result of transcription driven by upstream adenovirus promoters, either the E3 promoter or the major late promoter. In most of the vectors we have made and characterized, the gene to be expressed has been flanked by an upstream SV40 early promoter element and downstream poly A$^+$ addition sequences, but we and others *(10)* have found that promoterless inserts in the E3 region also express protein in some vectors. Currently, obtaining expression of inserts in E3 is largely an empirical process and it is not yet possible to predict, *a priori*, the expression levels for any given insertion in E3. When inserts are located in E1, the use of a strong promoter upstream of the coding sequences is more-or-less essential, and a number of studies have been done with various promoters driving various genes inserted into the E1 region. The reader is referred to ref. *2* for further details and additional references.

Acknowledgments

Work carried out in the authors' laboratories was supported by grants from the Medical Research Council, National Science and Engineering Council, and the National Cancer Institute of Canada. FLG is a Terry Fox Research Scientist of the National Cancer Institute of Canada.

References

1. Ginsberg, H. S. (1984) *The Adenoviruses* (Plenum, New York).
2. Berkner, K. L. (1988) Development of adenovirus vectors for expression of heterologous genes. *BioTechniques* **6**, 616–629.
3. Jones, N. and Shenk, T. (1979) Isolation of adenovirus type 5 host range deletion mutants defective for transformation of rat embryo cells. *Cell* **16**, 683–689.
4. Graham, F. L., Smiley, J., Russell, W. C., and Nairn, R. (1977) Characteristics of a human cell line transformed by DNA from human adenovirus type 5. *J. Gen. Virol.* **36**, 59–72.
5. Ghosh-Choudhury, G., Haj-Ahmad, Y., and Graham, F. L. (1987) Protein IX, a minor component of the human adenovirus capsid, is essential for the packaging of full length genomes. *EMBO J.* **6**, 1733–1739.
6. Berkner, K. L. and Sharp, P. A. (1983) Generation of adenovirus by transfection of plasmids. *Nucleic Acids Res.* **11**, 6003–6020.
7. Haj-Ahmad, Y. and Graham, F. L. (1986) Development of a helper independent human adenovirus vector and its use in the transfer of the Herpes Simplex Virus thymidine kinase gene. *J. Virol.* **57**, 267–274.
8. Johnson, D. C., Ghosh-Choudhury, G., Smiley, J. R., Fallis, L., and Graham, F. L. (1988) Abundant expression of Herpes Simplex Virus glycoprotein gB using an adenovirus vector. *Virology* **164**, 1–14.
9. Schneider, M., Graham, F. L., and Prevec, L. (1989) Expression of the glycoprotein of VSV by infectious adenovirus vectors. *J. Gen. Virol.* **70**, 417–427.
10. Davis, A. R., Kostek, B., Mason, B. B., Hsiao, C. L., Morin, J., Dheer, S. K., and Hung, P. P. (1985) Expression of hepatitis B virus surface antigen with a recombinant adenovirus. *Proc. Natl. Acad. Sci. USA* **82**, 7560–7564.
11. Spessot, R., Inchley, K., Hupel, T. M., and Bacchetti, S. (1989) Cloning of the herpes simplex virus ICP4 gene in an adenovirus vector: Effects on adenovirus gene expression and replication. *Virolology* **168**, 378–387.
12. Ruben, M., Bacchetti, S., and Graham, F. L. (1983) Covalently closed circles of human adenovirus type 5 DNA. *Nature* **301**, 172–174.
13. Graham, F. L. (1984) Covalently closed circles of human adenovirus DNA are infectious. *EMBO J.* **3**, 2917–2922.
14. Ghosh-Choudhury, G., Haj-Ahmad, Y., Brinkley, P., Rudy, J., and Graham, F. L. (1986) Human adenovirus cloning vectors based on infectious bacterial plasmids. *Gene* **50**, 161–171.
15. McGrory, J., Bautista, D., and Graham, F. L. (1988) A simple technique for the rescue of early region I mutations into infectious human adenovirus type 5. *Virology* **163**, 614–617.

16. Graham, F. L. (1987) Growth of 293 cells in suspension culture. *J. Gen. Virol.* **68,** 937–940.
17. Sharp, P. A., Moore, C., and Haverty, J. L. (1976) The infectivity of adenovirus 5 DNA–protein complex. *Virology* **75,** 442–456.
18. Chinnadurai, G., Chinnadurai, S., and Green, M. (1978) Enhanced infectivity of adenovirus type 2 DNA and a DNA–protein complex. *J. Virol.* **26,** 195–199.
19. Graham, F. L. and van der Eb, A. J. (1973) A new technique for the assay of infectivity of human adenovirus 5 DNA. *Virology* **52,** 456–467.

CHAPTER 12

Manipulation
of Vaccinia Virus Vectors

Michael Mackett

1. Introduction

Vaccinia virus has been used to express many diverse genes, such as pro-karyotic enzymes, eukaryotic growth factors, protozoan structural proteins, and >50 different virus gene products (for reviews, *see* refs. *1–3*). The wide-spread use of vaccinia virus as a vector owes much to the ease of generating recombinants, the authenticity of the foreign gene product, and the wide variety of uses to which they have been put. For example, HIV 1 (human immunodeficiency virus) envelope glycoprotein expressed by a vaccinia re-combinant is biologically and antigenically indistinguishable from the au-thentic glycoprotein *(4–7)*. Recombinants have been used to generate HIV-neutralizing antibody *(4–6)* to immunize animals and humans *(8–10)*, and to analyze cytotoxic T-cell and antibody-dependent cellular cytotoxicity *(11–13)*. Furthermore, the antigenicity of HIV *env* has been improved by site-directed mutagenesis of protease cleavage sites *(14)*.

Vaccinia virus is the prototype orthopoxvirus and has a large double-stranded DNA genome of approx 180 kbp. Virus particles have a complex architecture with a basic oval or brick-shaped structure of approx 200×300 nm. The outer protein coat of the virus houses an inner dumbell-shaped core that is capable of synthesizing functional capped, methylated, and poly-adenylated mRNA, using vaccinia DNA as its template. This ability, along

From: *Methods in Molecular Biology, Vol. 7: Gene Transfer and Expression Protocols*
Edited by: E. J. Murray ©1991 The Humana Press Inc., Clifton, NJ

with other virus-encoded functions, such as a DNA polymerase, allows the virus to replicate exclusively in the cytoplasm of the infected cell. Thus, pox-viruses have a number of unconventional biological properties *(for review, see* ref. *15)* that need to be taken into account when using them as cloning and expression vectors. Since eukaryotic promoters, such as the SV40 late promoter and retrovirus long terminal repeats, do not function in vaccinia virus, the strategy for construction of recombinants has generally involved a two-step procedure utilizing vaccinia promoters.

The first step involves assembling a plasmid with a chimeric gene flanked by vaccinia virus DNA. The chimeric gene is constructed to contain a vaccinia virus transcriptional start site and upstream regulatory sequences, referred to here as the promoter, adjacent to the protein-coding sequences of the foreign gene. When inserted into the virus, the chimeric gene should be transcribed by the vaccinia DNA-dependent RNA polymerase from the natural vaccinia RNA start site, and the mRNA produced should be translated into the authentic foreign protein. Efficient expression of genes has been obtained with mRNA leader sequences varying from a few to several hundred nucleotides. If desired, the plasmid can be constructed so that translation is initiated from the authentic vaccinia translational start. However, this has the disadvantage of producing hybrid proteins and requires precise engineering in order to maintain the open reading frame during translation of the recombinant mRNA. The second stage of the process is the insertion of the chimeric gene into vaccinia virus. This is achieved by the transfection of vaccinia virus infected cells with the constructed plasmid DNA, which allows homologous recombination to occur between the sequences flanking the chimeric gene and the corresponding sequences in virus genomic DNA. The result is that at low frequency, the chimeric gene is inserted into virus DNA, is packaged, and yields infectious recombinant virus.

The recombinant viruses can then be detected by a variety of methods. This is usually achieved either by screening selected or unselected recombinant viruses for the foreign gene using DNA hybridization or by screening for the gene product with an immunological detection method. In order to screen fewer viral plaques, several methods for increasing the relative frequency of specific recombinants have been devised by including a preselection screen for the recombinant event.

The site at which the foreign gene is inserted into vaccinia virus DNA is determined by the sequences flanking the chimeric gene. Obviously, this site must be nonessential for growth in tissue culture. The thymidine kinase *(tk)* gene locus is the most frequently used, although a number of different sites have been used. Interruption of the *tk* gene coding sequence by foreign DNA generates recombinant viruses that are *tk* negative *(tk⁻)*, and allows them to grow in a *tk⁻* cell line (such as HTK⁻143) in the presence of 5-bromo-deoxyuridine (BUdR). Wild-type parental virus is *tk* positive *(tk⁺)*and will not grow. However, spontaneous *tk⁻* mutants arise at a frequency that necessitates secondary DNA or immunological screens to distinguish recombinant from spontaneous *tk⁻* viruses.

1.1. Design of Plasmid Vectors

To allow and simplify the rapid construction of recombinant viruses expressing foreign genes, a series of plasmid vectors, termed insertion or coinsertion vectors, have been developed (Fig. 1, refs. *16–19*). The essential feature of insertion vectors is a vaccinia virus promoter with multiple unique restriction endonuclease sites adjacent to the RNA start site translocated within vaccinia virus DNA, usually the virus *tk* gene. DNA fragments coding for any continuous protein-coding sequences can then easily be inserted adjacent to the vaccinia virus promoter. Since vaccinia virus does not splice genes, it is necessary to use cDNA.

Coinsertion vectors contain two vaccinia virus promoters; one is used to express a marker gene, the second is used to express the foreign gene. The marker gene can be a dominant selectable gene, such as *E. coli gpt (16,17)*, or an enzyme, such as β-galactosidase *(18)*. Recombinants are selected by using the dominant selectable marker, and the resultant drug-resistant viruses should also express the coinserted gene. Alternatively, incorporation of 5-bromo-4-chloro-3-indoyl-β-D-galactopyranoside (X-gal) in the agarose overlay allows visual detection of recombinants expressing β-galactosidase as blue plaques. Plasmids that contain the β-galactosidase gene driven by one promoter and a foreign gene linked to a second virus promoter can be used to generate easily identifiable recombinant viruses, which should also express the gene of interest. Any of these basic vectors can be modified with a minimum of effort by the use of synthetic oligonucleotides.

2. Materials

2.1. Virus Stocks

Many vaccinia virus strains are available; however, the most commonly used strains are WR, Copenhagen, and Wyeth. The laboratory strains WR and Copenhagen give higher titers in tissue culture than does Wyeth. However, Wyeth (New York City Board of Health strain) is a licensed vaccine strain. Both crude and concentrated virus stocks are stable at –20 or –70°C for many years. For long-term storage, repeated freeze-thawing should be avoided; if possible, stocks should be stored at –70°C.

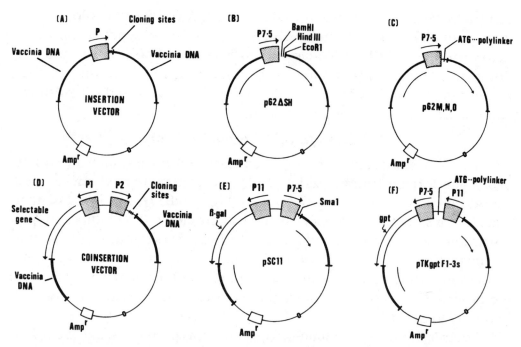

Fig. 1. Plasmid vectors for insertion and expression of foreign genes in vaccinia virus. (A) A generalized plasmid insertion vector; vaccinia sequences flanking the cloning sites can be from any nonessential region of the virus genome. (B), (C) Specific examples of insertion vectors. In both cases, the virus *tk* gene flanks the sites for insertion of genes *(19* and unpublished); p62M, N, and O contain a polylinker consisting of HindIII, BamHI, SmaI, and EcoRI sites, and differ only in that these sites are in three different open reading frames. Similarly, the three *gpt* coinsertion vectors (F) contain a polylinker, each of the three being in different open reading frames. A generalized coinsertion vector is shown in (D). Flanking vaccinia DNA is indicated by thick lines, plasmid DNA by a thin line, and vaccinia promoters (P) by open boxes. The direction of transcription from these promoters is indicated by external arrows. $P_{7.5}$ is a vaccinia promoter expressed throughout the replicative cycle; P_{11} is a late vaccinia virus promoter of a structural phosphoprotein. The direction of transcription and position of the vaccinia virus *tk* coding sequences is indicated by internal arrows. Amp^r, plasmid ampicillin resistance gene; β-gal, *E. coli* β-galactosidase; *gpt*, *E. coli* guanine phosphoribosyl transferase gene.

2.2. Cell Lines

Although traditionally grown on the chorioallantoic membrane of fertile hens' eggs, vaccinia virus will grow well in the majority of tissue culture cell lines, e.g., RK13, BHK, MRC5, and Hep2. Monolayers of primate cell lines, such as CV1, Vero, HeLa, have also been used extensively to contain plaques and grow reasonable amounts of virus. For large-scale production of virus, cells in spinner culture or microcarrier culture can be used. HeLaS3 spinner cells have been routinely used since they will also grow in monolayer.

2.3. Assay of Virus Infectivity, Plaque Purification, and Production of Virus Stocks

1. Recently confluent monolayers of CV1, Vero, or similar cell line. Murine cells give smaller plaques than primate cells.
2. Dulbecco's Modified Eagle's Medium (DMEM) containing 5% fetal calf serum (FCS) or (DMEM) with 5% FCS, depending on cell type.
3. Virus diluent: Phosphate-buffered saline (PBS) sterilized by autoclaving, containing 0.05% BSA (1 mL of a 5% stock of BSA filter-sterilized/100 mL PBS).
4. Sterile 2.5 mg/mL Trypsin.
5. PBS.
6. Stock of 1% crystal violet in 50% ethanol, working strength 0.2% in 20% ethanol.
7. Water bath sonicator (Megasonic 80kc).
8. 2% Noble agar or 2% low-gelling-temperature agarose (BRL) in H_2O, sterilized by autoclaving.
9. A 2× concentrate of (sterile) DMEM.
10. 1% neutral red, sterilized by filtration.
11. Fetal calf serum.
12. Hypotonic buffer: 10 mM Tris-HCl, pH 9, 1 mM EDTA; (TE) or 5 mM citrate phosphate buffer, pH 7.4.
13. Dounce homogenizer (tight-fitting).
14. 36% w/v sucrose buffered by 10 mM Tris-HCl, pH9.0.
15. 1 mM Tris-HCl, pH 9.0; 0.1 mM EDTA.
16. 20, 30, 40, and 50% w/v sterile sucrose in 10 mM Tris-HCl, pH 9.0; 1mM EDTA.

2.4. Generation and Selection of Recombinant Viruses

2.4.1. Transfection Protocol (see Chapter 2)

1. Stock virus, 25 cm² of monolayer cells, such as CV1 (HTK⁻143 cells will also act as hosts), and appropriate media containing 5% FCS.
2. Sheared calf thymus DNA (stock 10 mg/mL in H_2O).
3. 2.5M CaCl$_2$ (sterilized by filtration).
4. 2× HEPES buffered saline (also sterile): 280 mM NaCl, 50 mM HEPES, 1.5 mM NaH$_2$PO$_4$ (pH 7.12). Adjust pH accurately with 1M NaOH.

2.4.2. Selection of tk⁻ Phenotype

1. HTK⁻143 cells. Other *tk*⁻ monolayer cell lines can be used, but these don't form virus plaques as efficiently.
2. Stock 25 mg/mL sterile filtered BUdR. Store at –20°C.
3. Agar overlay, as in Section 3.

2.4.3. Selection of β-Galactosidase Positive Phenotype

1. Any cell type used for forming virus plaques is appropriate (*see* Note 4).
2. Stock 2% X-gal solution in dimethyl formamide.
3. Agar overlay, as in Section 3.

2.4.4. Selection for E. coli gpt Gene (see Note 3)

1. *See* plaque purifying virus. Any cell type is appropriate (*see* Note 4).
2. Mycophenolic acid (Sigma): 10 mg/mL in 0.1 M NaOH, sterile-filtered. Store at –20°C.
3. Xanthine: 10 mg/mL in 0.1 M NaOH, sterile-filtered. Store at –20°C.
4. 50× HAT: 700 mg/mL hypoxanthine, 10 μg/mL aminopterin in 0.1 M NaOH, 200 μg/mL thymidine in H_2O, sterile-filtered. Store at –20°C.

2.5. Detection of Nonselected Recombinants

2.5.1. DNA Dot-Blot Hybridization

1. Nitrocellulose (Schlier and Schull, 0.45 μm).
2. 50 mM Tris-HCl, pH 7.5; 100 mM NaCl.
3. 0.5 M NaOH.
4. 1 M Tris-HCl, pH 7.
5. 2× SSC: 300 mM NaCl, 0.03 M sodium citrate.

2.5.2. Immunologically Based Screen

1. Methanol or formaldehyde (37% stock).
2. PBS/BSA: PBS containing 4% BSA, 0.02% sodium azide.
3. Primary antibody diluted to working strength in PBS/BSA solution.
4. Either enzyme-conjugated secondary antibody or ^{125}I staphylococcal A protein diluted to working strength in PBS/BSA solution. Phosphatase or peroxidase secondary conjugates can be used (*see* Note 8). (If a phosphatase conjugate is used, Tris-buffered saline/BSA solutions should be adopted).
5. TBS: 0.1 M Tris-HCl, pH 8.0; 0.1 M NaCl.
6. TBS lysis mix: TBS plus 0.5% NP40 and 0.1% aprotinin.

3. Methods

The initial requirement for the procedure is to generate a stock of vaccinia virus of known titer that is to act as the recipient of the cloned foreign gene. This is necessary for later steps that involve transfection with recombinant vaccinia virus insertion vectors (*see* Note 1). This chapter will not cover the steps involved in constructing the plasmid insertion vectors. Comprehensive protocols for these procedures can be found in Vols. 2 and 4, this series. *See* Fig. 2 for a flow diagram of the methodology.

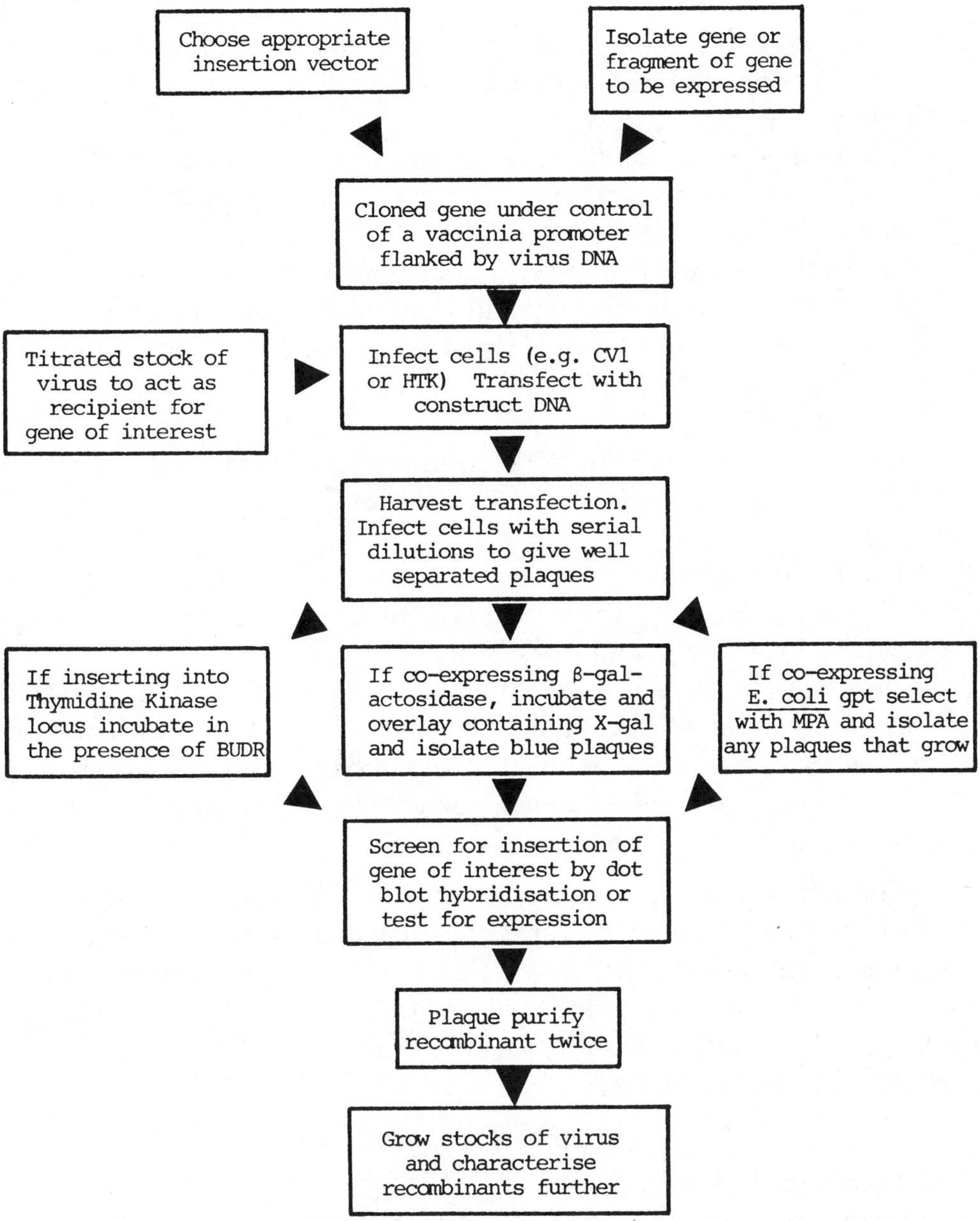

```
┌─────────────────────┐              ┌─────────────────────┐
│ Choose appropriate  │              │ Isolate gene or     │
│ insertion vector    │              │ fragment of gene    │
│                     │              │ to be expressed     │
└─────────────────────┘              └─────────────────────┘
             ◄                              ►
              ┌─────────────────────────────┐
              │ Cloned gene under control   │
              │ of a vaccinia promoter      │
              │ flanked by virus DNA        │
              └─────────────────────────────┘
                            ▼
┌─────────────────┐  ┌─────────────────────────┐
│ Titrated stock  │  │ Infect cells (e.g. CV1  │
│ of virus to act │►│ or HTK)  Transfect with │
│ as recipient for│  │ construct DNA           │
│ gene of interest│  │                         │
└─────────────────┘  └─────────────────────────┘
                            ▼
              ┌─────────────────────────────┐
              │ Harvest transfection.       │
              │ Infect cells with serial    │
              │ dilutions to give well      │
              │ separated plaques           │
              └─────────────────────────────┘
        ◄                   ▼                   ◄
┌──────────────────┐ ┌──────────────────────┐ ┌──────────────────┐
│ If inserting into│ │ If co-expressing β-gal│ │ If co-expressing │
│ Thymidine Kinase │ │ -actosidase, incubate │ │ E. coli gpt select│
│ locus incubate in│ │ and overlay containing│ │ with MPA and iso-│
│ the presence of  │ │ X-gal and isolate blue│ │ late any plaques │
│ BUDR             │ │ plaques               │ │ that grow        │
└──────────────────┘ └──────────────────────┘ └──────────────────┘
        ◄                   ▼                   ◄
              ┌─────────────────────────────┐
              │ Screen for insertion of     │
              │ gene of interest by dot     │
              │ blot hybridisation or       │
              │ test for expression         │
              └─────────────────────────────┘
                            ▼
                  ┌───────────────────┐
                  │ Plaque purify     │
                  │ recombinant twice │
                  └───────────────────┘
                            ▼
              ┌─────────────────────────────┐
              │ Grow stocks of virus        │
              │ and characterise            │
              │ recombinants further        │
              └─────────────────────────────┘
```

Fig. 2. Flow diagram for construction of vaccinia virus recombinants.

3.1. Assay of Virus Infectivity

1. Harvest infected cells in hypotonic buffer (either 10 mM Tris-HCl, pH 9.0, or 5 mM phosphate-citrate pH 7.4) and freeze and thaw twice in order to burst the cells and release the virus.
2. Thaw an aliquot of virus stock to be titered, and disperse any aggregated cell debris by using a mild waterbath sonicator for 15–30 s (Megasonic 80kc).

3. Add 0.1 vol of 2.5 mg/mL trypsin solution and incubate at 37°C for 30 min. This step can be left out, but doing so will decrease the titer two- to fivefold.

4. Make tenfold serial dilutions of virus in PBS + 0.1% BSA at 4°C. To minimize pipeting errors, dilutions can be done in duplicate and each dilution titrated on several monolayers.

5. Remove the medium from a cell monolayer that has just reached conflu-ence, wash once with PBS, and add 1 mL of virus dilution for a 60-mm² tissue culture dish or 0.2 mL of virus dilution for 15 mm² monolayers in 24-well dishes (*see* Note 6).

6. Incubate for 1–2 h at 37°C.

7. Add 5 mL of the appropriate medium (i.e., DMEM) containing 5% FCS for a 60-mm² plate; 1 mL for a 15-mm² well. Incubate at 37°C for 36–48 h.

8. Remove the medium, wash twice with PBS, and then add 1 mL of 0.2% crystal violet (in 20% ethanol), and incubate for 5 min at room temp-erature. Remove the stain and air-dry.

9. A focus of infection spreads outward from the cell initially infected. Infected cells round up and may become detached. As a consequence, a hole appears in the monolayer. These holes, referred to as plaques, are counted. (To avoid random sampling errors, monolayers with approx 100 plaques are counted.)

Knowing the dilution used to produce a certain number of plaques and assuming that a single infectious virus particle is responsible for each plaque allows one to calculate the infectivity of the stock. The infectivity is usually expressed as plaque-forming units/mL (PFU/mL) and will depend on the cell line used to titrate the virus. Titers can vary as much as five-fold when plaqued on different cell lines.

3.2. Plaque Purification

1. Follow steps 1–6 in Section 3.1.

2. Remove the virus inoculum and overlay the monolayer with MEM con-taining 1% Noble (or low gelling temperature agarose) and 5% FCS. Melt the 2% stock agarose and add an equal vol of 2× MEM + 10% FCS. Do not overlay when agar plus medium is >45°C. If a selective medium is required, this can be incorporated into the overlay.

3. Let the agar set on a level surface and incubate at 37°C for 36–48 h.

4. Stain the cells by overlaying the agarose with 1% Noble agarose contain-ing 0.01% neutral red. Incubate at 37°C until virus plaques are seen as clear areas in the monolayer (only living cells take up the neutral red).

5. Pick well-isolated plaques, using a Pasteur pipet with a small bulb attached. Put the Pasteur pipet into the agarose directly over a plaque so that the pipet is in contact with the monolayer. By suction, remove the agarose plug. This inevitibly removes the majority of the infected monolayer in the region of the plaque.
6. Transfer the plug and virus monolayer to 0.5 mL of MEM containing 5% FCS.
7. Release the virus by three cycles of freeze-thawing.
8. To replaque, follow steps 4–6 of Section 3.1., and 2–6 above.

3.3. Production of Virus
3.3.1. Small Virus Stocks

1. Use half the virus recovered from a plaque to infect a 25-cm² monolayer of cells that have just reached confluency (steps 5–7 in Section 3.1.).
2. Incubate at 37°C for 48–72 h or until the majority of cells show a cytopathic effect from virus infection.
3. Scrape the cells into the medium and recover them by pelleting at low speed in a bench-top centrifuge.
4. Resuspend the cells in hypotonic buffer, e.g., 10 mM Tris-HCl, pH 9.0, 1mM EDTA, and release the virus by three cycles of freeze-thawing.

3.3.2. Crude, Larger Stocks

1. Seed 5–10 bottles (150 cm²) with 5×10^7 HeLa S3 spinner cells each (in MEM). Allow the cells to settle overnight. Alternatively, use 10 monolayers (150 cm² each) of cells, such as CV1 or HTK⁻143.
2. Take half the progeny from a small stock (or approx 1 PFU/cell). Disperse any cell aggregation by mild sonication, then incubate with 0.1 vol of 2.5 mg/mL trypsin (Difco 1:250) for 30 min at 37°C.
3. Dilute the virus stock in PBS/0.05% BSA to give 2 mL/150-cm² bottle.
4. Add 2 mL of virus dilution/bottle and incubate for 1–2 h at 37°C. Add 25 mL MEM plus 5% FCS and incubate for a further 48–72 h.
5. Recover the infected cells by scraping into the medium and pelleting at low speed in a bench top centrifuge. Resuspend the cells in 2 mL/monolayer of 10 mM Tris-HCl, pH 9, 1 mM EDTA, and subject the suspension to three cycles of freeze-thawing to release the virus.
6. The virus stock is titrated to determine its infectivity (*see* Section 3.1.).

3.3.3. Purified Stocks

1. Grow 2–10 L of HeLa S3 spinner cells to a density of 5×10^5 cells/mL or grow 10–20 monolayers (150 cm²) or roller bottles of the appropriate cell type.

2. Incubate the crude virus stock with 0.1 vol of 2.5 mg/mL trypsin at 37°C for 30 min. The amount of stock should be sufficient to infect the cells at a multiplicity of 5 PFU/cell. For monolayer cells and roller bottles, follow steps 3 and 4, Section 3.2.2.

3. Concentrate the spinner cells to 5×10^6 cells/mL by low-speed centrifugation, and resuspend the cells in culture medium containing 5% FCS.

4. Add the trypsin-treated crude virus stock to the concentrated spinner cells and incubate in suspension for 1 h at 37°C. Dilute with culture medium to give 5×10^5 cells/mL. Incubate for a further 48 h.

5. Harvest the infected cells and resuspend them in 10 mM Tris-HCl, pH 9.0, at 4°C. Use 2 mL/2×10^7 infected cells from a monolayer or 2 mL/100 mL of suspension culture. This and subsequent steps should be carried out on ice.

6. Homogenize with 15–20 strokes of a tight-fitting Dounce homogenizer. Check for complete cell lysis by microscopy.

7. Pellet the nuclei by centrifugation at 750 g for 5 min at 4°C. Resuspend the pellet in 10 mM Tris-HCl, pH 9.0. Repeat step 6, recentrifuge, and combine the supernatants.

8. Add 0.1 vol of 2.5 mg/mL trypsin and incubate at 37°C for 30 min with frequent vortexing.

9. Layer onto an equal vol of 36% (w/v) sucrose in 10 mM Tris-HCl, pH 9.0, in a Beckman SW27 tube or equivalent. Centrifuge at 13,500 rpm in the SW27 rotor or equivalent ($25,000g$) for 80 min at 4°C (*see* Note 7).

10. Discard the supernatant and resuspend the pellet (virus and debris) in 2 mL of 1 mM Tris-HCl, pH 9.0. Add 0.1 vol of 2.5 mg/mL trypsin and incubate at 37°C for 30 min.

11. Overlay 2 mL of virus suspension onto continuous sucrose gradients (20–50% in 1 mM Tris-HCl, pH 9.0) in Beckman SW27 tubes or their equivalent. Centrifuge at 12,000 rpm in the SW27 rotor ($18,750g$) for 45 min at 4°C.

12. Collect the banded virus with a syringe through the side of the tube. Dilute 1:3 with 1 mM Tris-HCl, pH 9.0, and pellet the virus by centrifugation at $25,000g$ for 60 min at 4°C.

13. Occasionally, when using large vols of spinner cells, significant amounts of virus and debris pellet in the gradients. It can be valuable to retrypsinize these pellets and band on a second gradient.

14. Resuspend the virus in 1mM Tris-HCl, pH 9.0. Freeze aliquots at –70°C.

15. Thaw an aliquot and titrate, following the protocol described previously.

16. These virus stocks are stable for many years at –20°C or, preferably, at –70°C.

3.4. Generation of Recombinants

3.4.1. Transfection Protocol (see Note 5)

1. Infect a recently confluent 25 cm² monolayer of CV1 cells (or another cell line that can be transfected efficiently) at a multiplicity of 0.05 PFU/cell of purified virus (see Section 3.1., steps 2–7; at step 4, dilute the virus to give the desired amount).
2. Add 1 µg of the plasmid transfer vector to 19 µg of sheared calf thymus DNA in 1 mL of HEPES buffered saline (see Chapter 2).
3. Form coprecipitates by addition of 2.5 M CaCl$_2$ to a concentration of 125 mM. Leave at room temperature for 20–30 min.
4. Two hours after infection of the monolayers, remove the virus inoculum and wash thoroughly three times in PBS or serum-free MEM. Add 0.5 mL of the DNA suspension and incubate at room temperature for 20 min.
5. Add 8 mL of DMEM plus 5% FCS and incubate at 37°C for 4–6 h.
6. Replace the medium with 5 mL of DMEM plus 5% FCS and incubate at 37°C for 48 h.
7. Recover the cells by scraping into the medium and pelleting at low speed in a bench centrifuge. Resuspend in 10 mM Tris-HCl, pH 9, 1 mM EDTA; release virus by three cycles of freeze-thawing.

3.5. Selection of Recombinant Viruses

3.5.1. Selection of tk⁻ Phenotype

1. Approximately one-fifth of a transfection experiment is used to infect recently confluent HTK⁻143 cells at 10^{-1}, 10^{-2}, and 10^{-3} dilutions. (steps 1–5 of Section 3.2.), using an overlay containing 25 mg/mL BUdR).
2. At 48 h postinfection, cells are stained with neutral red and well-isolated plaques picked (steps 5 and 6 of Section 3.2.). These *tk⁻* viruses can then be tested for the presence or expression of the foreign gene of interest.

3.5.2. Selection of β-Galactosidase Positive Virus

1. Approximately one-fifth of a transfection experiment is used to infect recently confluent HTK⁻143 cells (steps 2–5 of Section 3.1.).
2. Forty-eight hours postinfection, the liquid overlay is replaced with 1% agarose in half-strength MEM containing 20 µg/mL X-gal (1:100 dilution of 2% X-gal in dimethyl formamide). Allow to set and incubate at 37°C (2.5 mL/60-mm² dish is sufficient.)

3. After 4–6 h, plaques that are positive for β-galactosidase expression can be seen as discrete blue foci.

4. Pick blue plaques (steps 5 and 6 of Section 3.2.) into 0.5 mL MEM containing 5% FCS.

5. Virus from the plaque can then be further plaque-purified using an overlay containing X-gal or grown in small wells to test for insertion and expression of the gene of interest.

3.5.3. Selection of E. coli gpt Positive Viruses (see Note 3)

Mycophenolic acid (MPA) blocks the salvage pathway that leads to production of GMP by inhibiting the enzyme IMP dehydrogenase that produces XMP from IMP. Mammalian cells cannot utilize xanthine to overcome this block unless the cells express the *E. coli gpt* gene. This is the basis of the extensive use of the *gpt* gene, a dominant selectable marker in eukaryotic cells. Recent reports *(16,17)* have shown that MPA will block the growth of vaccinia virus and that expression of the *gpt* gene from a vaccinia promoter will relieve this block. Consequently, transfer vectors have been designed (Fig. 1) that express the gene of interest from one promoter and the *E. coli gpt* gene from a second promoter. Selection for *gpt* expression allows identification of recombinant viruses that will coexpress the gene of interest. Two procedures have been described *(16,17)*. One *(16)* uses aminopterin in addition to MPA as part of the selective procedure. The protocol below outlines this strategy rather than using MPA alone.

1. Approximately one-fifth of a transfection experiment is used to infect recently confluent cell monolayers (all cell lines so far tested that will plaque vaccinia well are appropriate). Use steps 1–5, Section 3.2., with an overlay containing MEM, 5% FCS, 2.5 µg/mL MPA, 250 mg/mL xanthine, 14 µg/mL hypoxanthine, 0.2 mg/mL aminopterin, and 4 µg/mL thymidine.

2. At 48 h postinfection, cells are stained with neutral red and well-isolated plaques picked (steps 4 and 5 of Section 3.2.). These isolated MPA-resistant viruses can then be tested for the presence or expression of the foreign gene.

3.6. Detection of Unselected Viral Recombinants

3.6.1. DNA Dot-Blot Hybridization

1. Infect *tk⁻* 143 cells growing in 15-mm² wells (1–2×10^5 cells) with half the progeny of an isolated plaque (Section 3.1., steps 5 and 6). This can be *tk⁻*, β-gal positive, or MPA-resistant virus, i.e., putative recombinants from a transfection (24-well plates are ideal for this purpose.)

2. Incubate at 37°C for 36–48 h with medium containing 5% FCS and the appropriate selective agent. Harvest the infected cells by scraping into the medium. This can be achieved conveniently by using the plunger from a 1 mL syringe.
3. Collect one-fifth of the recovered material on nitrocellulose sheets by filtration, using a dot-blot manifold. If this is not available, up to 50 μL can be applied directly to the nitrocellulose using a micropipet.
4. Wash the nitrocellulose filter with 100 mM NaCl, 50 mM Tris-HCl, pH 7.5.
5. Place the filter for three 1-min intervals alternating between Whatman 3MM paper and Whatman 3MM paper saturated with each of the following: (a) 0.5M NaOH; (b) 1M Tris-HCl, pH 7; and (c) 2× SSC.
6. Air-dry and bake the filter at 80°C in a vacuum oven for 2 h. The filter can then be hybridized with a radioactively labeled foreign gene DNA probe (*see* Vol. 2, this series). Hybridization using probes with a specific activity of 10^7 cpm/μg DNA give a strong signal on overnight exposure of the filter to X-ray film.

3.6.2. Immunological Detection of Recombinants

Antisera specific for the foreign gene product can also be used to detect recombinant viruses, either directly on fixed infected monolayers or using extracts of monolayers. Binding of the antibody to infected cells or extracts can be detected by using either ^{125}I staphylococcal A protein or an enzyme-conjugated secondary antibody.

3.6.2.1. PLAQUE SCREEN

1. See step 1 of DNA dot-blot hybridization.
2. Wash infected monolayers well with PBS and fix by adding 1 mL of cold methanol for 10 min.
3. Wash the fixed infected monolayers with PBS and block nonspecific binding sites by incubation at room temperature for 1 h with PBS containing 4% BSA and 0.02% sodium azide.
4. Wash the monolayers once with PBS and incubate for a further 2 h at room temperature with PBS containing 4% BSA, 0.02% sodium azide, and the appropriate dilution of antibody.
5. Wash the cell monolayer five times with PBS.
6. Incubate the monolayers for 2 h at room temperature with PBS containing 4% BSA, 0.02% sodium azide, and a stock peroxidase-conjugated antispecies antibody (1:500 or higher dilution). For example, if a monoclonal antibody is used in the first antibody step, then the secondary antibody should be a peroxidase-conjugated antimouse antibody. Dako D314 at 1:500 works well (*see* Note 8).

7. Wash the monolayers with PBS and add peroxidase substrate (*see* Chapter 26, this vol.). After a few min, color will develop where the primary antibody has bound to the recombinant infected cells of a plaque. At lower dilutions, all the cells may be infected and the whole monolayer may react. Recombinants can then be plaque-purified further and the procedure repeated to check that all virus plaques in a stock are expressing the recombinant gene product.

3.6.2.2. DOT-BLOT SCREEN

Under some circumstances, a dot-blot screen might be more appropriate. This has the advantage of testing for gene expression, rather than simply testing for insertion of the foreign DNA into the virus (as in Section 3.6.1.). The following procedure works well with proteins expressed at the cell surface and reasonably well with proteins located in the cytoplasm. For nuclear proteins, a total cell extract should be transferred to the nitrocellulose. Where the foreign gene product is secreted from the cell into the supernatant, it is clear that this procedure will not work.

1. Remove the medium from the cells, wash twice with PBS, and lyse with 100 µL of a solution containing 0.1 M Tris-HCl, pH 8.0; 0.1 M NaCl; 0.5% NP40 and 0.1% aprotinin.
2. Spot 25 µL of lysate from each monolayer onto nitrocellulose and leave it to air-dry.
3. Pretreat the filter with 50 mL of TBS containing 4% BSA and 0.02% NaN$_3$ for 2 h at room temperature on a rocking platform.
4. Add antiserum that will recognize the foreign gene product and incubate overnight at 4°C or for 2 h at room temperature on a rocking platform.
5. Wash the filter five times for 2 min each with 50 mL of TBS.
6. Incubate with gentle agitation for 1 h in PBS containing 4% BSA, 0.02% NaN$_3$, and 0.5 µCi of ^{125}I staphylococcal A protein.
7. Wash the filter five times, for 2 min each, in TBS. Allow to air-dry and expose to X-ray film. A positive result indicates which monolayers were infected with recombinant virus. Alternatively, an enzyme-conjugated secondary antibody can be used in place of the ^{125}I staphylococcal A protein (*see* Section 3.6.2.1.).

4. Notes

1. The choice of insertion vector is crucial (*see* Fig. 1). For ease of use, coinsertion vectors are preferable. However, the most important criterion for choosing a vector is the use to which the recombinant is to be

put. It is possible to use single-stranded vectors *(20)*, which have the advantage of increasing recombination frequencies and allow direct sequencing of the constructs. If high levels of expression are required, then either a vaccinia late structural promoter *(21)* or the T7 RNA polymerase system described by Fuerst et al. *(22)* should be used. If the recombinants are to be tested in immunological assays, early promoters are preferable. Under some conditions, foreign genes expressed by vaccinia late promoters do not stimulate cell-mediated immunity (specifically cytotoxic T-cells) and will not create target cells for cytotoxic T-cell lysis *(23)*.

2. A complication for expression of a foreign gene arises from the possibility of the foreign gene containing signals recognized uniquely by vaccinia for termination of transcription. The sequence TTTTTNT has been identified as an early transcriptional termination signal *(24)*. HIV 1 *env* has two such sequences, as does the human papillomavirus type 16 L1 gene. Both of these genes have been expressed in vaccinia using the 7.5K promoter, which has early and late transcriptional elements *(4–6,25)*. The L1 gene was expressed much more efficiently by using a late promoter.

3. Recent reports *(16,17)* of the use of the *E. coli gpt* gene and MPA as a dominant selectable marker have indicated some advantages over other procedures devised to isolate recombinant vaccinia viruses. One-step plaque isolation with the absence of spontaneous selectable mutants, an ability to use a variety of cell lines, and the use of alternative insertion sites within the vaccinia genome are all distinct advantages. In addition, BUdR used for *tk⁻* selection is highly mutagenic, whereas MPA is not. Avoidance of mutagens should ensure a greater virus stability.

4. Many cell lines, other than CV1, have been used successfully to generate recombinants, e.g., MRC5, HTK143, and chick embryo fibroblasts.

5. Increasing wild-type virus input in the transfections tends to decrease the percentage of recombinants produced (even though total overall yield may be increased). Thus, it is better to use relatively low input of virus; 0.05 PFU/cell works well. Often, over 50% of *tk⁻* viruses from a transfection are recombinant, whereas the rest are spontaneous *tk⁻* mutants. We have also noticed that when very large fragments are inserted, the percentage of recombinant *tk⁻* viruses decreases.

6. Virus yields at various stages of growth vary depending on the cell type used for growth, the parental vaccinia strain, and, possibly, the recombinant gene product expressed. Vaccinia strain WR grown in HeLa S3 give approx 100 PFU/cell. As a rough guide, between 10^2 and 10^4 PFU

can be recovered from a plaque, 10^8 PFU can be recovered from a small bottle, and as much as several milliliters of 10^{10} PFU/mL can be recovered from ten 150 cm² bottles of HeLa S3. Purified stocks should be in the region of $1–5 × 10^{10}$ PFU/mL/L of suspension cells.

7. Virus recovered after pelleting through a sucrose cushion is suitable for most required recombinant uses, and a subsequent banding step is necessary only to give a purer stock for immunization.

8. An alternative to step 6 is to incubate with PBS containing 4% BSA, 0.02% sodium azide, and 0.1–0.5 µCi of ^{125}I staphylococcal A protein for 1 h at room temperature.

Wash five times with PBS. Air-dry and expose the monolayer to film. (This may necessitate removing the rims of Petri dishes.) Development of X-ray film will indicate whether the primary antibody bound.

A further alternative to using peroxidase-conjugated secondary antibodies is to use alkaline phosphatase conjugated secondary antibodies. These have the advantage of giving a more sensitive assay; however, TBS should be used throughout the procedure, instead of PBS. For step 7, dissolve 10 mg of naphthol AS-MX phosphate (free acid Sigma N4875) in 1 mL N-N dimethylformamide. Add 49 mL of 0.1 M Tris-HCl, pH 8.2. Immediately before use, add 50 mg of fast blue BB salt (purified grade, Sigma F3378).

Acknowledgment

I would like to thank Wendy Pelham for excellent secretarial help. I am supported by the Cancer Research Campaign.

References

1. Mackett, M. and Smith, G. L. (1986) Vaccinia virus expression vectors. *J. Gen. Virol.* **67,** 2067–2082 .

2. Mackett, M., Smith, G. L., and Moss, B. (1985) The construction and characterisation of vaccinia virus recombinants expressing foreign genes, in *DNA Cloning: A Practical Approach* (Glover, D. M., ed.), IRL, Oxford, pp. 191–211.

3. Moss, B. and Flexner, C. (1987) Vaccinia virus expression vectors. *Annu. Rev. Immunol.* **5,** 305–324.

4. Chakrabarti, S., Robert-Guroff, M., Wong-Staal, F., Gallow, R. C., and Moss, B. (1986) Expression of the HTLV-III envelope gene by a recombinant vaccinia virus. *Nature* **320,** 535–537.

5. Hu, S.-L., Kosowski, S. G., and Dalrymple, J. M. (1986) Expression of AIDS virus envelope gene in recombinant vaccinia virus. *Nature* **320,** 537–540.

6. Kieny, M. P., Rautmann, G., Schmitt, D., Dott, K., Wain-Hobson, S., Alizon, M., Girard, M., Chamaret, S., Laurent, A., Montagnier, L., and Leoocq, J.-P. (1986) AID Virus *env* protein expressed from a recombinant vaccinia virus. *Biotechnology* **4,** 790–795.

7. Lifson, J. D., Feinberg, M. B., Reyes, G. R., Rabin, L., Banapour, B., Chakrabarti, S., Moss, B., Wong-Staal, F., Steiner, K. S., and Engleman, E. G. (1986) Induction of CD4-dependent cell fusion by the HTLV III/LAV envelope glycoprotein. *Nature* 323, 725–728.

8. Hu, S.-L., Fultz, P. N., McClure, H. M., Eichberg, J. W., Thomas, E. K., Zarling, J., Singhal, M. C., Kosowski, S. G., Swenson, R. B., Anderson, D. C., and Todaro, G. (1987) Effect of immunization with a vaccinia-HIV *env* recombinant on HIV infection of chimpanzees. *Nature* 328, 721–723.

9. Zagury, D., Leonard, R., Fouchard, M., Reveil, B., Bernard, J., Ittele, D., Cattan, A., Zirimwabagabo, L., KaLumbu, M., Justin, W., Salaun, J.-J., and Goussard, B. (1987) Immunization against AIDS in humans. Scientific correspondence. *Nature* 326, 249,250.

10. Zagury, D., Bernard, J., Chenier, R., Desportes, I., Leonard, R., Fouchard, M., Reveil, B., Ittele, D., Lurhuma, Z., Mbayo, K., Ware, J., Salaun, J.-J., Goussard, B., Dechazal, L., Burny, A., Nara, P., and Gallow, R. C. (1988) A group specific anamnestic immune reaction against HIV 1 induced by a candidate vaccine against AIDS. *Nature* 332, 728–731.

11. Zarling, J. M., Eichberg, J. W., Moran, P. A., McClure, J., Sridhar, P., and Hu, S.-L. (1987) Proliferative and cytotoxic T-cells with AIDS virus glycoproteins in chimpanzees immunized with a recombinant vaccinia virus expressing AIDS virus envelope glycoproteins. *J. Immunol.* 139, 988–990.

12. Walker, B. D., Chakrabarti, S., Moss, B., Paradis, T. J., Flynn, T., Dumo, A. G., Blumberg, R. S., Kaplan, J. C., Hirsch, M. S., and Schooley, R. T. (1987) HIV-specific cytotoxic T-lymphocytes in seropositive individuals. *Nature* 328, 345–348.

13. Walker, B. D., Flexner, C., Paradis, T. J., Fuller, T. C., Hirsch, M. S., Schooley, R. T., and Moss, B. (1988) HIV-1 reverse transcriptase is a target for cytotoxic T-lymphocytes in infected individuals. *Science* 240, 64–66.

14. Keiny, M. P., Lathe, R., Riviere, X., Dott, K., Schmitt, P., Girard, M., Montagnier, L., and Lecocq, J.-P. (1988) Improved antigenicity of the HIV *env* protein by cleavage site removal. *Protein Eng.* 2, 219–225.

15. Moss, B. (1985) Replication of poxviruses, in *Virology* (Fields, B. N., Knipe, D. M., Chanock, R. M., Melnick, J. L., Roizman, B., and Shape, R. E., eds.), Raven, New York, pp. 658–703.

16. Boyle, D. B. and Coupar, B. E. H. (1988) A dominant selectable marker for the construction of recombinant poxviruses. *Gene* 65, 123–128.

17. Falkner, E. G. and Moss, B. (1988) *Eschericia colic gpt* gene provides dominant selection for vaccinia virus open reading frame expression vectors. *J. Virol.* 62, 1849–1854.

18. Chakrabarti, S., Brechling, K., and Moss, B. (1985) Vaccinia virus expression vector: Coexpression of β-galactosidase provides visual screening of recombinant virus plaques. *Mol. Cell. Biol.* 5, 3403–3409.

19. Mackett, M., Smith, G. L., and Moss, B. (1984) General method for production and selection of infectious vaccinia virus recombinants expressing foreign genes. *J. Virol.* 49, 857–864.

20. Wilson, E. M., Hodges, W. M., and Hruby, D. E. (1986) Construction of recombinant vaccinia virus strains using single-stranded DNA insertion vectors. *Gene* 49, 207–213.

21. Stunnenberg, H. G., Lange, H., Philipson, L., van Miltenburg, R. T., and Van der Vliet, P. C. (1988) High expression of functional adenovirus DNA polymerase and precursor terminal protein using recombinant vaccinia virus. *Nucleic Acids Res.* 16, 2431–2444.

22. Fuerst, T. T., Earl, P. L., and Moss, B. (1987) Use of a hybrid vaccinia virus-T7 RNA polymerase system for expression of target genes. *Mol. Cell. Biol.* **7,** 2538–2544.
23. Coupar, B. E. H., Andrew, M. E., Both, G. W., and Boyle, D. B. (1986) Temporal regulation of influenza hemagglutinin expression in vaccinia virus recombinants and effects on the immune response. *Eur. J. Immunol.* **16,** 1479–1487.
24. Rohrmann, G., Yuen, L., and Moss, B. (1986) Transcription of vaccinia virus early genes by enzymes isolated from vaccinia virions terminates downstream of a regulatory sequence. *Cell* **46,** 1029–1035.
25. Browne, H. M., Churcher, M. J., Stanley, M. A., Smith, G. L., and Minson, A. C. (1988) Analysis of the L1 gene product of human papilloma virus type 16 by expression in a vaccinia virus recombinant. *J. Gen. Virol.* **69,** 1263–1273.

CHAPTER 13

Manipulation
of Baculovirus Vectors

Mark J. Bailey and Robert D. Possee

1. Introduction

The development of expression vectors from baculoviruses has provided molecular biologists with one of the most efficient and effective ways of synthesizing foreign gene products in a heterologous system. In contrast to the other recent excellent reviews on the subject *(1,2)*, this contribution aims to explore the various practical aspects of the system, and in consequence, to highlight particular difficulties that may be encountered by workers new to the field. However, before describing the methodology peculiar to baculovirus expression vectors, it is of value to briefly consider the isolation, structure, and replication strategy of this unique group of viruses. Detailed and more comprehensive reviews that describe the biology of baculoviruses are available *(3–5)*.

1.1. Isolation and Characterization

Baculoviruses have been isolated only from invertebrates and, in particular, from insect species. This latter observation may simply reflect the interests of invertebrate pathologists and virologists, and not reflect the true species distribution. However, what has been clearly established is that baculoviruses do not infect vertebrate species or plants. Therefore, baculoviruses present few safety problems when used as expression vectors. The viruses are currently classified according to their structure and are included in three

From: *Methods in Molecular Biology, Vol. 7: Gene Transfer and Expression Protocols*
Edited by: E. J. Murray © 1991 The Humana Press Inc., Clifton, NJ

subgroups: (a) nuclear polyhedrosis viruses (NPVs), (b) granulosis viruses (GVs), and (c) nonoccluded viruses (NOV). Each virus is named after the species from which it was first isolated. This review addresses only the first category and uses as its primary example the *Autographa californica* (Ac NPV). This is regarded as the prototype baculovirus, has been the focus for molecular studies, and is the virus most widely used for expression work.

1.2. Structure

Most baculoviruses produce two structurally distinct forms. Both have as their core a nucleocapsid containing the double-stranded, covalently closed, circular DNA genome (AcNPV; ca. 130 kbp). This is surrounded by a lipoprotein envelope that delineates the virus particle. In some viruses, multiple nucleocapsids are enclosed within the envelope (MNPVs); in others, such as the *Heliothis zea* baculovirus, only a single nucleocapsid is thus packaged (SNPVs). Depending on the ultimate fate of the virus particle, the envelope is acquired in one of two ways. In the first, extracellular virus particles (ECVs) are formed as nucleocapsids bud through the plasma membrane of infected cells. During this process, the 64 kDa glycoprotein (gp64) surface antigen (probably the ECV cell attachment protein) is acquired, and antisera to this polypeptide is neutralizing *(6)*. In the second process, nucleocapsids are enveloped within the infected cell nucleus to form occluded virus particles (OCVs). These apparently lack gp64, since antiserum to this protein fails to neutralize OCV. The virus particles are further packaged into polyhedra or occlusion bodies comprising a single virus encoded polypeptide (polyhedrin) of ca. 30 kDa. The relevance of these two structural forms will be discussed below.

1.3. Replication In Vivo and In Vitro

Polyhedra serve to protect the virus particles from adverse environmental conditions and allow the virus to persist on leaf surfaces or in soil before encountering a susceptible host. The major target for the virus in the insect life cycle is the larval or caterpillar stage. The normal route of transmission is *per os*, since polyhedra are acquired while the insect feeds on contaminated foliage. Following ingestion, the occlusion body passes undamaged through the acid foregut into the midgut. Here, the alkaline pH causes the polyhedrin protein to solubilize, releasing the virus particles. These attach to gut epithelial cells, pass through, and replicate in the basal lamella before establishing a systemic infection. Therefore, whereas the polyhedra facilitate horizontal transmission, the ECV disseminates the virus infection throughout the insect.

Baculoviruses may also replicate in cultures of insect cells. However, it should be noted that intact polyhedra are noninfectious for these cells, unless the packaged virus particles are released *via* alkali treatment prior to inoculation; the culture medium is too acidic (pH 6.2) for this to occur spontaneously. The ECV subsequently produced by these infected cells is responsible for spreading the infection; the polyhedra take no part in continuing propagation of the virus, although they continue to be synthesized.

It is from experiments in cell culture that we have started to understand the biochemical events in the replication strategy of the virus. Essentially, after the virus DNA has reached the nucleus, the genome is expressed in four temporally distinct phases. These are the immediate early (α), delayed early (β), late (γ), and very late (δ) phases. In the a phase, genes are expressed using the host transcriptional machinery. They apparently do not require the synthesis of other virus gene products, since they are produced in cells treated with cycloheximide. In the β, γ, and δ phases, genes that require prior synthesis of virus encoded cofactors are expressed. The last two phases describe the production of ECV (γ), which bud from infected cells, and, subsequently, mature polyhedra containing virus particles (δ). During the δ phase, two virus proteins are produced in copious quantities, eventually accounting for some 50% of the total cell protein. These are the polyhedrin protein, described above, and the p10 gene product, which is a nonstructural polypeptide of 10 kDa, thought to play some role in the formation of the polyhedra. Both proteins are nonessential for the replication and formation of virus particles *(7–9)*, and therefore, have been targeted for use in expression vectors.

1.4. The Development of Baculovirus Expression Vectors

The baculovirus most commonly used for expression work is AcNPV, although the *Bombyx mori* (silkworm) NPV has been similarly exploited to a lesser extent *(10)*. All the baculovirus vectors freely available at present use the promoter region of the polyhedrin gene to drive the expression of foreign genes.

It is important to appreciate that, unlike simple prokaryotic vectors based on plasmids, it is not yet possible to directly ligate foreign genes into the baculovirus genome. The DNA is very large (ca. 130 kbp), and unique restriction enzyme sites have not been reported. Therefore, the strategy for using baculoviruses as vectors involves manipulation of a portion of the virus genome in a bacterial plasmid; typically one of the pUC series. This type of plasmid is designated the transfer vector and, as implied by its name, it serves as a vehicle for inserting the foreign gene into the virus genome.

1.5. Vector Construction

The derivation of baculovirus vectors is a matter of record and will not be discussed here in detail. The reader is referred to the papers of Smith et al. *(11)*, Pennock et al. *(12)*, Possee *(13)*, and Matsuura et al. *(14)* for a full account. Essentially, as described above, most vectors have been based on the polyhedrin gene of AcNPV. This was located by several workers within a 7.3-kbp fragment generated by digestion of the virus genome with EcoRI and is designated "I" in accordance with the proposal of Vlak and Smith *(15)*. The complete sequence of this fragment has been determined and will be reported shortly (Possee and coworkers, unpublished data). A partial restriction map of the fragment is presented in Fig. 1. The vectors produced in our laboratory *(13,14)* were constructed as follows: The EcoRI fragment I was subcloned into a derivative of pUC8 lacking all of the polylinker region except the EcoRI site. Thereafter, the polyhedrin coding sequences were removed using Bal31 exonuclease. In some vectors, only the amino terminal coding sequences were deleted *(13);* in others, such as pAcYM1 *(see* listing of vectors *(14))*, the entire coding region was removed. The yield of foreign gene products is the same with both types of vector. The promoter region of the polyhedrin gene was retained together with the 3' noncoding sequences containing the transcription termination signals *(see below)*. The deleted coding sequences were replaced with a synthetic oligonucleotide linker, usually BamHI, to facilitate insertion of foreign genes into the vector. The use of this linker also necessitated deleting a BamHI site downstream from the polyhedrin gene in the EcoRI fragment. It is also possible to insert a polylinker containing multiple cloning sites, which is advantageous when working with a variety of foreign gene cassettes lacking BamHI-compatible ends.

1.6. Features of the Transfer Vectors Important in Expression

The polyhedrin gene transcription initiation site was determined by mRNA sequencing *(16)*, and those flanking regions essential to transcription were elucidated by deletion mutagenesis *(14,17)*, and linker scan mutagenesis *(18)*. Transcription is dependent on the integrity of the complete 49-nucleotide untranslated 5' leader sequence before the polyhedrin ATG and 15–20 nucleotides upstream from the mRNA initiation site; reduced levels of foreign gene expression resulted if any of these nucleotides were removed. Sequence comparisons between different baculovirus polyhedrin (and p10) genes have identified a highly conserved region of 12 nucleotides spanning the transcription start site *(19)*. Site directed mutagenesis of this sequence has revealed that the central TAAG motif, where transcription initiates, is

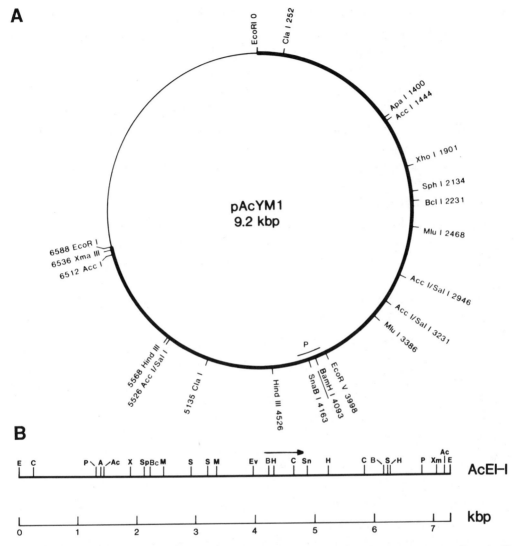

A

B

Fig. 1. (a) Restriction map of the baculovirus vector pAcYM1 (narrow line indicates the position of the plasmid vector pUC8 into which the baculovirus fragment was inserted). Restriction sites unique to the baculovirus DNA and their relative positions are given. A unique BamHI site has been created after the adenine in the polyhedrin transcriptional initiation codon (ATG); the entire open reading frame of polyhedrin has been deleted in pAcYM1. The line over the BamHI site indicates the position of the polyhedrin gene 3' and 5' noncoding regions. Inserts must be correctly oriented.

Fig. 1. (b) Restriction map of the EcoR I fragment of the AcNPV genome. All the polyhedrin baculovirus vectors are based on this fragment. Arrow indicates the position of the polyhedrin open reading frame (ORF).

Key to the restriction enzyme sites: Ac, Acc I; A, Apa I; B, Bam HI; Bc, Bcl I; C, Cla I; E, Eco RI; Ev, Eco RV; H, Hind III; M, Mlu I; P, Pvu III; S, Sal I; Sn, Sna BI; Sp, Sph I; X, Xho I; Xm, Xma III.

absolutely required for expression (K. Gearing and R. D. Possee, unpublished data). Therefore, any transfer vector to be used for deriving recombinant virus must have a complete copy of the 5' noncoding sequence included in its structure; some of the earlier vectors, e.g., pAc373 *(20)*, and pAcRP5 *(13)*, lack these sequences and consequently express less efficiently.

The transcription termination site for the polyhedrin gene has been determined by S1 nuclease analysis *(16)*. The 3' noncoding region of the polyhedrin gene must also be retained in the transfer vector, since deletions or insertions in this sequence will produce a nonviable virus (Possee, unpublished data).

The vectors pAcYM1 *(14)*, pVL941 *(1)*, and pEV55 *(2)* all satisfy these critera and should give optimal yields of foreign protein. However, the foreign gene must donate its own translation initiation codon. A variety of other useful vectors that supply translation initiation codons and thus permit the expression of foreign genes as fusion products are also available; other vectors have signal peptide sequences that direct the secretion of the gene product. These are given in Table 1.

1.7. Preparation of Recombinant Viruses

After insertion of the foreign gene, the transfer vector is coprecipitated with infectious AcNPV DNA and added to *Spodoptera frugiperda* cells (Sf-21AE *(21)*) to initiate virus replication. Within the nucleus of the infected cell, recombination takes place between the homologous sequences flanking the polyhedrin gene in the normal virus and the foreign gene in the transfer vector (*see* Fig. 2). The result is the replacement of the polyhedrin gene with the foreign gene, thus deriving a polyhedrin-negative mutant unable to produce polyhedra. These viruses are detected by visual observation of plaque assays of the progenyvirus.

The efficiency of recombination is difficult to assess, since recording such events depends on the skill of the operator in finding polyhedrin-negative plaques; generally efficiencies of 0.1–0.01% are observed. However, many recombinant plaques will be masked by polyhedrin positive viruses. When the reverse experiment was done, i.e., rescuing polyhedrin-negative virus with a plasmid containing the polyhedrin gene, recombination frequencies of up to 10% were observed *(7)*. Similar high values were obtained when producing viruses containing the β-galactosidase gene that facilitates the production of easily identifiable blue plaques (Possee, unpublished data). The minimum length of AcNPV DNA flanking the foreign gene in the transfer vector that is required for recombination has not been determined. However, a new vector, pAcCL29, which contains an M13IG sequence to facilitate single stranded

Table 1
Some Useful Baculovirus Vectors[a]

Vector	Description
pAcYM1	High-level expression vector, BamHI cloning site, retains complete 5' leader sequence and first nucleotide of polyhedrin ATG. Polyhedrin coding sequences are completely deleted *(14)*. Foreign gene must donate ATG.
pAcRP23.lacZ	Used to generate virus recombinants able to stain blue in the presence of X-gal. Potential as blue/white selectable marker for transfection; unfortunately, lacZ gene may mutate spontaneously and produce white plaques. Very useful as a control for efficient transfection/recombination.
pAcRP14	Retains polyhedrin ATG, which is immediately followed by BamHI linker to minimize extra sequence when expressing gene fusions (Possee, unpublished data).
pAc360	Fusion protein (11 *N*-terminal amino acids of polyhedrin remain) BamHI site (+34) *(1)*.
pAc373	Bam HI site located 8 bp before polyhedrin ATG *(20)*.
pAcVC3	Dual expression vector. AvaII fragment of pAcYM$_1$ removed, BamHI site converted to a BglII site and cloned in reverse orientation into the EcoRV site of pAcYM$_1$ *(23)*. Expression of at least two proteins.
pAcVC$_1$	As pAcVC3 except polyhedrin gene retained in AccII fragment from pEcoRI "I," result, dual expression vector (polyhedrin and insert), progeny virus particles are occluded and used to infect larvae. This system is of use only if you have access to an insectory, but has great potential for the commercial exploitation of baculovirus expressed products from a cheap source, i.e., the caterpillar factory.
pAcJM25	Contains VSV glycoprotein leader sequence in pAcYM1. Cloning in phase results in processing of signal peptide and membrane deposition of product. Export and secretion dependent on insert proteins (J. Millard, personal communication).
pAcCL29	Vector able to produce single stranded DNA in *E. coli* for site directed mutagenesis *(22)*.

[a]These are based on plasmids containing a selectable marker, β lactamase, and replicate to high copy number in *E. coli.* Those generated in Summers' laboratory are well described in his excellent baculovirus manual *(29)*.

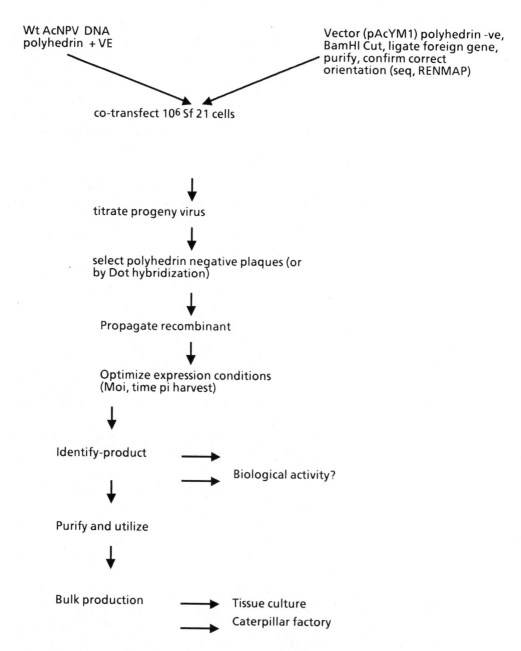

Fig. 2. Diagram of the steps involved in the construction of the recombinant plasmid vector, the transfection of insect cells, and isolation and identification of recombinant virus. Purified wild-type virus genomic DNA, containing the polyhedrin ORF (polyhedrin +ve), is mixed with the recombinant plasmid vector. After transfection of the insect cells, homologous recombination occurs between the virus genome and the regions flanking the insert in the vector DNA. Progeny replicate and possess the polyhedrin-negative phenotype, which is the basis of selection. Recombinant virus express the insert via the polyhedrin transcriptional and translational machinery.

DNA generation in *E. coli,* performs efficiently in the production of virus recombinants, and contains only 5 kbp of AcNPV DNA derived from pAcYM1 *(22);* pAcYM1 has approx 7 kbp of virus sequences.

1.8. Processing of Foreign Genes in Insect Cells

Proteins expressed by baculoviruses in insect cells appear to be biologically active and undergo correct posttranslational modification, including low-order glycosylation, phosphorylation, palmitylation, myristylation, signal peptide cleavage, and intracellular transport. However, the level of expression of some proteins may be affected by the ability of the insect cells to correctly process them. A full review of the processing of foreign gene products by baculoviruses has been published recently *(2).*

1.9. Future Developments

Our understanding of the molecular biology of baculoviruses is in its infancy. It must be emphasized that we do not understand why the very late genes of these viruses are so well expressed or, more important, why some foreign genes are poorly produced, whereas others match the level of polyhedrin. Further basic research is required to investigate these observations and permit the coherent design of better expression vectors.

Currently, the scope of AcNPV as an expression vector is being extended by utilizing strong promoter, the p10 gene that, like polyhedrin, is expressed during the δ phase *(8,9).*

The use of early promoters is also envisaged, and these may enable the production of a cascade of gene products throughout the replication cycle, thus allowing the construction and expression of metabolic pathways important in a number of industrial processes. Dual expression systems are already available *(23),* based on the duplication, in opposite orientations in the vector, of the polyhedrin transcription and translation machinery. The dual expression vector has been successfully exploited to evaluate the role of two different Blue tongue virus gene products in capsid morphogenesis and particle maturation *(24);* we envisage that multiple expression systems will be a great asset for both research and commercial purposes.

In a number of laboratories, developments are under way that will exploit alternative baculovirus vectors by including toxinogenic genes to enhance the virulence of virus destined for the field control of specific insect pests.

A further area for future development concerns the scale-up of methods for growing the recombinant viruses, thus deriving large quantities of expressed proteins; two options are available. The first concerns the use of suspension cultures grown in simple spinner flasks or air-lift fermenters and has been addressed in two recent reviews *(25,26).* The second option involves the use of insect larvae. One of the principal reasons for using the silkworm NPV as an expression vector was that there is a long history of domestic cultivation of this insect (10). Although an attractive method, insect culture has yet to be adopted by many workers, presumably because of a reluctance to work with the whole animal. It is easier for most laboratories to use cell culture.

1.10. Advantages of Baculoviruses as Expression Vectors

The baculovirus system has a number of advantages in that it is relatively simple to use, is nonpathogenic to animals or plants, and is a helper independent recombinant expression system that is capable of producing protein in large quantities (>100 mg/L). The single expression vectors can accept large inserts to allow the expression of complex genes, operons, and even, viral genomes.

The decision to use baculovirus vectors for the expression of functional gene(s) must be dependent on the availability of resources in a given laboratory. It is assumed that the operator has a basic knowledge of virology, tissue culture techniques, and molecular biology. Access to a 28°C incubator, laminar flow cabinet, and media preparation facilities will also be necessary.

2. Materials

2.1. Cell Culture—General

1. TC-100 medium; 10% FCS; Penicillin, streptomycin, and kanamycin.
2. *Spodoptera frugiperda* cells (Sf 21/Sf 9).
3. PBS (Dulbecco's A).
4. Trypan blue 0.05% in PBS.
5. DMSO and liquid nitrogen for cell storage.
6. Inverted microscope (must be of high quality).
7. Tissue culture hood.
8. 28°C incubator.
9. Tissue culture plasticware.
10. Hemocytometer.

2.2. Titration, Propagation, and Purification of Viral DNA

1. 3% low-gelling temperature agarose (Sea Plaque, FMC) in distilled water.
2. Neutral red 0.01% in PBS.
3. TE: 10 mM Tris-HCl, pH 8.0; 1 mM EDTA.
4. 10 and 50% sucrose in TE.

5. Virus lysis buffer: 2% sodium *N*-lauryl sarcosine, 1 m*M* EDTA.

6. 50% w/w CsCl solution TE containing ethidium bromide (25μg/mL). CAUTION: Ethidium bromide is mutagenic.

7. Cell lysis buffer: 50 m*M* Tris-HCl, pH7.8; 5% 2-mercaptoethanol; 10 m*M* EDTA; 0.4% SDS.

8. Ribonuclease.

9. Proteinase K.

10. Phenol:chloroform (50:50), equilibrated with 100 m*M* Tris-HCl, pH 8.0.

11. 3*M* sodium acetate, pH 5.2.

12. 100 and 70% ethanol.

2.3. Transfection and Generation of Recombinant Virus

1. Transfection mix: HEPES buffer; 40 m*M* HEPES, 2 m*M* sodium phosphate, 10 m*M* potassium chloride, and 280 m*M* sodium chloride (pH 7.5).

2. 0.1*M* D-glucose.

3. 2.5*M* calcium chloride.

2.4. DNA Dot-Blot Analysis

1. 0.2*M* sodium hydroxide.

2. 10 m*M* ammonium acetate.

3. 20× SSC (saline sodium citrate): 175.3 g sodium chloride; 88.2 g sodium citrate, pH 7.0; with 10*M* sodium hydroxide.

4. 100× Denhardt's solution: Ficoll, 10 g; Polyvinylopyrrolidine, 10 g; BSA (fraction V); 10 g distilled water to 500 mL.

5. Hybridization buffer: 10 mL deionized formamide, 1.0 mL of 100× Denhardt's solution, 1.0 mL of 2 mg/mL denatured salmon sperm DNA, 1.0 mL of 20 × SSC, and 7.0 mL distilled water.

6. Nick translation kit.

7. Dot transfer apparatus.

8. Nylon membrane.

2.5. Immunoblot Analysis
of Recombinant Virus-Infected Cells

1. RIPA buffer: 1% Triton X-100; 1% sodium deoxycholate; 0.5*M* sodium chloride; 0.05*M* Tris-HCl, pH 7.4; 0.01*M* EDTA; and 0.1% SDS.

2. PAT buffer: 0.1% BSA, 0.01% Tween-20 in PBS.

3. Phosphatase-conjugated antibody.

4. Phosphatase substrate: 44 μL NBT (nitro blue tetrazolium) in 10 mL of 0.1*M* Tris-HCl, pH 9.5; 0.1*M* NaCl; 0.05*M* MgCl$_2$. Add 33 μL BCIP (5-bromo-4-chloro-3-indolyl phosphate).

3. Methods

Lepidopteran insect cells are routinely grown in TC100 medium. This is a complex medium requiring skill and experience to prepare; GIBCO-BRL now conveniently sell this product in powder form, which can be prepared, filter-sterilized, and stored at 4°C for some months. It is supplemented before use with 5 or 10% fetal calf serum (FCS); penicillin (50 U/mL), streptomycin (50 µg/mL), and kanamycin (50 U/mL) may be added if desired. The complete medium is stable for at least 3 mo at 4°C. The FCS should be tested for cell viability before purchasing in bulk; it may have to be heat-inactivated (56°C/30 min) prior to use.

3.1. Maintenance of Insect Cells

Spodoptera frugiperda IPLB-Sf-21AE cells (Sf21) *(21)* were originally derived from insect pupal ovaries and have been used for all our work. (A cloned version of this cell line (Sf9) was derived in Max Summer's laboratory and is available from the American Tissue Culture Collection; it is unclear which cell line is the best to use.) We commonly use Sf21 cells between passage 150 and 180 for our work. The higher level is not a limiting factor to cell growth; with care, cells can be maintained indefinitely. However, we have observed a decrease in virus production when cells of high passage number are used and, for reproducibility, prefer to use a defined passage range. Cells may be grown as either monolayer or suspension culture at 28 or 21°C in atmospheric air. The doubling time is 18–24 h, depending on culture conditions and temperature. Cells may be counted in an improved Neubauer chamber by diluting in medium and trypan blue (final concentration, 0.05% w/v). It is essential to keep cells in a healthy condition prior to use in transfection experiments and plaque assays (*see below*).

3.1.1. Monolayer Culture

In general, it is advisable to seed cells at a density of 2×10^4 cm^2 and allow them to become confluent before subculturing. However, the cells can be seeded at lower densities to permit the maintenance of cells at room temperature for up to 10 d. The cells are harvested by gently scraping them, with a sterile rubber policeman, from the flask into fresh medium. It is imperative that the cells are not subjected to trypsin, since this will severely reduce viability.

3.1.2. Suspension Culture

This system is particularly useful for growing larger stocks of virus or recombinant protein. Cells are seeded at 10^5/mL in TC100/5% FCS in round-bottomed flasks and stirred with a magnetic bar at 100 rpm. It is essential to maintain the supply of oxygen to the cells; hence, the surface area exposed to the atmosphere should be maximized. Therefore, it is advisable that only 50% of the available vol in a flask be used (e.g., 500 mL in a 1000-mL flask). Cultures of up to 2000 mL can be grown in this way, but with some reduction in total cell number attributable to oxygen limitation, unless air is bubbled through the medium. The maximum cell number obtained is usually between 2 and 4×10^6.

3.1.3. Storage of Cells in Liquid Nitrogen

Cells should be harvested when they are in their exponential phase of growth and diluted into TC100 medium containing 10% FCS and 10% DMSO (final concentration, $1–4 \times 10^6$/mL. Cryotubes are filled with 1–2 mL and chilled on ice before placing in gaseous nitrogen for approx 2 h. The cells are subsequently immersed in liquid nitrogen for long-term storage. In this state, they remain viable indefinitely. The cells are revived by thawing rapidly at 37°C, diluting 1:5 in fresh medium, and dispensing into a 25-cm² flask. After incubation at 28°C for 24 h, the medium should be changed and the cells incubated further until ready for subculture.

3.2. Titration of Virus in a Plaque Assay

This is possibly the most critical technique to master when using the baculovirus expression system for the first time. The production of clear, well-defined plaques is vital, since this permits the easy identification of recombinant virus lacking polyhedra. Furthermore, accurate titers of virus stocks are required for the calculation of the multiplicity of infection (moi; infectious virions per cell) to be used when optimizing expression and comparing yields from different viruses. In our experience, workers new to the field have more difficulty with this method than any other. The stages involved are described below.

1. Actively growing (subconfluent) cells should be harvested and accurately counted as described above; viability must exceed 98% (*see* Note 1).
2. Dilute the cells to a concentration of 0.75×10^6/mL and dispense 2 mL into each 35-mm tissue culture dish). Before use, incubate at 28°C for 1–3 h on a level, vibration-free surface. Alternatively, the cells may be seeded at a concentration of 10^6/dish and used the following day (*see* Note 2).
3. Remove all media and add, drop-wise, 100 μL of appropriately diluted virus to the center of the dish. Gently rock the plate to ensure even distribution of the virus; then incubate at room temperature for 1 h.
4. The virus inoculum must be removed with a Pasteur pipet after tilting the dish to one side to facilitate drainage.

5. Prepare overlay medium by mixing sterile 3% low-gelling temperature agarose, cooled to 37°C with an equal vol of TC100/5% FCS, prewarmed to the same temperature. Add 1.5 mL overlay medium to the side of each dish, allow to set for 20 min, and then supplement with 1.0 mL TC100/5% FCS as a liquid feeder layer (plaques do not form well unless this extra medium is added). Incubate dishes in a humid environment at 28°C for 72–96 h.

6. Plaques may be observed without staining by directing a light source to the side of each dish and viewing against a black background. Alternatively, the cells may be stained by adding 1.0 mL neutral red (0.01% w/v in PBS) directly to the dishes and incubating for 2 h at 28°C. Thereafter, all liquid is removed by inverting the dish over a sterile beaker and then blotting residual stain with a paper towel. Allow to destain, by standing for at least 5 h (preferably overnight) at 21°C. Uninfected cells retain the red stain; infected areas (plaques) appear clear. By viewing the stained monolayer over a light box, plaques can be counted and the titer of the virus stock easily calculated. The selection of recombinant virus lacking the polyhedrin gene will be described below.

3.3. Virus Propagation

The propagation of AcNPV in insect cells will be described from the isolation of a single plaque to a large (1000 mL) suspension culture.

1. With a sterile Pasteur pipet, remove the agarose from a clear, well-isolated plaque and disperse into 0.5 mL of TC100/5% FCS containing antibiotics. The recovery of virus varies but should be about 10^4–10^5 PFU/mL.

2. This stock is amplified by inoculating 100 µL of the virus onto 5×10^5 cells in 35-mm culture dishes after removal of the medium. After 1 h at room temperature, TC100/5% FCS is added and the cells incubated at 28°C for 3–4 d until the cells display cytopathic effect. The harvested medium is clarified by low-speed centrifugation ($1000g$) and the virus stock titrated as described above; the titer should be 10^6–10^7 PFU/mL.

3. To amplify the stock further, prepare 80-cm² flasks with 5×10^6 cells and inoculate with virus at a moi of 0.1–0.5 PFU/cell; incubate as before until all cells are infected. This virus stock should be 5×10^7–10^8 PFU/mL.

4. Virus stocks of the highest titer (>10^8 PFU/mL) may be produced by inoculating 50–1000 mL suspension cultures (5×10^5 cells/mL with 0.1–0.5 PFU/cell, and incubating at 28°C for 3–4 d.

3.4. Purification of Virus DNA

The quality and purity of this DNA is essential if successful transfection of insect cells is to be achieved. For the majority of procedures, wild-type AcNPV DNA will be required; however, if you choose to use dual vectors containing the polyhedrin gene (i.e., pAcVC$_1$), then viral genomic DNA lacking the polyhedrin gene must be prepared.

1. It is usually necessary to have a total of 0.5–1.0×10^9 infected cells to permit purification of useful quantities of virus. This quantity of cells should be prepared using a suspension culture, as described above.

2. The cells are pelleted at 1000g for 10 min and then the virus particles are pelleted at 75,000g for 1 h at 4°C. The pellets are conveniently resuspended in 10 mL TE and residual cell debris removed using low-speed centrifugation (1000g).

3. The virus is then applied to a 20 mL 10–50% (w/v) discontinuous sucrose gradient and sedimented to the interface (25,000g Beckman SW41) for 1 h at 4°C.

4. The thick white virus band is harvested by downward displacement, diluted with TE, and pelleted at 75,000g for 1 h at 4°C.

5. The pellet is resupended in approx 1.6 mL of TE. The virus is disrupted by the addition of 0.4 mL of virus lysis buffer (20% [w/v] sodium-*N*-lauryl sarcosine, 10 m*M* EDTA) and incubation at 60°C for 30 min.

6. The lysate is added to the top of a 50% (w/w) CsCl gradient in TE containing ethidium bromide (25 µg/mL). Spin at 45,000 rpm at 20°C for 24 h (Beckman Ti70). The virus DNA may also be purified using a swing-out titanium rotor (e.g., Beckman SW41); in this case, the lysed virus is applied to the top of a 5 mL 50% (w/w) CsCl cushion and the DNA sedimented at 45000g for 16 h at 20°C.

7. Harvest the lower (supercoiled) and upper (nicked circular and linear) bands and pool prior to extraction with butanol to remove ethidium bromide.

8. Dialyze extensively against TE before measuring the concentration and then store at 4°C; do not freeze the DNA, since this destroys infectivity. The yield should be about 100–200 µg. Throughout the purification, it should be remembered that the genome is large and easily damaged by pipeting and other harsh mechanical treatment.

3.5. Insertion of Foreign Genes into the Transfer Vector

The use of a transfer vector, such as pAcYM1, requires that the foreign gene be excised with a restriction enzyme that produces BamHI-compatible sticky ends. Alternatively, the insert and digested vector must be treated with a suitable enzyme to produce flush ends for blunt-end ligation. The gene must also have its own translation, initiation, and termination codons. If only part of a coding sequence is to be expressed, then synthetic signals must be added prior to insertion. Vectors retaining the polyhedrin ATG may also be used (e.g., pAcRP14). In our experience, the amount of 3' noncoding sequence retained after the translation stop codon is not important. However, it is advisable to remove the 5' noncoding region before the ATG of the foreign gene, particularly if it is GC-rich; Bal31 or exonuclease III digestion are very effective for this purpose. Such manipulations are adequately described elsewhere *(27,28)*. Once the foreign gene has been inserted into the transfer vector, it is advisable to sequence across both ends of the gene either by the Maxam and Gilbert chemical degradation method from a suitable restriction endonuclease site in the insert and EcoRV in the vector (90 bp from the adenine at +1), or, more conveniently, by double-stranded dideoxy plasmid sequencing, using primers generated to complement sequences at each end of the inserted gene.

It is also advisable to use very pure DNA for transfection. Therefore, plasmids should be prepared according to Chapter 1 and purified by CsCl gradient centrifugation.

3.6. Transfection of Insect Cells and the Generation of Recombinant Virus

The best results are often obtained by titrating the recombinant plasmid DNA against the viral genomic DNA; routinely we use 2, 10, and 25 μg of input plasmid DNA with 1 μg of virus DNA for reliable recombination. The quality of the cells is also very important: they must be in the exponential phase of growth and have a viability greater than 98% (*see* Note 4).

1. Seed 1.5×10^6 Sf21 cells in 2 mL TC100/5% FCS in a 35-mm dish and incubate at 28°C for 3 h; alternatively, seed the dishes with 10^6 cells and incubate at the same temperature overnight before using.
2. Make up transfection mix as follows, mix 475 μL HEPES buffer, 95 μL 0.1 M D-glucose, and 1 μg AcNPV DNA; add 1–10 μg plasmid DNA, and mix. Then add to 950 μL H_2O. Mix well.

3. Add 50 µL 2.5 M CaCl₂, dropwise, to the transfection mix while gently vortexing (this should take no longer than 10 s to avoid shearing the virus DNA). Incubate at room temperature for 30 min. This should produce a fine precipitate.

4. Remove all medium from the cells and add the transfection mix. Incubate at room temperature for 1 h. Add 2 mL TC100/5% FCS and incubate at 28°C for 2 h. Remove the transfection mix/medium and add a further 2 mL TC100/5% FCS; incubate at 28°C for 48–72 h.

5. Inspect the cells for the presence of polyhedra to confirm that the transfection has been successful. The infected cells should contain large "sugar cube-like" inclusions, which can be seen within the nucleus by direct observation using an inverted microscope. These are the occluded virus particles of the wild-type virus. It may also be possible to test for expression of the foreign gene using antibody assays *(see below)*. Harvest the cells and medium, and pellet the former using low-speed centrifugation. Titrate the virus in the supernatant fraction using the plaque assay technique previously described (appropriate dilutions to use are 10^{-1}–10^{-4}). Store unused undiluted virus at 4°C.

3.7. Recombinant Virus Selection

The isolation of recombinant viruses lacking the polyhedrin gene may be achieved using several methods. The first relies on observation of plaques with a light microscope, the others on detection of appropriate viruses with DNA or antibody probes.

3.7.1. Visual Identification of Plaques

The selection of a recombinant in the progeny virus from a transfection mix against the background of the polyhedrin-positive plaques requires patience and careful observation. The stained or unstained plaques may be viewed by directing light sideways on the dish and holding it against a dark background. Polyhedrin-negative plaques appear clear. On occasion, certain biological properties may facilitate the selection process. For instance, the fusogenic properties of the glycoprotein of VSV resulted in the pro-duction of giant cell syncytia when recombinant virus expressed the protein *(29)*. Ring with a fine felt-tip pen any putative polyhedrin-negative plaques and view under a good high-resolution inverted microscope. Isolate the plaques as described previously (Section 3.3.) and retitrate until the stock is clear of contaminating wild-type virus. Pick at least five clear plaques, since AcNPV sometimes mutates to a polyhedrin-negative phenotype.

3.7.2. Dot-Blot Hybridization (Modified from Ref. 30)

1. Titrate the transfection mix supernatant by standard plaque assay and dilute to 50 PFU/mL.
2. Seed a 96-well plate with 10^4 Sf cells/well and allow to settle for 1 h.
3. Aspirate culture fluid and add 200 µL (10 PFU) of diluted transfection mix. Incubate in a moist box at 28°C for 72 h.
4. With a multichannel pipet, transfer the culture fluid to a fresh 96-well plate, seal with parafilm, and store at 4°C.
5. To the cells, add 400 µL of $0.2M$ NaOH; incubate for 15 min at room temperature. Add 20 µL of $0.01M$ ammonium acetate and mix by pipeting up and down five to 10 times.
6. Transfer the lysate to a prewetted nylon membrane, using a Bio-Rad vacuum dot-blot apparatus. Wash out wells with lysis mix ($0.2M$ NaOH: $0.01M$ ammonium acetate) and aspirate.
7. Remove the filter and wash it twice, for 2 min each time, in 4× SSC and once in 2× SSC. Air-dry. Cover with cling film and UV-irradiate for 45 s on UV products transilluminator ($8 \mu W/cm^2$).
8. Treat at 42°C for 4 h in hybridization buffer. Add radioactively labeled probe in fresh buffer and incubate overnight at 42°C. Wash away unwanted, unbound probe three times for 5 min with 6× SSC at room temperature. Expose membrane to X-ray film.

3.7.3. Detection of Recombinant Virus
by Immunoblotting Techniques

1. Remove culture media from the microtiter plate and add 200 µL of RIPA buffer.
2. Incubate at 37°C for 15 min and freeze-thaw twice at −70°C.
3. After the final thaw, transfer lysed cells to dot-blot apparatus containing nitrocellulate membrane wet with RIPA buffer.
4. Aspirate and wash with RIPA buffer. Remove the membrane and wash in PAT.
5. Incubate with PAT-diluted antibody (dilution will depend on antibody titer and source) for 2 h at room temperature.
6. Wash 5 times for 2 min each in PBS 0.1% Tween 20.
7. Add antispecies alkaline phosphate conjugate (diluted 1:3000 in PAT) and incubate for 2 h at room temperature.
8. Wash away unbound conjugate and add substrate in the dark; NPT/ BCIP (GIBCO/BRL) is the most sensitive.
9. A positive reaction indicates the presence of recombinant virus. As many as five 96-well plates may be needed, since a low efficiency (<0.1%) would mean the probability of only one recombinant/plate of 1000 PFU.

10. Perform titrations (10^{-2}, 10^{-3}, and 10^{-4}) on positive wells, and select recombinants either by visual selection or by further rounds of limiting dilution hybridization.

3.8. Extraction of Recombinant Virus DNA from Infected Cells for Southern Blot Analysis

A useful and very rapid method for analyzing recombinant virus DNA is to extract nucleic acid from infected cell cultures.

1. Tissue culture dishes (35-mm diameter) are seeded with 10^6 cells as described previously and incubated for 3 h at 28°C. The medium is removed and virus added to the center of each dish at a moi of 10 PFU/cell. After 1 h at room temperature, the inoculum is removed and replaced with 2 mL of TC100/5% FCS.

2. The cultures are incubated at 28°C for 24 h, harvested, and the cells washed with PBS in 1.5-mL microfuge tubes using a low-speed spin in the centrifuge.

3. The cells are then resuspended in 250 μL of TE and 250 μL of cell lysis buffer added. Ribonuclease A is added to a final concentration of 40 μg/mL and the lysate incubated at 37°C for 30 min. Proteinase K is then added (to a final concentration of 100 μg/mL) and the incubation continued for a further 30 min at the same temperature.

4. The lysate is extracted twice with phenol/chloroform; vigorous shaking must be avoided to prevent shearing of the virus DNA. The DNA is precipitated from the final aqueous phase by the addition of sodium acetate (to $0.3M$) and 2 vol of ethanol. The nucleic acid is pelleted using a microfuge and washed twice with 70% ethanol, air-dried, and resuspended in 100 μL TE. The DNA may be more readily resuspended after storage at 4°C overnight.

5. A small quantity of this material (5–10 μL; equivalent to about 100 ng) is sufficient for digestion with restriction enzymes and subsequent analysis in agarose gels and Southern blot hybridizations. After staining the gel with ethidium bromide, the virus specific bands are readily apparent.

When working with dual vectors, it is obvious that two membranes need to be prepared for probing with either insert or antibody. Similar protocols can be adapted if cloning and expressing genes with functional activity, in which case lysed cells or tissue culture supernatants can be screened. Once the recombinant has been isolated, plaque-purified, and amplified, optimum conditions for expression can be determined by varying the moi, time of incubation, and product levels determined by SDS-PAGE.

To date, we have yet to completely fail to express a gene in the baculovirus system. However, we do know of a number of proteins that are very poorly produced. Evidence suggests that blocks that occur may be at the translational level, along with stability or toxic properties of the construct. Ways to circumnavigate these problems are being investigated, though significantly more knowledge of the processing events, and signal and indicator sequences of normal lepidoperteran genes and polypeptides needs to be elucidated to allow the directed targeting of chimeric protein in the cell. Such procedures would undoubtedly facilitate the purification of products on a commercial scale, certainly if the product could be exported into the culture fluid. The development of multiple expression vectors utilizing promoters other than the polyhedrin will allow the construction of vectors that can express important metabolic pathways. Today, however, some of these problems can be addressed by the coinfection of cells with two or more recombinant viruses.

Further commercial acceptance of this system will come with the development of serum-free, chemically defined media, which should dramatically reduce the cost of manufacture.

4. Notes

1. Cells must at all times be kept in a healthy ($1–20 \times 10^5$/mL) and viable state. They are the key to success.
2. Plaque assays need to be performed on level, vibration-free surfaces; do not add hot agarose (above 40°C), because it kills cells. Do not heat- or cold-shock cells with nonequilibrated media.
3. Ensure all materials are detergent-free, especially in cell culture.
4. DNA must be pure and uncontaminated for transfections.
5. Secreted proteins may be, and often are, present in small quantities in the culture supernatant; therefore, it may be necessary to concentrate by ammonium sulfate cutting. Growth in serum-free medium for 24–72 h postinfection may facilitate purification by removing contaminating serum albumin.

References

1. Luckow, V. A. and Summers, M. D. (1988) Trends in the development of Baculovirus expression vectors. *Biotechnology* **6,** 47–55.
2. Miller. L. K. (1988) Baculoviruses as gene expression vectors. *Annu. Rev. Microbiol.* **42,** 177–199.
3. Doerfler, W. and Bohm, P. (eds.) (1986) The molecular biology of baculoviruses. *Curr. Top. Microbiol. Immunol.* **131.**

4. Granados, R. R. and Federici, B. A. (eds.) (1986) *The Biology of Baculoviruses*, vol.1, *Biological Properties and Molecular Biology* (CRC, Boca Raton, FL).

5. Kelly, D. C. (1982) *Baculovirus* replication. *J. Gen. Virol.* **63**, 1–13.

6. Volkman, L. E., Goldsmith. P. A., Hess, R.T.D., and Faulkner, P. (1984) Neutralization of budded *Autographa californica* NPV by a monoclonal antibody: Identification of the target antigen. *Virology* **133**, 354–362.

7. Smith, G. E., Vlak, J. M., and Summers, M. D. (1983) Physical analysis of *Autographa californica* nuclear polyhedrosis virus transcripts for polyhedrin and 10,000-molecular weight protein. *J. Virol.* **45**, 215–225.

8. Vlak, J. M., Klinkenberg, F., Zaal, K. J. M., Usmany, M., Klinge-Roode, E. C., Geervliet, J. B. F., Roosien, J., and Van Lent, J. W. M. (1988) Functional studies on the p10 gene of *Autographa californica* nuclear polyhedrosis virus using a recombinant expressing a p10 Beta-galactosidase fusion gene. *J. Gen. Virol.* **69**, 765–776.

9. Williams, G. V., Rohel, D. Z., Kuzio, J., and Faulkner, P. (1989) A cytopathological investigation of *Autographa californica* nuclear polyhedrosis virus p10 gene function using insertion/deletion mutants. *J. Gen. Virol.* **70**, 187–202.

10. Maeda, S., Kawan, T., Obinata, M., Fujiwara, H., Horwich, T., Saeki, Y., Sato, Y., and Furusawa, M. (1988) Production of human interferon in silkworm using a baculovirus vector. *Nature* **315**, 592–594.

11. Smith, G. E., Summers, M. D., and Fraser, M. J. (1983) Production of human B interferon in insect cells with a baculovirus expression vector. *Mol. Cell. Biol.* **3**, 2156–2165.

12. Pennock, G. D., Shoemaker, C., and Miller, L. K. (1984) Strong and regulated expression of *E. coli* Beta-galactosidase in insect cells using a Baculovirus vector. *Mol. Cell. Biol.* **4**, 399–406.

13. Possee, R. D. (1986) Cell-surface expression of influenza virus hemagglutinin in insect cells using a Baculovirus vector. *Virus Res.* **5**, 43–59.

14. Matsuura, Y., Possee, R., Overton, H. A., and Bishop, D. H. L. (1987) Baculovirus expression vectors: The requirement for high level expression of protein, including glycoproteins. *J. Gen. Virol.* **68**, 1233–1250.

15. Vlak, J. M. and Smith, G. E. (1982) Orientation of the genome of *Autographa californica* nuclear polyedrosis virus: A proposal. *J. Virol.* **41**, 118–121.

16. Howard, C., Ayres, M. D., and Possee, R. D. (1986) Mapping the 5' and 3' ends of *Autographa californica* nuclear polyhedrosis virus polyhedrin mRNA. *Virus Res.* **5**, 109–119.

17. Possee, D. and Howard, S. C. (1987) Analysis of the polyhedrin gene promotor of AcNPV. *Nucleic Acid Res.* **15**, 10233–10248.

18. Rankin, C., Ooi, B. G., and Miller, L. K. (1988) Eight base pairs encompassing the transcription start point are the major determinants for baculovirus polyhedrin gene expression. *Gene* **70**, 39–49.

19. Rohrmann, G. F. (1986) Polyhedrin stucture. *J. Gen.Virol.* **67**, 1499–1513.

20. Smith, G. E., Ju, G., Ericson, B. L., Moschera, J., Lahm, H., Chizzonite, R., and Summers M. D. (1985) Modification and secretion of human interleukin-2 produced in insect cells by a baculovirus expression vector. *Proc. Natl. Acad. Sci. USA* **82**, 8404–8408.

21. Vaughn, L., Goodwin, R. H., Tompkins, G. L., and McCawley, P. (1977) The establishment of two cell lines from the insect *Spodoptera frugiperda* (lepidoptera: noctuidae). *In Vitro* **13**, 213–217.

22. Livingstone, C. and Jones, I. (1989) Baculovirus expression vectors with single strand capability. *Nucleic Acid Res.* **17**, 2366.

23. Emery, V. C. and Bishop, D. H. L. (1987) The development of multiple expression vectors for high level synthesis of eukaryotic proteins: Expression of LCMV-N and AcNPV polyhedrin proteins by a recombinant baculovirus. *Protein Eng.* 1, 359–366.

24. French, T. J. and Roy, P. (1990) Synthesis of Bluetongue virus (BTV) corelike particles by a recombinant baculovirus expressing the two structural core proteins of BTV. *J. Virol.* **64**, 1530–1536.

25. Maiorella, B., Inlow, D., Shauger, A., and Harano, D. (1988) Large scale insect cell-culture for recombinant protein production. *Biotechnology* **6**, 1406–1418.

26. Cameron, I. R., Possee, R. D., and Bishop, D. H. L. (1989) Insect cell culture technology in baculovirus expression systems. *Trends Biotechnol.* **7**, 66–70.

27. Maniatis, T., Fritsch, E. F., and Sambrook, J. (1982) *Molecular Cloning: A Laboratory Manual* (Cold Spring Harbor Laboratory, Cold Spring Harbor, NY).

28. Heinikoff, S. (1984) Unidirectional digestion with ExoIII creates targeted break points for DNA sequencing. *Gene* **28**, 351–359.

29. Bailey, M. J., Mcleod, D. A., Kang, C. Y., and Bishop, D. H. L. (1989) Glycosylation is not required for the fusion activity of the G Protein of VSV in insect cells. *Virology* **169**, 323–331.

30. Summers, M. D. and Smith, G. E. (1987) A manual of methods for baculovirus vectors and insect cell culture procedures. Texas Agricultural Experiment Station, Texas A&M University, Texas.

CHAPTER 14

Manipulation of SV40 Vectors

Marie-Louise Hammarskjöld

1. Introduction

SV40 is a small simian virus that has been extensively used as a viral vector in mammalian cells *(1–4)*. The viral genome is a double-stranded supercoiled DNA molecule of 5243 bp (Fig. 1A) that is packaged into a capsid containing the viral structural proteins VP1,VP2, and VP3. SV40 induces a lytic infection cycle in permissive cells. The first step in the replication cycle is synthesis of early mRNA. This is followed by DNA replication and expression of late mRNAs that encode the structural proteins. New virus particles are formed, and the infection ultimately kills the cells.

Early and late SV40 expression is directed by two different viral promoters (PE and PL) that function in opposite directions. Between these two promoters is a control region that contains a strong enhancer and binding sites for several different cellular transcription factors. The region between the two promoters also contains the origin of DNA replication. The SV40 early promoter is constitutively active, not only in monkey cells, but also in cells from several other species. When cells are infected with SV40, early transcription is tightly regulated by the major early gene product, large T-antigen. This protein binds to sites in the promoter to act as a feedback inhibitor of early transcription. In addition, T-antigen binds to the origin of replication, which promotes DNA replication.

From: *Methods in Molecular Biology, Vol. 7: Gene Transfer and Expression Protocols*
Edited by: E. J. Murray © 1991 The Humana Press Inc., Clifton, NJ

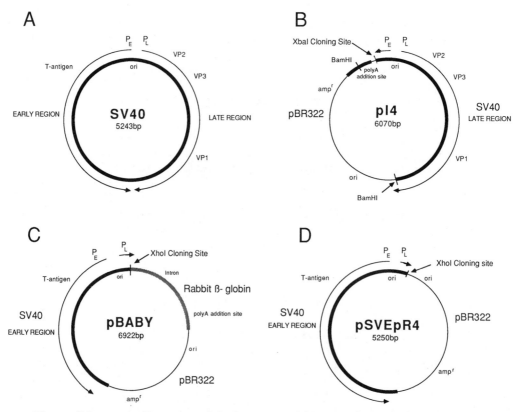

Fig. 1. Schematic diagrams of the genome of SV40 and the SV40 expression vectors pI4, pBABY, and pSVEpR4. The detailed maps and constructions of these vectors have been described elsewhere (8,11,12).

The SV40 late promoter is activated by the onset of viral DNA replication. It controls the synthesis of the viral capsid proteins that are made in very large amounts at late times after infection. This is a result of template amplification and the lack of feed back inhibition of the late promoter. Thus, this promoter is an excellent choice for transient expression of foreign genes in cells permissive of SV40 DNA replication, e.g., monkey cells and certain human cell lines. For a complete review of SV40 molecular biology, (see ref. 5).

SV40 vectors can be divided into two categories: early replacement vectors, in which the early region of SV40 is replaced by a foreign gene, and late replacement vectors, in which a foreign gene takes the place of the genes encoding the SV40 capsid proteins (1,2). In the first type of vector, the gene of interest is inserted downstream of the SV40 early promoter. Such constructs can be used in three different ways: to make stable cell lines expressing the gene, in transient transfection experiments, or to generate virus stocks containing the gene. For transient expression, the constructs are usually transfected into cells that constitutively express T-antigen. This enables the DNA to be replicated, leading to amplification of the transfected DNA. Several cell lines of this type are available. The original T-antigen-producing cell lines are called COS cells (for CV1 origin SV40) and were obtained by transfecting monkey CV1 cells with origin-defective variants of SV40 *(6)*. These cells produce enough T-antigen to promote DNA replication, but the levels are not high enough to cause inhibition of expression from the early promoter. More recently, cell lines (e.g., CMT) have been made that express T-antigen under control of the metallothionein promoter. In some of these cell lines, very high levels of T-antigen are produced when heavy metals are added to the culture medium *(7)*. These cells are especially useful for the generation of virus stocks containing foreign genes, since DNA replication is very efficient. For transient expression they may be less well suited, since inhibition of expression from the early promoter may occur. Virus stocks generated in CMT cells can be used for the infection of other cells (e.g., COS, CV1, HeLa) with high efficiency. Because of packaging restrictions, virus stocks can be obtained only if the inserted gene is <2.5 kbp.

In SV40 late replacement vectors, the late region of SV40 is removed and foreign genes are expressed under the control of the SV40 late promoter. These vectors have almost exclusively been used to express genes in cells permissive for SV40 replication, since efficient transcription from the late promoter occurs only after the onset of DNA replication. If the early region is kept intact, the vectors will make T-antigen, which permits their use in any cell line permissive for SV40 replication (i.e., monkey cells and several different human cell lines). In the case of late replacement vectors, foreign genes can be packaged into virus particles if the constructs are transfected into cells together with helper virus or a "helper" vector expressing the SV40 capsid proteins. The same size restrictions apply for both early and late replacement vectors.

This chapter describes how late and early SV40 replacement vectors can be used to express transiently large amounts of foreign gene products using a modification of the DEAE-dextran method to transfect cells *(8,9,10; see also* Chapter 3). It also describes how a virus stock can be obtained after transfection of COS or CMT cells with an early replacement vector and how expression of foreign gene products can be monitored using indirect immunofluorescence staining.

Figures 1B, C, and D show the early replacement vector pI4 and the late replacement vectors pBABY and pSVEpR4 *(8,11,12)* that are used in these experiments. In addition to SV40 sequences, these vectors contain a region from pBR322 providing a bacterial origin of replication and an ampicillin-resistance gene. Thus, they can be used as shuttle vectors between *E. coli* and mammalian cells. This permits production of large amounts of vector DNA in *E. coli* which is then used to transfect mammalian cells. For the expression of genes containing their own polyA addition signals, pSVEpR4 was constructed. It contains the whole early region of SV40, the origin of replication, the enhancer sequences, and the late promoter sequences up to the KpnI site in SV40 (bp 294 in the SV40 genome). A unique XhoI site was created at this site, downstream of the late promoter for the cloning of foreign genes. The vector pBABY is similar to pSVEpR4, but, in addition to the SV40 and pBR322 sequences, it contains a segment from the rabbit β-globin gene that includes the second intron and polyA addition signal. This vector was made to allow expression of genes lacking such sequences. Both pBABY and pSVEpR4 were constructed specifically for use in transient experiments. Using these vectors, high-level expression of several different gene products has been obtained in monkey cells and in different human lymphoblastoid cell lines *(8,11–13)*.

The vector pI4 is an early replacement vector that contains the late region of SV40 as well as the SV40 control region. The vector contains a unique XbaI site for the insertion of foreign genes downstream of the early SV40 promoter and an additional segment of SV40 containing polyA addition signals is 3' of this site. This vector can be cotransfected together with a plasmid containing a selectable marker to generate stable cell lines expressing inserted genes *(14,15)*. Alternatively, it can be used in transient experiments. High levels of expression are obtained if CMT or COS cells are used for template amplification *(6,7,11)*. Virus stocks containing the gene of interest can also be produced. In this case the DNA is cleaved with BamHI, to remove the pBR322 sequences, circularized by ligation, and transfected into COS or CMT cells. The initial virus particles produced are used to infect new cells. After 2–3 passages, a high-titer stock is usually obtained. The "poison" sequences, composing a small region in pBR322 that has been shown to inhibit replication in mammalian cells *(16)*, are not contained in pSVEpR4, pBABY, and pI4.

2. Materials

1. COS-7 and CMT3 cells: The cells are maintained in Iscove's Modified Dulbecco's Medium containing 10% calf serum (HyClone defined, supplemented bovine calf serum, HyClone Laboratories, Logan, VT) and gentamicin sulfate (25 µg/mL). The cells are split (1/5) every

3–4 d. They should never be allowed to overgrow. COS-7 cells can be obtained from the American Type Culture Collection, Rockville, MD (ATCC cat. no. CRL 1651).

2. Plastic tissue-culture dishes (100 mm diameter).

3. TD: 140 mM NaCl, 25 mM Tris-HCl, 5 mM KCl, 0.5 mM Na$_2$HPO$_4$, pH 7.5. Dissolve 8 g NaCl and 380 mg of KCl in 300 mL of H$_2$O. In a separate bottle dissolve 100 mg of Na$_2$HPO$_4$ (anhydrous) and 3 g Tris base in 200 mL of H$_2$O. Mix the two solutions and add H$_2$O (to 1000 mL). Adjust to pH 7.5 with HCl. Autoclave.

4. TS: TD with MgCl$_2$ and CaCl$_2$ added (1 mM final concentration).

5. Versene solution: 500 mL TD, 2.5 mL 0.1M EDTA (neutralized).

6. Trypsin/versene: 0.05% trypsin in versene.

The following solutions (7–9) are made fresh on the day of transfection:

7. DEAE-dextran solution: Make a 1 mg/mL DEAE-dextran (mol wt 500,000; Pharmacia or Sigma) solution in TS at 37°C. Vortex well to make sure that the DEAE-dextran dissolves properly. Filter the solution through a 0.45-µm filter. Keep at room temperature.

8. Glycerol solution: Add 80 mL of TS to a clean bottle. Add 20 mL of pure glycerol (Sigma G-9012) by pipeting up and down in the TS until all the glycerol is removed from the pipet. Filter through a 0.45-µm filter and keep at room temperature.

9. Chloroquine solution: Make a 10 mM stock solution by dissolving 52 mg of chloroquine diphosphate (Sigma C-6628) in 10 mL of H$_2$O. Filter through a 0.45-µm filter and keep protected from light. Use 1 mL of this solution/100 mL of medium.

10. Ligase buffer: 50 mM Tris HCl, pH 7.5; 1 mM MgCl$_2$; 10 mM dithiothreitol (DTT); 50 µg/mL nuclease-free bovine serum albumin (BSA); 50 µM ATP.

11. T4 DNA ligase 2 U/µL.

12. ZnCl$_2$: Make a 100 mM solution by dissolving 1.36 grams of ZnCl$_2$ in 80 mL of H$_2$O. Adjust the vol to 100 mL with H$_2$O. Filter through a 0.22-µm filter.

13. CdSO$_4$: Make a 1 mM solution by dissolving 22.6 mg of CdSO$_4$ (1 H$_2$O) in 100 mL of H$_2$O. Filter through a 0.22-µM filter.

14. Microscope slides.

15. Acetone/methanol, 2:1. Keep at –20°C.

16. Evan's blue solution for counterstaining: Dissolve 100 mg of Evan's blue in 100 mL of H$_2$O.

3. Methods

3.1. Transfection of CMT3 Cells

A transfection efficiency of 25–50% is regularly obtained with this method (*see* Note 1).

1. Split 100 mm-plates containing COS approaching confluence cells the day before transfection. Remove the medium from the plates, wash twice with 10 mL TD, and add 2 mL trypsin/versene. Remove after 1 min and place the cells in a 37°C incubator until the cells come off (usually 5–10 min).
2. Disperse the cells in Iscove's medium (10% serum) to about 1.5×10^6 cells/10mL. Place the cell suspension in 100-mm plastic tissue-culture dishes (10 mL/plate). Put the plates in a 37°C CO_2 tissue-culture incubator. The next day, the plates should be 70–80% confluent.
3. The next morning, prepare the DNA for transfection. For each plate, that is to be transfected, dilute 5 μg of plasmid DNA (e.g., pSVEpR4, pBABY, or pI4 into which the genes to be expressed have been inserted at the unique cloning site) with TS to 75 μL.
4. Mix the DNA solution with 750 μL of the DEAE-dextran solution. Keep at room temperature.
5. Remove the medium from the plates containing the COS cells and wash the cells twice with 10 mL of room-temperature TS.
6. Add the DNA/DEAE-dextran solution (1.5 mL/plate) carefully to the middle of the plates without disturbing the monolayer.
7. Put the plates back into the incubator and leave them for 60 min, carefully tilting every 15 min.
8. Aspirate off the DNA/DEAE-extran solution and add 3 mL of 20% glycerol solution. Distribute immediately by careful tilting. Leave the glycerol on the cells for 1.5–2 min. (Time is critical; don't attempt this with more than 3 plates at a time!) (*see* Note 3).
9. Aspirate off the glycerol completely. Quickly add 10 mL of TS to each plate and carefully tilt the plates several times. Aspirate and wash once more with 10 mL of TS to remove every trace of glycerol.
10. Add 10 mL of room-temperature Iscove's medium with 10% calf serum and 100 μM chloroquine phosphate to each plate. Put the plates back into the incubator for 5 h.
11. Aspirate off the chloroquine-containing medium and wash the cells twice with 10 mL of TS. Replace the medium with 10 mL of fresh Iscove's medium with 10% calf serum.

12. If the product of the gene under study is secreted into the medium, the medium can be changed to serum-free medium 30 h posttransfection without negative effects on yields.

13. The cells are harvested at 60–70 h posttransfection. At this point, the cells can be removed from the plates by mild trypsin treatment or by scraping the cells off the plates with a rubber policeman after washing the cells twice with 10 mL of TS. The efficiency of transfection can be determined by indirect immunofluorescence staining, as described below.

3.2. Generation of Virus Stocks

For genes cloned into the vector pI4, virus stocks containing the gene can be obtained, provided that the size of the gene is <2.5 kbp. The following method can be used to generate high-titer stocks.

1. Cleave 2 μg of the vector with BamHI to completion to remove the pBR322 sequences (check that the inserted gene lacks BamHI sites). Clean the DNA by phenol/chloroform/isoamyl alcohol extractions and EtOH precipitation.

2. Dissolve the precipitated DNA in 750 μL of ligase buffer and add 5 μL of T4-DNA ligase. Incubate at 14°C for 4 h. Religation at this low concentration promotes recircularization. Heat at 65° for 10 min to inactivate the ligase.

3. Mix with 750 μL of DEAE-dextran (1 mg/mL) and use the DNA directly to transfect a 100-mm plate of COS or CMT3 cells, using the method described above. If CMT3 cells are used, add medium containing $ZnCl_2$ and $CdSO_4$ (1 mL of each solution/L of medium) after the chloroquine treatment to induce the expression of T-antigen.

4. After about 3–4 d, a cytopathic effect should be observed in some of the cells (usually 1–5 %). At first several small vacuoles can be observed in the cytoplasm of the cells; later the cells round up and detach from the surface of the plate.

5. After 7 d, scrape the cells off the plate into the medium with a rubber policeman, and freeze and thaw this material three times to release the virus from the cells. Vortex and use the material to infect COS or CMT3 cells.

6. For infection, use 100-mm plates of COS or CMT3 cells that are about 50% confluent and have been recently split. Remove the medium from the cells and wash once with 10 mL of TS. Add 1.5 mL of the freeze-thawed material to each plate, and place the plates in the 37°C incubator. Tilt every 15 min.

7. After 60 min of adsorption, add 10 mL of Iscove's medium containing 10% calf serum. If CMT3 cells are used, add heavy metals as above. Put the plates back in the incubator. A cytopathic effect should be observed in some of the cells after 2–3 d.

8. After 7 d, harvest the cells as above and freeze-thaw the material. Use 1.5 mL to infect fresh COS or CMT3 cells and harvest after 7 d. At this time, the majority of the cells should have detached from the plates. The resulting virus stock should have a relatively high titer. The efficiency of expression that can be obtained after infection with this stock can be determined by using different dilutions of the material to infect cells (e.g., COS, CVl, HeLa). The percentage of cells expressing the inserted gene can be determined by indirect immunofluorescence staining as described below. *(see* Notes 4 and 5*)*.

3.3. Detection of Expression Using Indirect Immunofluorescence
3.3.1. Preparation of Cell Smears

1. Wash the plate containing transfected or infected cells twice with TD.
2. Add 1 mL trypsin/versene solution. Disperse by tilting and leave on the plates for 1 min. Remove the trypsin and place the plates in the incubator. Wait until the cells detach from the surface of the plates.
3. Add 10 mL of Iscove's medium with 10% calf serum to each plate and disperse the cells carefully by pipeting up and down. This inactivates the trypsin.
4. Transfer the cells to a 15-mL centrifuge tube and spin at 2000 rpm for 10 mins without using a brake in a table-top centrifuge.
5. Remove the medium and resuspend the cells carefully in 10mL of TD.
6. Repeat step 4, then remove the TD and resuspend the cells in TD + 10% calf serum to a concentration of about $1–2 \times 10^6$ cells/mL. (If the cells are about 80% confluent at the time of harvesting, a 100-mm plate will contain about $4–5 \times 10^6$ cells). At first, it is better to dilute the cells too little rather than too much.
7. After suspending the cells, put one drop on an acetone-washed glass slide with a Pasteur pipet. Leave it on for a few seconds, and then, from the other side of the drop, suck the solution back. The cells are heavy enough to fall onto the glass and stay there. Examine the slide under the microscope. Ideally, you should see a large number of cells, but they should not be crowded. If they are, dilute further to reach an acceptable dilution.

8. Once the dilution is acceptable, repeat step 7 for all slides that you wish to make. Let the slides air-dry for 30–60 min at room temperature.

9. Fix the air-dried slides by immersing them into an ice-cold solution (–20°C) of acetone/methanol (2/1) for 5 min.

10. Dry in air for 5–10 min. The fixed slides can be stored at 4°C for about a week before staining.

3.3.2. Staining

1. Mark the area containing the cells with a marking pen. Wet the fixed slide by immersing it in TD for a couple of mins. Remove the slide and dry around the area containing the cells using a Kimwipe or Kleenex®. From this point on, the slides should never be allowed to dry, since this will lead to high background!

2. Add 50 µL of primary antibody (Ab) diluted in TD to the marked area. Incubate at 37° C for 1 h in a "humid box." This should be a container that seals airtight. A small plastic box with a tight-fitting lid works well. Put a piece of moistened filter paper at the bottom of the box. The box should be covered when not in use, and H_2O should be added to the filter paper whenever needed, to keep it moist. The primary antibody should be directed against the gene product that you expect to express. The optimal dilution depends on the antibody and has to be determined for each antibody by testing different dilutions (*see* Chapter 26).

3. After incubation, wash the slides three times by immersing in TD. Dry around the cells. Put the secondary Ab (50 µL) on the cells and incubate as above. The secondary antibody should be directed against immunoglobulin from the species from which the first antibody was derived (i.e., antirabbit Ig antibodies should be used if the first antibody was derived from a rabbit) and should be conjugated to a fluorescent dye (e.g., FITC or Texas red). Usually, a 1/40 dilution works well. Conjugated antibodies can be obtained from several different companies (e.g., Sigma, Fisher-Promega).

4. After incubation with the second antibody, wash three times with TD. Dry around the cells. Immerse the slide in Evan's blue solution (1/10 dilution of the stock solution in H_2O) for 3 min. This will stain the cells blue so that they will be easier to visualize under the microscope. After staining wash the slides four times in TD.

5. Add a drop of TD/Glycerol (1/1) to the marked area and put on a coverslip. Keep stained slides, protected from light, at 4°C if they cannot be viewed immediately.

6. View the slides under a fluorescence microscope using an appropriate filter. Count fluorescent cells to determine the efficiency of expression. Nonfluorescent cells are clearly visible because of the counterstaining. Examples of fluorescence obtained using early and late replacement vectors are shown in Fig. 2.

4. Notes

1. COS and CMT cells can also be efficiently transfected by methods other than the one described above. Cells can be transfected by electroporation after trypsinization (*see* Chapter 5). Trypsinized cells can also be transfected with DEAE-dextran in solution using the above-described method. Using that method, we have sometimes been able to get transient expression in 80% of the cells. However, this method gives more variable results than transfecting the cells on the plates. For large-scale transient experiments, cells can be grown in roller bottles and transfected by the DEAE-dextran method described above.

2. The DEAE-dextran method does not work well for stable transfections. For such experiments, electroporation or the $CaPO_4$ method should be used.

3. Glycerol and chloroquine treatment help to increase the transfection efficiency *(8,9,17)*. The effect of the glycerol on the cells varies, depending on the general condition of the cells. It is therefore important to monitor this step carefully. This can be done by viewing the cells under the microscope during the shock. The cells should contract on the plate during the treatment, but should not start to come off the plates. If the cells are overtreated, they will lyse, releasing nuclei into the medium. It is important to use glycerol of high quality. Alternatively, the cells can be shocked with 10% DMSO for 2–5 min *(17,18)*. In our hands, however, DMSO is not as efficient as glycerol on either COS or CMT cells.

4. When making virus stocks, it is important not to grow the virus in multiple passages; this will lead to the generation of defective particles that will decrease the efficiency of expression of inserted genes. Two passages are usually enough to obtain a stock with a high titer. If fluorescent staining shows that the titer of the virus stock is low, the material should be passaged one more time and tested again.

5. Some sera give high backgrounds when used directly in immunofluorescence experiments. If this is a problem, the serum can be absorbed with nontransfected cells. For this purpose, the cells are scraped off plates

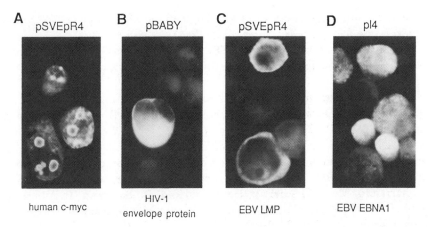

Fig. 2. Examples of immunofluorescence in COS cells transfected with different SV40 vector constructions. The cells were transfected with (A) a pSVEpR4 construct expressing the human c-*myc* protein *(17)* (B) a pBABY construct expressing the HIV envelope protein *(12)*, (C) a pSVEpR4 construct expressing the Epstein-Barr virus (EBV) latent membrane protein (LMP), and (D) a pI4 construct expressing the EBV EBNA1 protein.

and freeze-thawed twice. The cells are then added to serum, diluted (1/10) with TD (usually 10^6 cells/mL of diluted serum is enough), and the serum is incubated at room temperature with intermittent mixing for 60 min. After incubation, the cell debris is removed by centrifugation.

References

1. Gething, M. J. and Sambrook, J. (1981) Cell-surface expression of influenza hemagglutinin from a cloned DNA copy of the RNA gene. *Nature* **293,** 620–625.
2. Gluzman, Y. (1982) *Eukaryotic Viral Vectors* (Cold Spring Harbor Laboratory, Cold Spring Harbor, NY).
3. Mulligan, R. C. and Berg, P. (1981) Factors governing the expression of a bacterial gene in mammalian cells. *Mol. Cell. Biol.* **1,** 449–459.
4. Mulligan, R. C. and Berg, P. (1981) Selection for animal cells that express the *Escherichia coli* gene coding for xanthine-guanine phosphoribosyltransferase. *Proc. Natl. Acad. Sci. USA* **78,** 2072–2076.
5. Tooze, J. (1981) *DNA Tumor Viruses: Molecular Biology of Tumor Viruses, 2nd ed.* (Cold Spring Harbor Laboratory, Cold Spring Harbor, NY).
6. Gluzman, Y. (1981) SV40-transformed simian cells support the replication of early SV40 mutants. *Cell* **23,** 175–182.
7. Gerard, R. D. and Gluzman, Y. (1985) New host cell system for regulated simian virus 40 DNA replication. *Mol. Cell. Biol.* **5,** 3231–3240.
8. Hammarskjöld, M.-L., Wang, S.-C., and Klein, G. (1986) High-level expression of the Epstein-Barr virus EBNA1 protein in CVl cells and human lymphoid cells using a SV40 late replacement vector. *Gene* **43,** 41–50.

9. Luthman, H. and Magnusson, G. (1983) High efficiency polyoma DNA transfection of chloroquine treated cells. *Nucleic Acids Res* **11**, 1295–1308.
10. McCutchan, J. H. and Pagano, J. S. (1968) Enchancement of the infectivity of simian virus 40 deoxyribonucleic acid with diethylaminoethyl-dextran. *J. Natl. Cancer Inst.* **41**, 351–357.
11. Classon, M., Henriksson, M., Sumegi, J., Klein, G., and Hammarskjöld, M.-L. (1987) Elevated c-*myc* expression facilitates the replication of SV40 DNA in human lymphoma cells. *Nature* **330**, 272–274.
12. Rekosh, D., Nygren, A., Flodby, P., Hammarskjöld, M. L., and Wigzell, H. (1988) Coexpression of human immunodeficiency virus envelope proteins and tat from a single simian virus 40 late replacement vector. *Proc. Natl. Acad. Sci. USA* **85**, 334–338.
13. Hammarskjöld, M.-L., Heimer, J., Hammarskjöld, B., Sangwan, I., Albert, L., and Rekosh, D. (1989) Regulation of human immunodeficiency virus *env* expression by the rev gene product. *J. Virol.* **63**, 1959–1966.
14. Miller, C. K. and Temin, H. M. (1983) High-efficiency ligation and recombination of DNA fragments by vertebrate cells. *Science* **220**, 606–609.
15. Wigler, M., Sweet, R., Sim, G. K., Wold, B., Pellicer, A., Lacy, E., Maniatis, T., Silverstein, S., and Axel, R. (1979) Transformation of mammalian cells with genes from procaryotes and eucaryotes. *Cell* **16**, 777–785.
16. Lusky, M. and Botchan, M. (1981) Inhibition of SV40 replication in simian cells by specific pBR322 DNA sequences. *Nature* **293**, 79–81.
17. Lopata, M. A., Cleveland, D. W., and Sollner, W. B. (1984) High level transient expression of a chloramphenicol acetyl transferase gene by DEAE-dextran mediated DNA transfection coupled with a dimethyl sulfoxide or glycerol shock treatment. *Nucleic Acids Res.* **12**, 5707–5717.
18. Sussman, D. J. and Milman, G. (1984) Short-term, high-efficiency expression of transfected DNA. *Mol. Cell. Biol.* **4**, 1641–1643.

CHAPTER 15

Choice and Manipulation
of Retroviral Vectors

Jay P. Morgenstern and Hartmut Land

1. Introduction

During the past few years, retroviral vectors have become a very important and widely used means of gene transfer. In the laboratory, their use has expanded the capabilities of investigators to perform important experiments that have solved previously unanswerable biological questions. Retroviral vectors exploit the inherent capacity of retroviruses to transfer genetic material stably into a cell's genome and subsequently express it in a manner that is generally not detrimental to the host-cell. Initial entry of genetic material into cells via retroviral vectors is so efficient that it permits successful transfer of genes into limiting numbers of cells, such as hematopoietic stem cells in explanted bone marrow, and transfer approaching 100% in tissue-culture experiments. In comparison, chemical and electrical means of gene transfer require large initial numbers of cells and, under optimal circumstances, function at efficiencies several orders of magnitude lower than retroviral vectors, and only in a limited number of specific cell types.

1.1. Replication-Competent Retroviruses

All recombinant retroviral vector systems are based on the principles involved in the biology of retroviruses. These simple viruses consist of an encapsidated ribonucleoprotein core ensheathed by a membrane envelope.

From: *Methods in Molecular Biology, Vol. 7: Gene Transfer and Expression Protocols*
Edited by: E. J. Murray © 1991 The Humana Press Inc., Clifton, NJ

Each virus particle contains two copies of genomic RNA as well as the virus-specific RNA-dependent DNA polymerase or reverse transcriptase. Upon entry into a new host-cell, viral genomic RNA is copied into DNA, and the resulting proviral DNA is integrated into the host genome. The site of its integration within the host-cell genome is for the most part random, but the structure of the integrated provirus is invariant *(1)*. The proviral genome carries three genes: *gag, pol,* and *env.* The *gag* and *pol* genes encode constituents that form the viral core and the RNA-dependent DNA polymerase, respectively. The *env* gene encodes a glycosylated envelope protein that determines the viral host range. The structural genes are flanked by the so-called long-terminal-repeats (LTRs), which contain *cis*-acting sequences required to regulate proviral transcription.

Replication initially involves transcription of the proviral genome into RNA, which is initiated by the enhancer/promoter elements within the U3 region of 5' LTR and terminated by polyadenylation signals in the 3' LTR *(2,3)*. The basic structure of retroviral genomic RNA is indistinguishable from that of mammalian mRNA. The proviral DNA gives rise to two transcripts, namely, the genomic RNA (covering a full single complement of the proviral sequences) and a subgenomic RNA, which encodes the *env* gene product. This molecule is generated by splicing out *gag* and *pol*-specific sequences from the larger mRNA. Encapsidation of the genomic mRNAs in the form of a dimer is mediated through the packaging signal, or ψ (psi) site, beginning near the splice donor and extending downstream into the first few hundred basepairs of *gag* coding sequences *(4–6)*. *See* Fig. 1.

1.2. Replication-Defective Retroviruses

Replication-defective retroviruses can arise from replication-competent viruses as a consequence of recombination, by which host-cell-DNA sequences are gained at the expense of portions of the coding regions of their *gag, pol* or *env* genes. Nearly all of the acutely transforming retroviruses carrying oncogenes are viruses of this type. The propagation of defective retroviruses relies on the presence of a replication-competent helper virus. While the helper virus supplies the viral structural and replicative proteins within the same cell in *trans,* the defective viruses remain transmissible because they have retained all the necessary *cis*-acting retroviral sequences. Hence, acutely transforming retroviral stocks are composed of two complementing working parts that cooperate to transmit viral oncogenes into cells.

1.3. Retroviral Vector Systems

Recombinant retroviral vector systems mirror the two-part composition of acutely transforming retroviral stocks. The vector is an analog of the de-

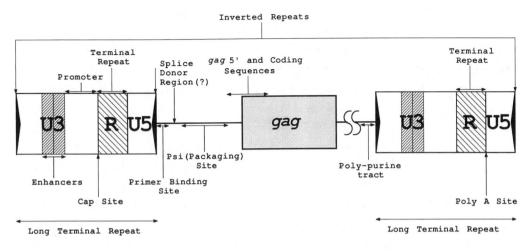

Fig. 1. *Cis*-acting signals in the retroviral genome.

fective transforming virus, with exogenous genes inserted in place of the excised coding sequences, and producer cell lines provide the full complement of viral polypeptides for packaging of vector proviruses, just as the helper virus does for defective transforming proviruses.

Retroviral vector systems have been established using both avian and murine retroviruses. However, the description that follows will concentrate on Moloney murine leukemia virus (Mo MuLV) based systems, since they are most applicable for gene-transfer experiments with mammalian cells.

In general, all retroviral vector constructs are derived from molecular proviral clones of replication-competent retroviruses in which segments of the *gag, pol,* and *env* coding regions have been excised and subsequently replaced with one or more genes that the experimenter wishes to deliver and express within a cell. Recombinant vector design can tolerate removal of all endemic replicative genes; however, the *cis*-acting signals for replication during the normal course of the retroviral life cycle, shown in Fig. 1, must be maintained. As long as these *cis*-acting sequences are maintained, retroviral vectors will generally tolerate insertion of most genes between their LTRs and transmit them in lieu of the normal viral genes. Unlike λ phage vectors, there appears to be no minimum size requirement for the retroviral genome, and the maximum size permitted, though not rigorously determined, is limited to approx 10 kb. Since proviral vector structures as small as 2.5 kb exist, genes as large as 7.5 kb can be utilized in the context of a retroviral vector.

Retroviral vectors have been designed that express either a single exogenous gene or multiple genes, with one generally being a dominant selectable marker. Vectors that transmit a single gene usually rely on the promoter residing within the 5' LTR for transcription of the gene *(7,8)*. The inherent simplicity of single-gene vectors has both advantages and liabilities. To their credit, single-gene vectors often avoid the diminished expression or low titer often encountered when utilizing complicated vector designs that deviate from the structure of wild-type or naturally occurring defective acutely transforming retroviruses *(9)*. However, the main disadvantage of single-gene vectors is that they require the insertion of genes that induce a readily identifiable cell phenotype, since otherwise infected cells cannot be easily identified. For these reasons, the use of single-gene vectors has been limited to transmission of oncogenes, growth factors, or drug-resistance genes (e.g., *8,10*).

Double-gene vectors expressing dominantly acting drug-resistance markers, together with any other gene of interest, are of greater utility. Hence any gene can be transmitted, irrespective of foreknowledge of its potential phenotypic effects, because its presence within the cell can be inferred by the cell's ability to survive in selective medium. Any novel phenotype subsequently exhibited by the drug-resistant cell can then be ascribed to the concomitantly inserted gene of interest. An alternative selection scheme has also been reported for a two-gene retroviral vector utilizing a cell-surface antigen as a marker that can be selected for by FACS sorting *(11)*.

1.3.1. Splicing-Competent Vectors

Two strategies have been devised for simultaneous expression of a drug-resistance gene and an exogenous gene in a retroviral vector. The first type, embodied by the vector pZIPneo SV(X) *(12)*, mimics the scheme employed by replication-competent retroviruses, whereby the *gagpol* open reading frame is expressed from unspliced mRNA, and the *env* gene from a singly spliced mRNA, both of which are transcribed from the LTR. In the specific case of the splicing vector pZIPneo SV(X), the exogenous gene is cloned 5' of the Mo MuLV splice acceptor(s), so that its expression relies on translation of nonspliced transcripts from the LTR. The drug-resistance gene *neo* is positioned 3' of the Mo MuLV splice acceptor(s), so that expression of the gene is directed by the spliced mRNA (Fig. 2). A difficulty encountered when using splicing vectors is the unpredictable nature of the splicing. Cryptic splice acceptors within genes, even when they are inserted in the form of cDNAs, can deleteriously interact with the viral splice donor to excise the transcript's Ψ site. As a consequence, transmission of recombinant virus is reduced. Another problem has been the alteration of the ratios of spliced to unspliced mRNA as a function of sequences within the exogenous genes. In extreme cases, this can lead to the predominance of one mRNA species at the total expense of the other *(9,13,14;* C. Cepko, personal communication). In order to circumvent these uncertainties, direct orientation vectors were developed.

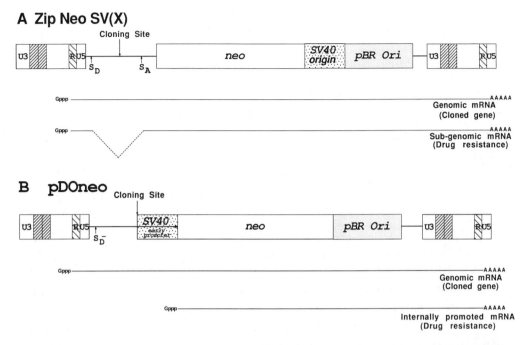

Fig. 2. Retroviral vectors and expression strategies. (A) pZIPneo SV(X) splicing vector and its derived mRNA transcripts. (B) pDOneo direct orientation nonsplicing, internal promoter vector and its derived mRNA transcripts.

1.3.2. Direct Orientation Vectors

Direct orientation (DO) vectors achieve expression of two genes by utilizing the LTR's promoter as the source of one transcript and an internal promoter inserted between the LTRs for initiation of a second. Generally, the LTR has been used in vectors such as pDOneo (Fig. 2) to drive expression of the exogenous genes and the internal promoter to express the drug-resistance marker *(15)*. Although no naturally occurring retroviruses with internal promoters have been isolated, they appear relatively inert to promoter insertion. Indeed, DO-type vectors have been used successfully many times (e.g., *16–18)*. There has even been a report of a vector with two internal promoters that successfully expresses two exogenous genes and a selective marker. However, the internal promoters gave rise to only low levels of expression *(19)*.

In cases in which a gene of interest, rather than the selectable marker, is controlled by an internal promoter, one should be aware that often expression from the internal promoter is suppressed by the flanking LTRs. The degree of this suppression varies with different internal promoter/LTR combinations or cell types and, in the extreme, the levels of expression can be reduced up to 50-fold *(20–22)*. However, in the general configuration of DO vectors *(see above)* the described promoter interference phenomenon is of no concern, since expression of drug resistance does not require very high levels of mRNA expression.

1.3.3. Self-Inactivating Vectors

To eliminate the influence of the LTRs on the regulation of internal promoters, a variation of the DO-vector approach was developed. In the so-called self-inactivating (SIN) vectors, the LTR is rendered transcriptionally inactive and gene expression is placed under the sole control of internal promoter(s) *(23–25)*. Operationally, this is achieved by deleting the enhancer/promoter sequences from the 3' LTR of a vector construct (Fig. 1). Though deleted of 3' LTR sequences, transcripts originating from the intact 5' LTR still maintain the *cis*-acting signals necessary for packaging, reverse transcription, and integration. However, as a result of the asymmetric nature of retroviral replication *(2,3,26)*, only the U3 repeat of the 3' LTR is transmitted and duplicated in the progeny proviruses. Hence, a deletion of the enhancer/promoter in the 3' U3 repeat will result in a provirus lacking transcriptional signals in both LTRs after one round of replication in SIN vectors.

1.3.4. Heterologous LTR Vectors

An approach to expand the host range of expression of the LTR in retroviral vectors is represented by the heterologous LTR (HL) vectors, whose usage to date has been limited, but holds significant potential. The promoter within the Mo MuLV LTR has a limited ability to function in certain cell types, such as embryonal carcinoma cells *(27,28)*. However, variant virus strains with mutated LTRs that work efficiently in these cells have been isolated *(29,30)*. Also, related strains of MuLVs possess enhanced transcriptional tropism for cell types of specific lineages, such as the erythroid and myeloid specificity of Friend virus (Fr-MuLV) or myeloproliferative sarcoma virus (MPSV), respectively. In all cases, these transcriptional characteristics have been mapped to the enhancer sequences within the viruses' LTRs *(31–34)*. In light of these findings, standard Mo MuLV based vectors have been modified as HL vectors to allow or enhance expression of exogenous genes in embryonal carcinoma or erythroid cells, respectively *(9,10,30,35,36)*. Work with HL vectors is carried out in similar fashion to work with SIN vectors, except that, rather than the enhancer sequences within the 3' LTR being deleted, they are exchanged with analogous sequences from a different viral strain. Just as with SIN vectors, these newly inserted transcriptional signals conferring altered transcriptional specificity will eventually appear in both flanking LTRs of progeny virus, and will henceforth be stably transmitted to subsequent generations.

1.4. Virus Packaging Cell Lines

Helper function, be it from replication competent virus or from a packaging cell line *(see below)*, is basically to furnish functional *gag, pol,* and *env* proteins to replication defective proviruses in *trans*. Although the role of the helper virus and the packaging cell line is identical, the manner in which the two carry out this task is different. Unlike cells infected with acutely transforming viral stocks, packaging cell lines in retroviral vector systems have been modified to yield defective recombinant virus in the absence of wild-type virus. This ability ascribed to producer cell lines is attractive for several reasons. In the absence of wild-type virus, defective recombinant proviruses will not spread, and will therefore remain permanently within the initially infected host-cell. This unidirectional gene transfer allows the experimenter to control the number of infected cells by manipulation of the multiplicity of infection *(e.g., 37,38)*. Helper-free recombinant retroviruses also circumvent the problem of viral interference associated with the *env* gene product of helper viruses *(see below)*, permitting multiple infections of a single cell. This lack in interference allows sequential introduction of multiple genes into cells and, for example, has been exploited to express heterodimeric proteins *(15,16)*. In addition, for applications in gene therapy it would be imperative to avoid the introduction of wild-type virus into a patient, since these viruses would be able to propagate and potentially contribute to the induction of neoplasias via insertional activation of cellular protooncogenes *(e.g., 39)*.

The creation of helper-free packaging cell lines became possible with the discovery of a virus-specific nucleotide sequence required for the encapsidation of viral RNA into virions. This sequence, or Ψ site, was localized between the splice donor and the *gag* initiator codon of Mo MuLV (Fig. 1). Upon transfection of a proviral construct devoid of the Ψ site into NIH 3T3 cells, the resultant cells, designated cells Ψ-2, were shown to package none of the proviral mRNAs lacking the packaging signal, yet they were able to efficiently transmit *gag, pol,* and *env*-defective, Ψ site$^+$ retroviral vector genomes *(5)*.

1.4.1. Varying Vector Host Range

The host range of recombinant virus budded from a producer cell line is a function of the *ENV* product encoded by its Ψ-producer construct, in a manner analogous to the formation of pseudotypes of defective proviral genomes by wild-type helper virus. The producer construct in Ψ-2 cells was based on a Mo MuLV proviral clone bearing an ecotropic *env* gene *(40)*, hence it yields recombinant virus of ecotropic host range, capable of infecting rodent cells exclusively. Cell lines that produce recombinant virus of the broader amphotropic host range, Ψ-am and PA12, have been assembled in much the same manner as Ψ-2 cells *(41,42)*, based on a proviral clone of an amphotropic isolate of Mo MuLV *(43)*. Amphotropic recombinant virus can infect most mammalian cells by virtue of the presence of its putative receptor on their cell surface. For this reason, cell lines producing viruses of this host range have been designated for use in human gene therapy. Xenotropic pseudotyped vectors recently have been shown to infect human hematopoietic progenitor cells at a higher efficiency than amphotropic controls *(44)*, suggesting that a producer cell line conferring xenotropic host range may prove useful in gene-transfer experiments with cell types previously found to be refractory to gene transfer via retroviral vectors.

1.4.2. Packaging Cell Lines with Reduced Probability to Yield Replication-Competent Helper

Although "first-generation" packaging lines, such as Ψ-2, Ψ-am, and PA12, generally performed their function well, it became apparent that, given a sufficient number of passages, wild-type virus would arise as a contaminant in their supernatants. Given the observation that this process is accelerated by the presence of a vector provirus, it has been assumed that the mechanism for helper formation is some form of homologous recombination that results in transfer of the vector's Ψ site to the producer construct. In theory, a single recombination event between a retroviral vector and a first generation Ψ-minus producer construct would result in the restoration of a wild-type proviral structure. In recent years, additional helper-free producer cell lines have been generated in an effort to minimize this problem. These second- and third-generation producer cell lines were designed to incorporate several lesions within their proviral producer constructs, so that multiple recombination events would have to take place between the producer constructs and vector sequences to recreate an intact provirus. Specifically, in addition to the requisite deletion of the Ψ site, a nonretroviral polyadenylation signal is substituted for the 3' LTR in the second-generation producer cell line PA317 *(39)*, while, in addition to the above lesions, third-generation producer cell lines have their *gagpol* open reading frame and *env* gene separated onto two separate expression plasmids *(46–48)*. To date, tests on third-generation producer cell lines harboring vector proviruses for replication-competent virus have proved negative under conditions where replication-competent virus has been detected in first- and second-generation cell lines.

1.5. Introduction of Genes into Retrovirus Vectors

1.5.1. Drug-Resistance Genes

Drug-resistance markers utilized in multiple-gene vectors are usually either metabolic genes that complement a defect (inherent or drug-induced) within a biosynthetic pathway of the recipient cell or antibiotic-resistance genes from procaryotic sources that have been adapted for function in eucaryotes. The most popular marker is the *neo* gene derived from the Tn5 transposon that operates dually to confer resistance to the aminoglycoside G418 (Geneticin®) in mammalian cells, and to kanamycin sulfate in *E. coli* (*see* Chapter 19) *(49)*. As an alternative, the *hph* gene from *Streptomyces hygroscopicus*, conferring resistence to hygromycin B in both mammalian cells and bacteria, has been used *(16,50)*.

1.5.2. cDNA Copies

Most investigators insert cDNA copies into the recombinant retroviruses. This usually represents the most straightforward way to construct the virus of choice. However, it is important to realize that the efficiency of retroviral replication can be affected by the introduced cDNA sequence (perhaps because of strong secondary structure present in RNA transcripts of these genes). As a consequence, one will be unable to generate high-titer recombinant viral stocks from viruses containing certain cDNA sequences.

1.5.3. Intron-Containing Genes

Genes can also be inserted into retroviral vectors in the form of genomic DNA. Introns within genes will be removed after a single round of replication if the gene is inserted in the "sense" orientation relative to the LTRs *(51)*. In fact, this aspect of the retroviral life cycle can be used to the experimenter's advantage in order to generate cDNAs from whole genes (e.g., *52*). Retroviruses have been invaluable tools in this respect, aiding in the elucidation of complex alternative splicing patterns of papova viruses, adenoviruses, and fibronectin genes *(7,53–55)*.

To ensure efficient virus transmission, the inserted DNA sequences should lack any transcriptional terminators, since premature termination of genomic retroviral transcripts will result in decreased vector titers. Although elimination of the polyadenylation signal may not be an absolute necessity, with existing precedence for efficient passage of certain genes with inactive terminators in retroviral vectors *(56,57)*, it is preferable to avoid the presence of such signals.

If one wishes to introduce a gene harboring essential regulatory elements within its introns, insertion of the gene is restricted to the antisense orientation. With a gene in this configuration, the introns are maintained, but an appropriate promoter has to be provided *(58,59)*.

2. Materials

2.1. Retrovirus Vectors

Examples include the following:
1. Splicing vector: pZipSV(X) *(12)*.

2. Direct orientation vectors: DOneo, pMZhyg-1 *(15,16)*, pXT1 *(17)*, LN series *(42)*, and pBabe series *(43)*.

2.2. Cells

Examples for packaging cell lines include:

1. First generation: Ψ-2 (ecotropic, ref. *5*), PA12 (amphotropic, ref. *42*), Ψ-am (amphotropic, ref. *41*).
2. Second generation: PA 317 (amphotropic, ref. *45*).
3. Third generation: GP+E (ecotropic, ref. *47*), ΨCRE (ecotropic, ref. *48*) and ΨCRIP (amphotropic, ref. *48*), and ΩE (ecotropic, ref. *50*).
4. Indicator cells: NIH 3T3 cells, XC-cells *(60)*.
5. Cells permissive for SV40: COS cells.

2.3. Tissue Culture

1. For all procedures, except when stated differently, use Dulbecco's Modified Eagle's Medium with high glucose concentration (DMEM) supplemented with 10% fetal bovine serum.
2. Phosphate-buffered saline (PBS): 1% NaCl, 0.025% KCl, 0.14% Na_2HPO_4, 0.025% KH_2PO_4 (all w/v), pH 7.2. Autoclave to sterilize.
3. Versene: 0.54 m*M* EDTA in PBS. Filter-sterilize (0.22-µm-filter).
4. Transfection buffer: 0.5% HEPES, 0.8% NaCl, 0.1% dextrose, 0.01% Na_2HPO_4 (anhydrous), 0.37% KCl (all w/v), pH 7.05, exact adjustment required. Filter-sterilize (0.22-µm-filter).
5. Polybrene (100×): 800 µg/mL dissolved in PBS. Filter-sterilize (0.22-µm-filter).
6. Tunicamycin (10,000×): 300 µg/mL dissolved in PBS. Caution: Extremely toxic. Filter-sterilize (0.22-µm-filter).
7. Mitomycin (100×): 2 mg/mL dissolved in PBS; store protected from light in 100-µL aliquots at −20°C (compound is light-sensitive). Filter-sterilize (0.22-µm).
8. Geneticin (G418) (100×): 100 mg/mL dissolved in 10 m*M* HEPES, pH 7.9. Filter-sterilize (0.22-µm-filter).
9. Crystal violet stain: 2% crystal violet in 20% methanol.
10. Glycerol shock solution: PBS containing 15% glycerol (v/v); sterilize by autoclaving.
11. 2.5*M* $CaCl_2$: Filter-sterilize (0.22-µm-filter).
12. Silicone vacuum grease: Sterilize by autoclaving.
13. Cloning rings.
14. Dimethyl sulfoxide (DMSO).

2.4. Reverse Transcription Assay

1. Reverse transcriptase assay mix (1.25×). Use 40 μL of the following mix per sample: 63 m*M* Tris-HCl, pH 8.3; 15.6 m*M* DTT; 750 μ*M* MnCl$_2$; 75 m*M* NaCl; 0.0625% v/v NP-40; 6.25 μg/mL oligo dT12-18; 12.5 μg/mL polyA; 12.5 μ*M* [^{a}-32P] dTTP, specific activity 1 Ci/mmol.
2. DE 52 anion exchange paper.
3. 2× SSC: 20× SSC is 3*M* sodium chloride, 0.3*M* sodium citrate.
4. 95% ethanol.

2.5. Rescue of Recombinant Retroviruses via Hirt Extraction

1. Hirt extraction buffer: 2% SDS, 10 m*M* Tris-HCl (ph 7.4), 10 m*M* EDTA.
2. Polyethylene glycol (PEG) 1000: diluted 50% (w/v) with serum-free DMEM. (Heat PDG to 40°C to dissolve.)
3. 5*M* sodium chloride.
4. Phenol chloroform: Melt redistilled phenol (GIBCO/BRL) at 60°C. (TAKE CARE!) Add an equal vol of chloroform (analytical grade).
5. Chloroform.
6. Isopropanol.
7. 0.3*M* ammonium acetate.
8. PBS: *see above.*
9. 95% ethanol.
10. TE: 10 m*M* Tris-HCl (pH 7.5), 1 m*M* EDTA.
11. NACS prepac column (GIBCO/BRL).
12. Glycogen.
13. 2% agar plates containing 50 μg/mL kanamycin sulfate.

3. Methods

3.1. Generation of Cell Lines Stably Producing Recombinant Helper-Free Retroviruses (see Note 1)

Highly efficient stable retrovirus-producer cell lines can be generated by infection of packaging cell lines with viral titers obtained from transiently transfected packaging cells. However, since packaging cells expressing a viral *env* gene are normally refractory to infection with retroviruses containing the same *env* gene product in their membrane the infection of packaging cell lines has to follow one of two protocols in order to circumvent this viral interference. Experimentally, the most simple way to proceed is to generate the transient virus stock by transfecting a packaging cell line of different tropism (expressing a different *env* gene). For example, stable producers of ecotropic viruses would then result from infection of ecotropic packaging cell lines (e.g., Ψ-2, GP+E, ΨCRE, ΩE) with amphotropic virus derived from the transfection of an amphotropic packaging cell line (e.g., Ψ-am, PA317, ΨCRIP). On the other hand, in order to avoid the potential hazard of amphotropic retroviruses harboring oncogenes or other pathogens, viral interference can be overcome by blocking the maturation of the *env* protein by treating ecotropic packaging cells with tunicamycin prior to retroviral infection. As an example, the latter protocol is described in detail.

3.1.1. Transfection of an Ecotropic Packaging Cell Line with Plasmids Containing Proviral DNA

1. The night before transfection, seed the packaging cells at a density of 7.5×10^5/9-cm tissue-culture dish (*see* Note 2).
2. Before transfection, remove the old medium and replace with 5 mL of fresh medium. Allow the newly added media to equilibrate in the incubator.
3. Place 0.5 mL of transfection buffer in a clear tube, and then add 10 μg of a plasmid containing the desired proviral DNA to the buffer (*see* Note 3).
4. Gradually add 25–30 μL of $2.5 M$ CaCl$_2$ (the amount one adds depends on the transfection buffer and must be titrated empirically) to initiate the formation of the DNA/CaPO$_4$ coprecipitate. Allow 20–30 min for complete precipitation (*see* Note 4).
5. Slowly drip the precipitate over the entire area of cells on the dish; then gently mix it using a rocking motion before returning the dish to the incubator. At this stage, one can look at the precipitate under the microscope (use 100–200× magnification; *see* Note 4).
6. Allow the precipitate to incubate for 4–6 h.
7. Remove the precipitate and wash the cells twice with prewarmed serum-free medium.
8. Glycerol-shock the cells for 4 min at 37°C in 3–5 mL of PBS containing 15% glycerol.
9. Remove the PBS/glycerol and wash twice with prewarmed serum-free medium.
10. Add 5 mL of medium containing serum and incubate the transfected cells for 24–48 h.

11. On the day the transfection is performed, plate an additional aliquot of packaging cells at 3×10^5 cells/9-cm dish, and incubate these cells overnight.
12. Add tunicamycin, to a final concentration of 0.03 µg/mL.
13. Incubate the cells in tunicamycin for 18 h.
14. Shortly before the end of the 18-h tunicamycin treatment, remove the medium containing the transiently produced virus from the transfected cells with a 5-mL syringe and filter through a microfilter (pore size 0.22 or 0.45 µm) to remove any floating cells in the supernatant.
15. Add 1/100 vol of 800-µg/mL polybrene to the viral supernatant and keep this solution on ice until needed (*see* Note 5).
16. Remove the medium from the tunicamycin-treated cells and wash once with PBS.
17. Add 2 mL of the viral supernatant to each dish of tunicamycin-treated cells, and allow the infection to proceed for 90–120 min at 37°C in the incubator.
18. Remove the virus-containing supernatant, add 10 mL of fresh medium and leave in the incubator overnight.
19. Trypsinize the culture and split it (1:10) into selection medium containing the appropriate drug (e.g., 1 mg/mL Geneticin® or G418, *see also* Note 14).
20. Refeed the cultures every 3–4 d until drug-resistant colonies grow out and can be ring-cloned.
21. Following this procedure, depending on the vector construct used, you can expect a total of 10–100 colonies (*see* Notes 6, 7, and 8).

3.1.2. Ring-Cloning of Cell Colonies Producing Recombinant Retrovirus

1. For each recombinant retrovirus construct, choose at least 12 colonies to be picked and circle them with a marker on the bottom of the tissue-culture dish.
2. Remove medium and wash once with PBS.
3. Place glass cloning rings (5 mm diameter, 8 mm height) dipped in autoclaved silicon grease over each of the selected clones to seal them from the remaining cells on the dish.
4. Add 200 µL of trypsin/versene (1:1) to the ringed colony and incubate until the cells detach from the dish (can be monitored under the microscope).

5. Seed the trypsinized cells into 24-well tissue-culture dishes containing 1 mL of the appropriate selection medium per well.

3.1.3. Selection of Producer Cell Clones with High Retrovirus Titers

The following procedure allows an estimation of retroviral titers between 10^4 and 10^6 colony-forming units (CFU)/mL.

1. Expand the isolated cell clones until they reach confluence in 6-well dishes.
2. Replace spent medium with 2 mL of new medium not containing any selective drug.
3. On the same day, split the recipient cells you wish to infect (usually NIH 3T3 cells) and seed them at 7.5×10^5 cells/9-cm dish. Prepare one dish per producer cell clone to be tested.
4. Incubate the producer and recipient cells overnight.
5. On the next day, remove the virus-containing medium from the producer cells with a 5-mL syringe and filter through a microfilter (pore size 0.22 or 0.45 μm) to remove any floating cells in the supernatant.
6. Take 20 μL of each producer clone supernatant (the rest can be kept frozen at –70°C) and add to 2 mL of medium containing 8 μg/mL of polybrene. Keep this dilution on ice until needed.
7. Remove the medium from the recipient cells and add the diluted viral supernatant.
8. Allow the infection to proceed for 90–120 min in the incubator.
9. Remove the virus and add 10 mL of fresh medium to remove the polybrene. Incubate overnight.
10. Freeze the producer cell clones in DMEM containing 40% fetal bovine serum and 10% DMSO (2 vials/clone).
11. The next day, split the infected cells (1:20) into medium containing the appropriate selective drug; keep at least two dishes (9-cm) for each producer cell clone to be assayed.
12. Feed the cells with selection medium every 3–4 d until the infected, drug-resistant colonies have become large enough to be counted.
13. Remove the medium, wash with PBS, and stain for at least 30 s in crystal violet stain.
14. Wash dishes in water, let them air-dry, and count colonies.

3.2. Preparation and Titration of Retroviral Stocks

Since retrovirus stocks stored at –70°C retain their activity for some years, it is useful to produce them in considerable quantities *(see* Note 9*)*. The scale of the virus preparation is not restricted (e.g., one 15-cm dish yields 10–15 mL/ harvest).

1. Grow the producer cell line to full confluency.
2. Remove spent medium and add half as much fresh medium to the producer cells.
3. Incubate the producer cells at least overnight. Depending on the packaging cell line, longer incubations (up to 3 d) may help to raise titers. On the other hand, if the incubation time is kept on the order of 20–24 h, a single culture can be used for at least two harvests.
4. After the appropriate incubation time, remove the medium containing the virus from the producer cells and filter through a microfilter unit with a pore size of 0.22 or 0.45 μm to remove any floating cells in the supernatant. Alternatively, this can be achieved by a 10-min spin at 2000–3000 rpm in a table-top centrifuge at 4°C under sterile conditions (*see* Note 10).
5. Aliquot the virus stock into appropriate amounts, quick-freeze in dry ice, and store at –70°C (*see* Note 11).
6. For titration of the virus stock, thaw a small aliquot and infect recipient cells (usually NIH 3T3 cells) with serial dilutions. Use 2 mL of medium containing 8 μg/mL of polybrene for a single 9-cm tissue culture dish in which 7.5×10^5 cells were plated on the previous day. Thereafter, continue as in Section 3.1.1. step 12.

3.3. Tests for Helper-Virus Contamination

To screen recombinant retrovirus stocks for the presence of replication-competent retroviruses, there are three assays that measure different helper-virus-specific parameters. If the absence of helper virus is crucial for the planned experiments, retrovirus stocks should be tested by at least the first two methods described here.

3.3.1. Detection of Wild-Type/Helper Virus by Serial Infection Assay Using NIH 3T3 Cells as Indicator Cells

1. Take 2 mL of undiluted virus stock containing 8 μg/mL polybrene and infect 10^5 NIH 3T3 cells on a 9-cm dish as described in Section 3.1.1.; however, rather than removing the producer supernatant after 90 min, add 6 mL of medium (this effectively keeps polybrene present in the medium at 2 μg/mL to enhance the spread of helper virus).
2. Maintain the infected NIH 3T3 cells in medium containing 2 μg/mL polybrene and no selective drugs until they reach confluence. Feed the cells every 3–4 d.

3. To determine the sensitivity of your assay conditions and as a positive control add a known amount of wild-type Mo MuLV (100 plaque-forming units) to an undiluted helper-free virus stock and test this sample in parallel.

4. Subsequently, harvest the supernatant from the previously infected cultures, filter to remove floating cells, and perform another retroviral infection with the undiluted supernatant on NIH 3T3 that were seeded at 7.5×10^5 cells/9-cm dish cells on the previous day.

5. On the next day, split the entire culture of newly infected NIH 3T3 cells (one 9-cm dish) onto four 15-cm dishes containing selection medium; keep these cultures for at least 14 d, feeding with selection medium every 3–4 d.

6. Any drug-resistant colonies found on the 15-cm dishes indicate the presence of helper virus.

3.3.2. XC-Cell Plaque Assay to Detect Wild-Type/Helper Virus

The XC-cell plaque assay measures the number of infectious Mo MuLV particles and was first described by Rowe et al. *(60)*. This assay is based on the observation that, unlike most rodent fibroblasts, XC cells fuse into syncytia upon infection with wild-type Mo MuLV. According to the specific requirements of individual experiments, the assay can be adapted for tissue-culture dishes of various sizes. With emphasis on high sensitivity in this particular context, conditions for 9-cm tissue-culture dishes are given.

1. Seed 10^5 NIH 3T3 cells/9-cm dish and incubate overnight.

2. Infect each of these cultures with 2 mL undiluted retrovirus stock containing 8 µg/mL polybrene. After 90 min, add 6 mL of medium; maintain the infected NIH 3T3 cells in medium containing 2 µg/mL polybrene and no selective drugs until they reach confluence. Feed the cells every 3–4 d.

3. As a positive control, infect parallel cultures with a serial dilution of a Mo MuLV stock. When choosing the appropriate dilutions, be aware that the assay can be quantified only in the range of 10–200 plaques/9-cm dish.

4. When the NIH 3T3 cells have grown to confluence, remove the medium and expose the cells directly (take lids off dishes) to UV irradiation. For this purpose it is most convenient to use the germicidal UV lamp in a laminar-flow hood for 30–40 s, with the dishes placed on the working surface.

5. Subsequently, overlay the irradiated cell cultures with 2×10^6 XC cells in 10 mL of medium containing 10% newborn bovine or horse serum (*see* Note 12).

6. Feed cultures with XC cell medium again the next day (add the medium, since XC cells usually are only loosely attached to the tissue-culture dish).

7. Two to three days after seeding the XC cells, plaques appear where syncytia had formed. Each plaque represents one infectious replication-competent virus particle in the original retrovirus stock. Stain carefully with crystal violet as described in Section 3.1.3. (remember, XC cells are only very loosely attached to the dishes) and count the plaques.

8. Helper-free retrovirus stocks should not give rise to any of such plaques. Therefore, to obtain a conclusive result, a positive control in each test series is essential.

3.5.3. Reverse Transcriptase Assay

This assay detects reverse transcriptase harbored by retroviral particles in the supernatant of producer cell lines or cells infected with replication-competent retroviruses. A modification of the method of Goff et al. *(61)* is decribed here. Together with the virus stocks or samples to be tested, supernatants from positive (e.g., Ψ-2 cells, which shed RNA-free retrovirus particles into the medium) and negative (e.g., NIH 3T3) control cells should be included in each assay.

1. Dispense 40 µL of 1.25× RT assay mix into individual wells of a 96-well tissue-culture dish (round bottom).

2. Add 10 µL of cell supernatant from cells that had reached confluence just 24–48 h earlier.

3. Seal the 96-well dish with parafilm; incubate at 37°C for 1–4 h.

4. Subsequently, spot 5–20 µL of each reaction onto DE 52 anion-exchange paper marked with a replica grid of a 96-well dish.

5. Remove unincorporated radioactivity by washing three times with 250 mL of 2× SSC at 22°C, with agitation. Then wash the DE 52 paper once with 95% EtOH and allow it to dry in a fume cupboard (do not handle the paper because, when wet, the paper is very fragile).

6. Reverse-transcriptase-positive supernatants can be seen by autoradiography for 2–48 h at –70°C with intensifying screens.

3.4. Infection of Target Cells with Retrovirus Stocks (see Note 13)

Infection of target cells with retrovirus stocks essentially follows the infection protocols described in Sections 3.1.1. (steps 15–21) and 3.2. Usually, undiluted virus stocks are used. However, when required, the virus concentration can either be diluted or be increased 10 to, maximally, 100-fold.

3.4.1. Concentrating Retroviruses

1. Spin the filtered supernatant in SW 28 rotor at 14,000 rpm (4°C) for <12 h (use sterile polyallomer tubes).
2. Gently resuspend the (invisible) pellet in 1/100 of the original vol in fetal bovine serum (undiluted); i.e., leave it on ice for 30–40 min without disturbing it, and then slowly pipet up and down a few times. Avoid foaming *(see also* Note 9).
3. Optional: Refilter through a 0.45-μm filter to sterilize the virus stock.
4. Store the concentrated virus stocks at –70°C.
5. It is important to titrate these concentrated stocks because the procedure of concentrating virus is not always reproducible Mo MuLV-based viruses are very fragile and requires practical experience.

3.4.2. Infection of Target Cells by Cocultivation with Retrovirus Producer Cells

1. Seed 10^6 retrovirus-producer cells/9-cm dish and incubate overnight.
2. Treat the cells for 2 h with 20–30 mg/mL of Mitomycin C in normal medium.
3. Wash the cells twice in medium without serum.
4. Trypsinize the cells, take them up in 10 mL of normal medium, and spin for 5 min at 1000 rpm in a table-top centrifuge at room temperature.
5. Resuspend the pellet in 5 mL of medium and count the cells.
6. Coseed producer cells, together with the recipient cells in a ratio of 2–3:1, and seed a total of 10^6 cells/9-cm dish into normal medium containing 2 μg/mL polybrene, but no selective drugs.
7. After 2–3 d, the cultures can be split according to the requirements of the individual experiment and drug selection can be applied *(see* Notes 14 and 15).

3.5. Retrieval of Retrovirus Vectors from Mammalian Cells via Plasmid Rescue

"Shuttling" of a retrovirus vector between mammalian cells and bacteria is made possible by placing drug-resistance markers, functioning in mammalian and in bacterial hosts as well as bacterial and SV40 origins of replication, between the retroviral LTRs. As a consequence, an integrated provirus derived from such a shuttle vector can be recovered from cellular chromatin in the form of plasmids that can be propagated in bacteria. These plasmids arise after induction of DNA replication at the viral origin by fusion of the cells harboring the provirus to COS cells (which are permissive for SV40 replication) and subsequent recombination between the LTRs or host-cell DNA sequences *(12,62)*. The protocol decribed below takes approx 1 wk and allows isolation of retroviral transferred genes as well as cellular DNA sequences specific for the locus of retroviral integration.

1. Seed COS cells and the cell line bearing the provirus to be rescued in a 1:1 ratio on a 9-cm dish at a density such that they will become confluent within 48 h.
2. Warm up polyethylene glycol (PEG) 1000 so that it is just melted and not hot (40°C). Dilute it to 50% (w/v) with serum-free DMEM.
3. Wash confluent cells three times in serum-free DMEM, with thorough draining of the final wash.
4. Fuse cells by carefully pipeting 2.0 mL of the PEG-DMEM (kept at 37°C) onto the cell monolayer and leave at room temperature for 60 s *(see* Note 16).
5. Gently but quickly wash the cells with 10 mL of serum-free DMEM. Then wash twice with serum-free DMEM, followed by two washes in DMEM + 10% serum.
6. Add back 10 mL of fresh DMEM + 10% serum.
7. Incubate cells for 1–3 d with medium changes each day. If you are trying to isolate cell-specific DNA sequences adjacent to the integrated provirus, incubate for only 24 h. If not, let cells incubate for 3 d.
8. To isolate low-mol wt episomal DNA, prepare a Hirt supernatant *(see also* Chapter 29) *(63)*. Wash cells twice in PBS, drain thoroughly, and lyse in 2 mL of Hirt extraction buffer. Scrape the lysate into an Oak Ridge tube and add NaCl from a 5 M stock solution to give a final concentration of 1.25 M NaCl.
9. Incubate at 4°C for 6 h and then spin at 18,000 rpm in a Sorvall SS34 rotor for 45 min.
10. Extract supernatant once with an equal vol of phenol/chloroform and once with 1 vol of chloroform.
11. Precipitate with 2 vol of isopropanol. Keep for 2 h at –20°C, or quick-freeze on dry ice. Pellet the precipitate at 15,000 rpm in a Sorvall SS34 rotor for 30 min at 4°C. If the pellet is white and fluffy (from SDS) resuspend it in TE, add ammonium acetate (to 0.3 M) and reprecipitate with 3 vol of ethanol.
12. Resuspend the final pellet in TE, and purify DNA on a NACS prepac column *(see* protocol of manufacturer, GIBCO/BRL).
13. Ethanol-precipitate the eluate in the presence of 1 µL of purified glycogen (Boehringer) as carrier. Quick-freeze, spin, and take up the pellet in 40 µL TE.

14. Transform 100 µL of competent recA⁻ bacteria with 1/4 of the prepared material *(see* Note 3). If the retrovirus to be rescued contains the *neo⁻* gene, plate the bacteria on agar plates containing kanamycin sulfate at 50 µg/mL. Several hundred drug-resistant colonies can be expected.

4. Notes

1. It is not always necessary to generate stable high-titer retrovirus-producer cell lines; i.e., for infection of established cell lines, the virus harvested 24–48 h after transfection of a retroviral vector into a packaging cell line often is of sufficient concentration to produce the required number of infectious events.

2. The Ψ-2 packaging cell line should be grown in newborn bovine serum.

3. For the genetic manipulation of plasmids containing proviral structures, it is essential to use bacterial hosts that are recA⁻ in order to avoid high recombination frequencies as a result of the presence of the two retroviral LTRs. In addition, if a retroviral plasmid contains two bacterial origins of replication (e.g., pZipSV(X)), it is advantageous to apply drug selection, at least for the selectable marker located between the LTRs.

4. A good DNA/CaPO4 precipitate will appear as a blue-grayhaze to the naked eye and as small black spots (even smaller than bacteria) under the microscope.

5. The retroviral stock, produced by the transient transfection, may be used to generate amphotropic retroviral stocks by infecting an untreated amphotropic packaging cell line instead of the tunicamycin-treated ecotropic cell line made in steps 11–12. (BEWARE! This protocol, although 100 times more efficient at producing retrovirus, requires a higher containment level because of the potential hazards of amphotropic recombinant retroviruses. Be aware of the regulations on biosafety.)

6. An alternative method of generating ecotropic recombinant retrovirus is as follows: Choose an amphotropic packaging cell line *(see* Section 2.2.) and proceed as in Section 3.1.1. steps 1–10, to generate amphotropic virus. The ecotropic stocks can be generated by subsequent infection of an ecotropic packaging cell line with the above amphotropic virus. The infection protocol is exactly as found in Section 3.1.1. steps 14–21. Note that no tunicamycin treatment of the packaging cell line is necessary. This method is 100 times more efficent at producing ecotropic stocks, but be aware of the increased hazard of amphotropic virus containing oncogenes or other pathogens! *See* the cautionary note in Note 5.

7. Producer cell lines that are generated by infection with retroviruses on average produce titers tenfold higher than cell lines that were constructed

by transfection. This probably results from the fact that retroviruses, in contrast to transfected DNA, integrate into actively transcribed regions of the chromatin.

8. Packaging cell lines producing recombinant retroviruses should be reselected from time to time with the drugs corresponding to (a) the resistance marker that was used to generate the packaging function, and (b) the marker contained in the respective retroviral vector. The reason for this is the genetic instability of rodent cell lines in culture, which can lead to loss of the introduced genes. Transfected DNA seems to be less stable than integrated proviruses.

9. The half-life of retroviruses at room temperature is approx 2 h. Keep stocks always on ice. Moreover, avoid foaming of the virus-containing solutions, since this will reduce the titer.

10. To remove living producer cells from retrovirus stocks, the harvested supernatants can either be spun at 2000–3000 rpm at 4°C or be filtered (pore size 0.45 µm). However, some filters may contain detergents, which will reduce the retrovirus titer. To counteract this problem, rinse the filter with a few mL of medium prior to filtering the virus stock.

11. Do not use polypropylene tubes. They will crack.

12. For a successful XC-plaque assay, it is essential to use XC-cell stocks that are subconfluent.

13. Since retroviral integration requires host-cell DNA synthesis, it is essential to keep the target cells in optimal growth conditions during and after the infection procedure. The cells of interest can be infected either by exposure to retrovirus stocks or by cocultivation with retrovirus-producing cells. With the latter procedure, the highest infection frequencies (up to 100%) can be achieved.

14. If you plan to use hygromycin B selection, it will be necessary to determine the dose–response relationship for each cell type that is to be exposed to the drug. Usually, cells can be selected at drug concentrations between 50 and 300 µg/mL.

15. Integrated proviruses present in the target cells, can rapidly and easily be characterized by analyzing restriction digests of the appropriate cellular DNAs by Southern blotting. By choosing three different restriction digests, the number of integrated virus copies, the integrity of the provirus, and the clonality of the infected cell population can be investigated.

    A digest with a restriction enzyme cutting once within the provirus will yield two DNA fragments, overlapping the boundaries between viral and cellular DNA. Therefore, the size of these fragments is dependent on and specific for the retroviral integration site. Usually, the labeled probe is chosen to hybridize with one-half of the proviral DNA, so that only one of the virus-specific fragments per virus integration site is visualized. Since infection with retrovirus stocks in most cases will lead to single virus insertions, specific retroviral integrations can also be used as convenient and conclusive markers to determine the clonality of a particular cell population.

A digest with a restriction enzyme cutting within each of the LTRs will yield a DNA fragment containing the entire provirus. By comparing the predicted and the experimentally determined size of this fragment, the integrity of the provirus can be controlled.

Similarly, a digest with a restriction enzyme releasing the gene inserted into the retroviral vector provides information on the integrity of the transferred gene of interest.

16. For different batches or brands of PEG, the optimum time may vary. As a start, try 45 and 90 s as well.

References

1. Varmus, H. E. (1982) Form and function of retroviral proviruses. *Science* **216,** 812–820.
2. Varmus, H. E. and Swanstrom, R. (1985) Replication of retroviruses, in *Molecular Biology of Tumor Viruses: RNA Tumor Viruses* (Weiss, R. A., Teich, N., Varmus, H., and Coffin, J., eds.) Cold Spring Harbor Laboratory, Cold Spring Harbor, NY, pp. 369–512.
3. Varmus, H. E. and Swanstrom, R. (1985) Replication of retroviruses, in *Molecular Biology of Tumor Viruses: RNA Tumor Viruses* (Weiss, R. A., Teich, N., Varmus, H., and Coffin, J., eds.) suppl., Cold Spring Harbor Laboratory, Cold Spring Harbor, pp. 75–134.
4. Bender, M. A., Palmer, T. D., Gelinas, R. E., and Miller, A. D. (1987) Evidence that the packaging signal of Moloney murine leukemia virus extends into the *gag* region. *J. Virol.* **61,** 1639–1646.
5. Mann, R., Mulligan, R. C., and Baltimore, D. (1983) Construction of a retrovirus packaging mutant and its use to produce helper-free defective retrovirus. *Cell* **33,** 153–159.
6. Mann, R. and Baltimore, D. (1985) Varying the position of a retrovirus packaging sequence results in the encapsidation of both unspliced and spliced RNAs. *J. Virol.* **54,** 401–407.
7. Kriegler, M., Perez, C. F., Hardy, C., and Botchan, M. (1984) Transformation mediated by the SV40 T antigens: Separation of the overlapping SV40 early genes with a retroviral vector. *Cell* **38,** 483–4891.
8. Eglitis, M. A., Kantoff, P., Gilboa, E., and Anderson, W. F. (1985) Gene expression in mice after high efficiency retroviral-mediated gene transfer. *Science* **230,** 1395–1398.
9. Bowtell, D. D., Cory, S., Johnson, G. R., and Gonda, T. J. (1988) Comparison of expression in hemopoietic cells by retroviral vectors carrying two genes. *J. Virol.* **62,** 2464–2473.

10. Laker, C., Stocking, C., Bergholz, U., Hess, N., De, L. J., and Ostertag, W. (1987) Autocrine stimulation after transfer of the granulocyte/macrophage colony-stimulating factor gene and autonomous growth are distinct but interdependent steps in the oncogenic pathway. *Proc. Natl. Acad. Sci. USA* **84,** 8458–8462.

11. Strair, R. K., Towle, M. J., and Smith, B. R. (1988) Recombinant retroviruses encoding cell surface antigens as selectable markers. *J. Virol.* **62,** 4756–4759.

12. Cepko, C. L., Roberts, B. E., and Mulligan, R. C. (1984) Construction and applications of a highly transmissible murine retrovirus shuttle vector. *Cell* **37,** 1053–1062.

13. Joyner, A. L. and Bernstein, A. (1983) Retrovirus transduction: Segregation of the viral transforming function and the herpes simplex virus tk gene in infectious Friend spleen focus-forming virus thymidine kinase vectors. *Mol. Cell. Biol.* **3,** 2191–2202.

14. Hwang, L. S., Park, J., and Gilboa, E. (1984) Role of intron-contained sequences in formation of Moloney murine leukemia virus *env* mRNA. *Mol. Cell. Biol.* **4,** 2289–2297.

15. Korman, A. J., Frantz, J. D., Strominger, J. L., and Mulligan, R. C. (1987) Expression of human class II major histocompatibility complex antigens using retrovirus vectors. *Proc. Natl. Acad. Sci. USA* **84,** 2150–2154.

16. Yang, Z., Korman, A. J., Cooper, J., Pious, D., Accolla, R. S., Mulligan, R. C., and Strominger, J. L. (1987) Expression of HLA-DR antigen in human class II mutant B-cell lines by double infection with retrovirus vectors. *Mol. Cell. Biol.* **7,** 3923–3928.

17. Boulter, C. A. and Wagner, E. F. (1987) A universal retroviral vector for efficient constitutive expression of exogenous genes. *Nucleic Acids Res.* **15,** 7194.

18. Miller, A. D. and Rosman, G. (1989) Improved retroviral vectors for gene transfer and expression. *Biotechniques* **7,** 980–990.

19. Overell, R. W., Weisser, K. E., and Cosman, D. (1988) Stably transmitted triple-promoter retroviral vectors and their use in transformation of primary mammalian cells. *Mol. Cell. Biol.* **8,** 1803–1808.

20. Emerman, M. and Temin, H. M. (1984) Genes with promoters in retrovirus vectors can be independently suppressed by an epigenetic mechanism. *Cell* **39,** 459–467.

21. Emerman, M. and Temin, H. M. (1986) Quantitative analysis of gene suppression in integrated retrovirus vectors. *Mol. Cell. Biol.* **6,** 792–800.

22. Emerman, M. and Temin, H. M. (1986) Comparison of promoter suppression in avian and murine retrovirus vectors. *Nucleic Acids Res.* **14,** 9381–9396.

23. Yu, S. F., von, R. T., Kantoff, P. W., Garber, C., Seiberg, M., Ruther, U., Anderson, W. F., Wagner, E. F., and Gilboa, E. (1986) Self-inactivating retroviral vectors designed for transfer of whole genes into mammalian cells. *Proc. Natl. Acad. Sci. USA* **83,** 3194–3198.

24. Hawley, R. G., Covarrubias, L., Hawley, T., and Mintz, B. (1987) Handicapped retroviral vectors efficiently transduce foreign genes into hematopoietic stem cells. *Proc. Natl. Acad. Sci. USA* **84,** 2406–2410.

25. Yee, J. K., Moores, J. C., Jolly, D. J., Wolff, J. A., Respess, J. G., and Friedmann, T. (1987) Gene expression from transcriptionally disabled retroviral vectors. *Proc. Natl. Acad. Sci. USA* **84,** 5197–5201.

26. Panganiban, A. T. and Fiore, D. (1988) Ordered interstrand and intrastrand DNA transfer during reverse transcription. *Science* **241,** 1064–1069.

27. Linney, E., Davis, B., Overhauser, J., Chao, E., and Fan, H. (1984) Nonfunction of a Moloney murine leukemia virus regulatory sequence in F9 embryonal carcinoma cells. *Nature* **308,** 470–472.

28. Gorman, C. M., Rigby, P. W., and Lane, D. P. (1985) Negative regulation of viral enhancers in undifferentiated embryonic stem cells. *Cell* **42**, 519–526.

29. Seliger, B., Kollek, R., Stocking, C., Franz, T., and Ostertag, W. (1986) Viral transfer, transcription, and rescue of a selectable myeloproliferative sarcoma virus in embryonal cell lines: Expression of the mos oncogene. *Mol. Cell. Biol.* **6**, 286–293.

30. Hilberg, F., Stocking, C., Ostertag, W., and Grez, M. (1987) Functional analysis of a retroviral host-range mutant: Altered long terminal repeat sequences allow expression in embryonal carcinoma cells. *Proc. Natl. Acad. Sci. USA* **84**, 5232–5236.

31. Chatis, P. A., Holland, C. A., Hartley, J. W., Rowe, W. P., and Hopkins, N. (1983) Role for the 3' end of the genome in determining disease specificity of Friend and Moloney murine leukemia viruses. *Proc. Natl. Acad. Sci. USA* **80**, 4408–4411.

32. Chatis, P. A., Holland, C. A., Silver, J. E., Frederickson, T. N., Hopkins, N., and Hartley, J. W. (1984) A 3' end fragment encompassing the transcriptional enhancers of nondefective Friend virus confers erythroleukemogenicity on Moloney leukemia virus. *J. Virol.* **52**, 248–254.

33. Stocking, C., Kollek, R., Bergholz, U., and Ostertag, W. (1985) Long terminal repeat sequences impart hematopoietic transformation properties to the myeloproliferative sarcoma virus. *Proc. Natl. Acad. Sci .USA* **82**, 5746–5750.

34. Stocking, C., Kollek, R., Bergholz, U., and Ostertag, W. (1986) Point mutations in the U3 region of the long terminal repeat of Moloney murine leukemia virus determine disease specificity of the myeloproliferative sarcoma virus. *Virology* **153**, 145–149.

35. Hariharan, I. K., Adams, J. M., and Cory, S. (1988) Bcr-abl oncogene renders myeloid cell line factor independent: Potential autocrine mechanism in chronic myeloid leukemia. *OncogeneRes.* **3**, 387–399.

36. Holland, C. A., Anklesaria, P., Sakakeeny, M. A., and Greenberger, J. S. (1987) Enhancer sequences of a retroviral vector determine expression of a gene in multipotent hematopoietic progenitors and committed erythroid cells. *Proc. Natl. Acad. Sci. USA* **84**, 8662–8666.

37. Turner, D. L. and Cepko, C. L. (1987) A common progenitor for neurons and glia persists in rat retina late in development. *Nature* **328**, 131–136.

38. Thompson, T. C., Southgate, J., Kitchener, G., and Land, H. (1989) Multistage carcinogenesis induced by *ras* and *myc* oncogenes in a reconstituted organ. *Cell* **56**, 917–930.

39. Hayward, W. S., Neel, B. G., and Astrin, S. M. (1981) Activation of a cellular onc gene by promoter insertion in ALV-induced lymphoid leukosis. *Nature* **290**, 475–480.

40. Jaenisch, R., Jahner, D., Nobis, P., Simon, I., Lohler, J., Harbers, K., and Grotkopp, D. (1981) Chromosomal position and activation of retroviral genomes inserted into the germ line of mice. *Cell* **24**, 519–529.

41. Cone, R. D. and Mulligan, R. C. (1984) High-efficiency gene transfer into mammalian cells: Generation of helper-free recombinant retrovirus with broad mammalian host range. *Proc. Natl. Acad. Sci. USA* **81**, 6349–6353.

42. Miller, A. D., Law, M. F., and Verma, I. M. (1985) Generation of helper-free amphotropic retroviruses that transduce a dominant-acting, methotrexate-resistant dihydrofolate reductase gene. *Mol. Cell. Biol* **5**, 431–437.

43. Chattopadhyay, S. K., Oliff, A. I., Linemeyer, D. L., Lander, M. R., and Lowy, D. R. (1981) Genomes of murine leukemia viruses isolated from wild mice. *J. Virol.* **39**, 777–791.

44. Eglitis, M. A., Kohn, D. B., Moen, R. C., Blaese, R. M., and Anderson, W. F. (1988) Infection of human hematopoietic progenitor cells using a retroviral vector with a xenotropic pseudotype. *Biochem. Biophys. Res. Commun.* **151,** 201–206.

45. Miller, A. D. and Buttimore, C. (1986) Redesign of retrovirus packaging cell lines to avoid recombination leading to helper virus production. *Mol. Cell. Biol.* **6,** 2895–2902.

46. Markowitz, D., Goff, S., and Bank, A. (1988) Construction and use of a safe and efficient amphotropic packaging cell line. *Virology* **167,** 400–406.

47. Markowitz, D., Goff, S., and Bank, A. (1988) A safe packaging line for gene transfer: Separating viral genes on two different plasmids. *J. Virol.* **62,** 1120–1124.

48. Danos, O. and Mulligan, R. C. (1988) Safe and efficient generation of recombinant retroviruses with amphotropic and ecotropic host ranges. *Proc. Natl. Acad. Sci. USA* **85,** 6460–6464.

49. Southern, P. J. and Berg, P. (1982) Transformation of mammalian cells to antibiotic resistance with a bacterial gene under control of the SV40 early region promoter. *J. Mol. Appl. Genet.***1,** 327–341.

50. Morgenstern, J. P. and Land, H. (1990) Advanced mammalian gene transfer: High titre retroviral vectors with multiple drug selection markers and a complimentary helper-free packaging cell line. *Nucleic Acids Res.* **18,** 3587–3596.

51. Shimotohno, K. and Temin, H. M. (1982) Loss of intervening sequences in genomic mouse alpha-globin DNA inserted in an infectious retrovirus vector. *Nature* **299,** 265–268.

52. Kaplan, P. L., Simon, S., Cartwright, C. A. and Eckhart, W. (1987) cDNA cloning with a retrovirus expression vector: Generation of a pp60c-src cDNA clone. *J. Virol.* **61,** 1731–1734.

53. Jat, P. S., Cepko, C. L., Mulligan, R. C., and Sharp, P. A. (1986) Recombinant retroviruses encoding simian virus 40 large T-antigen and polyomavirus large and middle T-antigens. *Mol. Cell. Biol.* **6,** 1204–1217.

54. Schwarzbauer, J. E., Mulligan, R. C., and Hynes, R. O. (1987) Efficient and stable expression of recombinant fibronectin polypeptides. *Proc. Natl. Acad. Sci. USA* **84,** 754–758.

55. Dostatni, N., Yaniv, M., Danos, O., and Mulligan, R. C. (1988) Use of retroviral vectors for mapping of splice sites in cottontail rabbit papillomavirus. *J. Gen. Virol.* **69,** 3093–3100.

56. Miller, A. D., Ong, E. S., Rosenfeld, M. G., Verma, I. M., and Evans, R. M. (1984) Infectious and selectable retrovirus containing an inducible rat growth hormone minigene. *Science* **225,** 993–998.

57. Tabin, C. J., Hoffmann, J. W., Goff, S. P., and Weinberg, R. A. (1982) Adaptation of a retrovirus as a eucaryotic vector transmitting the herpes simplex virus thymidine kinase gene. *Mol. Cell. Biol.* **2,** 426–436.

58. Cone, R. D., Weber, B. A., Baorto, D., and Mulligan, R. C. (1987) Regulated expression of a complete human beta-globin gene encoded by a transmissible retrovirus vector. *Mol. Cell. Biol.* **7,** 887–897.

59. Miller, A. D., Bender, M. A., Harris, E. A., Kaleko, M., and Gelinas, R. E. (1988) Design of retrovirus vectors for transfer and expression of the human beta-globin gene. *J. Virol.* **62,** 4337–4345.

60. Rowe, W. P., Pugh, W. E., and Hartley, J. W. (1970) Plaque assay techniques for murine leukemia viruses. *Virology* **42,** 1136–1139.

61. Goff, S., Traktman, P., and Baltimore, D. (1981) Isolation and properties of Moloney murine leukemia virus mutants: Use of a rapid assay for release of virion reverse transcriptase. *J. Virol.* **38,** 239–248.

62. Murphy, A. J. M. and Efstratiadis, A. (1987) Cloning vectors for expression of cDNA libraries in mammalian cells. *Proc. Natl. Acad. Sci. USA* **84,** 8277–8281.

63. Hirt, D. (1967) Selective extraction of Polyoma DNA from infected mouse cell cultures. *J. Mol. Biol.* **26,** 365–369.

SECTION 3
USE OF REPORTER GENES TO ASSAY
FOR TRANSFECTED GENE EXPRESSION

CHAPTER 16

Use of Tissue-Plasminogen Activator as a Reporter Gene

Nicholas C. Wrighton

1. Introduction

Throughout the past six or seven years, our ability to study and understand the process of eukaryotic gene expression has been greatly enhanced by the use of reporter genes. In essence, a reporter gene encodes a protein product for which a sensitive and convenient assay is available. Transcription of the reporter is driven by the control sequences of interest, so that the level of reporter protein reflects the transcriptional activity. Reporter genes in present usage include the chloramphenicol acetyltransferase (CAT) (ref. *1*; *see* elsewhere in this vol), β-galactosidase (β-gal) (ref. *2*) and, more recently, luciferase genes *(see* elsewhere in this vol).

This chapter describes the use of fibrin-agarose overlays to monitor *in situ* the expression of tissue-plasminogen activator (t-PA) when used as a reporter gene.

The t-PA enzyme is one of two major secreted serine proteases that initiate degradation of the fibrin network of blood clots *(4,* and ref. therein). It accomplishes this by its proteolytic conversion of the circulating proenzyme plasminogen into the active form, plasmin, which can then degrade fibrin via its serine protease activity. Because of the serine protease cascade controlling fibrinolysis, there exist extremely sensitive assays for t-PA, capable of detecting as little as 10^{-18} moles of activator *(4).*

From: *Methods in Molecular Biology, Vol. 7: Gene Transfer and Expression Protocols*
Edited by: E. J. Murray © 1991 The Humana Press Inc., Clifton, NJ

Cultured cells can be directly assayed for t-PA secretion by their overlay with, or their suspension within, a fibrin film containing plasminogen (5). Cells secreting the activator are detected by lysis of the milky fibrin clot, which forms a plaque. This *in situ* technique is sufficiently sensitive to detect expression in colonies, and even single cells, using the unaided eye. Furthermore, it is possible to recover such cells alive for additional characterization (5), since this assay is nondestructive.

Given a reliable protocol that allows unhurried and confident sample handling, fibrin-agarose overlays are very easy to perform. The resulting plaques can be scored readily with the unaided eye (unlike other potential single-cell assays, such as β-gal staining), and necessary incubation times can be determined by periodic examination of plates, i.e., the result develops in front of the researcher. Plates can also be stained with Coomassie blue or amido black (6) to enhance plaque detection, although this obviously results in cell death. After staining, plates can be fixed, dried down, and retained as a permanent record, still showing the correct plaque-to-cell spatial relationships.

The fibrin-agarose overlay assay is nonradiological and uses no other carcinogenic agents. Furthermore, the adoption from derived reagents of bovine plasma (fibrinogen, plasminogen, and thrombin) prevents possible exposure to hepatitis B and human immunodeficiency viruses. The assay therefore presents no occupational health hazards, except those normally associated with the culture of mammalian cell lines.

This chapter describes two *in situ* assays for t-PA. For both methods, it is assumed that cells have already been transfected with the relevant constructs between a t-PA cDNA and the transcriptional control regions of interest. Method A is used on adherent cells, which are washed free of serum-borne inhibitors of fibrinolysis while in a Petri dish and overlayed with fibrin-agarose. Method B is used when the cells to be assayed are suspension-growing. Here the cells must be washed by centrifugation and are actually resuspended in the fibrin–agarose. Nevertheless, the assay is still referred to as an "overlay."

The t-PA activity secreted from transfected cells can be quantified by counting the number of plaques or by measuring the overall extent of lysis of the overlay. This is based on the assumptions that a minimum level of t-PA is required to produce a plaque and that promoters of different strengths will then determine the number of cells secreting t-PA at or above this threshold level. The utility of t-PA as a reporter gene in transient transfection experiments has been demonstrated (7). The ranking of the activity of various promoters was shown to be the same when measured by fibrin–agarose overlays or CAT assays. However, CAT assays proved to be at least fivefold less sensitive.

A t-PA cDNA has also been used by the author as a reporter gene to study the elevation of transcription in vivo in response to the introduction of transcription factors (8). In this case, a stably transfected line was developed that secreted undetectable levels of t-PA before factor introduction, but produced dramatic fibrinolysis upon stimulation with the relevant factors. Quantification of the response in terms of transcription was based on a subsequent comparison with the plaque formation from a cell line secreting known quantities of t-PA (the Bowes melanoma line) and on a comparison of t-PA mRNA levels in the unstimulated cells with levels in the standard.

2. Materials

2.1. For Methods A and B

1. Bovine fibrinogen (Sigma F-4753); 10 mg/mL in sterile PBSA (Ca^{2+}- and Mg^{2+}-free). This will probably require considerable shaking to dissolve. Also, heating to 37°C may be necessary. Store frozen at –70°C in aliquots of 5–10 mL. PBSA is composed of 8g NaCl, 0.2 g KCl, 1.15 g Na_2HPO_4 and 0.2g KH_2PO_4 per liter distilled water.
2. Bovine plasminogen (Sigma P-6144): 1 U/mL in sterile PBSA. Snap-freeze in aliquots of 200 µL and store at –70°C.
3. Bovine thrombin (Sigma T-7513): 50 U/mL in sterile PBSA. Snap-freeze in aliquots of 25–50 µL and store at –70°C. Reagents 1, 2, and 3 under these conditions are stable for at least 3 m.
4. Low-melting-point agarose: 2.5% (w/v) in deionized distilled water (ddw). Make up in 50-mL lots in 100-mL glass bottles and autoclave to sterilize.
5. 1M $CaCl_2$: Filter-sterilize through a 0.45-µm membrane.
6. BME medium (GIBCO 073-1100), made up at 2× strength: Aliquot into 100-mL, bottles and supplement with 2× antibiotics (1.2% penicillin and 2% streptomycin, w/v) before use.
7. Serum-free tissue-culture medium for washing cells.

2.2. For Fixation and Staining

1. Glutaraldehyde: 0.125% (v/v) in ddw.
2. Methanol/acetic acid: 70%/10% (v/v) in ddw.
3. Amido black: 0.1% (w/v) in methanol/acetic acid.

3. Methods

3.1. Method A

1. Plate cells on 60-mm culture dishes. The assay as described here is sufficient for 10 dishes of this size (and can be scaled up for larger dishes) (*see* Note 2).

2. Melt a bottle of agarose, allow to cool, and then place in a 40°C water-bath situated in a tissue-culture hood. Also warm to this temperature a bottle of 2× BME and an aliquot of fibrinogen.

3. Thaw one aliquot each of plasminogen and thrombin. Keep on ice until use.

4. Pipet 10 µL of thrombin and 200 µL of plasminogen into the bottom of a 25-mL sterile plastic universal. Add 20 µL of $1 M$ $CaCl_2$ to the side of the tube (do not mix with thrombin/plasminogen).

5. Using a 10-mL plastic pipet add 10 mL 2× BME and mix by pipeting. Follow this with 10 mL of molten agarose, close the tube, and mix by inverting five times. Then place the universal in the 40°C waterbath, where the mixture will be stable for at least 30 min.

6. Remove the cells from the incubator and wash three times with warmed (37°C) serum-free culture medium in order to remove all traces of serum. Leave the dishes in the hood, but replace the lids to prevent drying out of the cells.

7. Add 2.5 mL of fibrinogen to the contents of the plastic universal, replace the cap, and mix by inverting five times. Then, using a 2-mL plastic pipet, transfer 2 mL of the mixture to each Petri dish. If necessary, gentle rocking can be used to promote even spreading of the mixture.

8. Allow the overlays to set in the hood for 10 min. Following this, return the dishes to the incubator, where clotting of the fibrinogen will occur in 5–10 min. Clotting is brought about by the action of the thrombin on the fibrinogen.

9. Incubate the cells at 37°C. Secretion of t-PA will give rise to clearings (plaques) in the milky fibrin–agarose overlay. Plaque formation is easily monitored by periodic examination of the dishes. Depending on the quantity of t-PA secreted, incubation times may be as short as a few hours or as long as 1–2 d (*see* Note 2).

3.2. Method B

1. This is also performed in 60-mm Petri dishes and, as is the case for method A, it is also sufficient for 10 assays of this size and can be scaled up.

2. Harvest suspension-growing cells and wash twice by centrifugation with warmed (37°C) serum-free culture medium. While cells are spinning, prepare the mix as in Section 3.1., steps 2–5, and place in the 40°C waterbath.

3. Count the cells and aliquot the desired quantity (usually 10^5) into a sterile plastic universal.

4. Pipet 2 mL of warmed serum-free medium into empty 60-mm tissue-culture dishes. Ensure that the medium wets the entire culture surface of each dish (*see* Note 3).

5. Pellet the cells (this counts as the third wash), aspirate all medium from the first tube, and resuspend the cells in 0.25 mL of fibrinogen using a 1 mL micropipetor.

6. Aspirate the medium from a wet tissue-culture dish.

7. Using a 2-mL plastic pipet, add 2 mL of the fibrinogen–agarose cocktail to the cells/fibrinogen, and mix by pipeting up and down five times. Be careful not to generate bubbles (*see* Note 1).

8. Transfer the cells to the empty Petri dish and spread evenly by gentle rocking.

9. Repeat steps 6–8 for the remainder of samples.

10. Allow agarose to set in the final dish as in Section 3.1., step 8, and then incubate cells as before.

3.3. Photography and Storage of Dishes

1. After the plaques have developed sufficiently, their growth is halted by flooding the Petri dishes with 0.125% (v/v) glutaraldehyde/ddw for 30 min. This treatment also serves to increase the contrast by enhancing the opacity of the fibrin.

2. The dishes can be photographed under dark-field illumination, i.e., they are placed above a dark background that is surrounded by the light source. This arrangement further increases the contrast between the plaques and the undigested fibrin, and produces striking pictures.

3. To further increase contrast, stain with 0.1% (w/v) amido black in 70% methanol/10% acetic acid in ddw (v/v/v) for 30 min. Destain using the methanol/acetic acid solvent alone.

4. Dishes can be dried down for storage. This provides a permanent record in which the original plaque-to-cell spatial relationships are retained. To do this, wash once with 5 mL of ddw; then remove all liquid above the fibrin–agarose overlay and leave uncovered in a dust-free room. Drying will be complete in about 2 d.

5. Vacuum-drying is not advisable, since bubbles, which destroy the overlay, often form in the fibrin–agarose during this process.

4. Notes

1. Petri dishes larger than 60 mm can be used (use appropriately larger volume), but it is more difficult to obtain even overlays using these.
2. The incubator must not vibrate excessively, since this can cause the overlays in dishes larger than 60 mm to rotate. If adherent cells are involved, any plaques will be streaked.
3. Petri dishes *must* be wet prior to pouring overlays, otherwise the fibrin–agarose mixture will not spread evenly.
4. Do not shake the fibrin–agarose mixture when mixing (in Method B), since this can cause rapid clotting. Also, do not jolt newly poured dishes; this may have the same effect and produce coarse, streaky clots.
5. Certain cell types secrete endogenous plasminogen activators that can interfere with the assay of the transfected t-PA. For instance, the author has found such activities in K562 cells, EJ bladder carcinoma cells, various hybridomas, and, when at high concentration, L cells (10^7 suspended in a 60-mm culture-dish overlay). Other authors have reported the induction of t-PA secretion in differentiating teratocarcinoma cells *(9)*. It may be possible to find an antibody that selectively blocks such endogenous activities when incorporated into the overlay. For this, the identity of the endogenous activity would need to be determined (*see* Note 6). If it turned out to be t-PA, the transfected cell line could not be of the same species as the cDNA.
6. Fibrin zymography *(6)* can be used to accurately determine the amount of t-PA secreted in absolute terms. It can also be used to determine the identity of an endogenous plasminogen activator.
7. Endogenous plasminogen activators can be induced by certain physical and chemical treatments. For instance, UV irradiation induces secretion of a plasminogen activator in chick and human fibroblasts *(10)*.
8. Suspension-growing cells that tend to clump upon washing with serum-free medium must be dissociated before resuspension in fibrin–agarose overlays.
9. Small numbers of suspension-growing cells are difficult to spin down accurately. In this case, resuspend the cells at high concentration after washing and incorporate a small aliquot into the overlay.

References

1. Gorman, C. M., Moffat, L. F., and Howard, B. H. (1982) Recombinant genomes which express chloramphenicol acetlytransferase in mammalian cells. *Mol. Cell. Biol.* **2,** 44–51.

2. Hall, C., Jacob, E., Ringold, G., and Lee, F. (1983) Expression and regulation of *E. coli* LacZ gene fusions in mammalian cells. *Mol. Appl. Genet.* **2,** 1–9.

3. de Wet, J. R., Wood, K. V., deLuca, M., Helinski, D. R., and Subramani, S. (1987) Firefly luciferase gene: Structure and expression in mammalian cells. *Mol. Cell. Biol.* **7,** 725–737.

4. Dano, K., Andreasen, P. A., Grondahl-Hansen, J., Kristensen, P., Nielsen, L. S., and Skriver, L. (1985) Plasminogen activators, tissue degradation, and cancer. *Adv. Cancer Res.* **44,** 137–266.

5. Jones, P., Benedict, W., Strickland, S. and Reich, E. (1975) Fibrin overlay methods for the detection of single transformed cells and colonies of transformed cells. *Cell* **5,** 323–329.

6. Granelli-Piperno, A. and Reich, E. (1978) A study of proteases and protease–inhibitor complexes in biological fluids. *J. Exp. Med.* **148,** 223–234.

7. Kenten, J. H., Wood, C. R., Stephens, P. E., Bendig, M. E., Boss, M. A., and Hentschel, C. C. (1986) Laboratory methods. A sensitive, nondestructive assay for transfected genes. *DNA* **5,** 257–262.

8. Wrighton, N. C. and Grosveld, F. G. (1988) A novel *in vivo* transcription assay demonstrates the presence of globin-inducing *trans*-acting factors in uninduced murine erythroleukemia cells. *Mol. Cell. Biol.* **8,** 130–137.

9. Strickland, S. and Mahdavi, V. (1978) The induction of differentiation in teratocarcinoma stem cells by retinoic acid. *Cell* **15,** 393–403.

10. Miskin, R. and Reich, E. (1980) Plasminogen activator: Induction of systhesis by DNA damage. *Cell* **19,** 217–224.

CHAPTER 17

Use of *E. coli lacZ* (β-Galactosidase) as a Reporter Gene

Grant R. MacGregor, Garry P. Nolan, Steven Fiering, Mario Roederer, and Leonard A. Herzenberg

1. Introduction

Our understanding of the molecular mechanisms that govern gene expression has been facilitated by the ability to introduce recombinant DNA molecules into heterologous cellular systems both in vitro and in vivo. One approach to defining DNA sequences important in the regulation of gene expression is to place controlling elements (e.g., promoter/enhancer sequences) upstream of a DNA coding sequence, introduce these constructs into transgenic animals or cells in culture, and analyze the levels of gene product produced by the introduced construct. Ideally, such a reporter gene should encode a product that is stable, innocuous to the cell or organism in which it is being expressed, and should be readily detectable, even when present in small quantities.

Extensive genetic and biochemical characterization of the *Escherichia coli* (*E. coli*) *lacZ* gene, which encodes the glycoside hydrolase, β-D-galactosidase (β-gal) (EC 3.2.1.23), makes it an ideal choice for use as a reporter gene; *lacZ* has been used in a variety of systems, including bacteria and yeast *(1);* cultured cells from mammals *(2–8),* avians *(9),* and insects *(10);* nematodes *(11);* adult mice

From: *Methods in Molecular Biology, Vol. 7: Gene Transfer and Expression Protocols*
Edited by: E. J. Murray © 1991 The Humana Press Inc., Clifton, NJ

(12); developing insect larvae *(13–15);* and murine embryos *(16–19).* The 3081-bp sequence of the bacterial *lacZ* gene has been determined *(20).* The first 27 amino acids of the protein can be replaced without affecting enzyme activity *(1),* allowing translational fusions to be made between either *N*-terminal eukaryotic translation initiation signals, or heterologous gene sequences encoding extensive protein domains, and the truncated β-gal gene product. Commercially available antibodies to β-gal allow immunochemical localization and detection of β-gal (and β-gal fusion proteins) in fixed cells and cell extracts. Finally, there are a number of chromogenic and fluorogenic substrates and biochemical assays that enable rapid and sensitive detection of β-gal (as few as 5 mol of β-gal in a single viable cell).

Four assays for biochemical detection of β-gal are presented in detail here. The choice of the particular assay system is dependent on experimental need and instrumentation available. The first two assays are used to measure β-gal activity in cell extracts (Table 1). A third assay is presented for histochemical localization of β-gal activity in fixed cells or tissue sections by either light microscope visualization or transmission electron microscopy. Finally, we detail the previously published FACS-gal assay *(6, 7)* which can quantitate β-gal expression with great sensitivity in viable cells on a cell-by-cell basis. FACS-gal quantitation of *lacZ* expression in single viable cells can be performed in concert with all the standard features of the fluorescence-activated cell sorter (FACS): cloning, sorting, analysis of the distribution of gene expression within a population of cells, and multiparameter analysis.

1.1. Spectrophotometric Assay Using ONPG

A simple and rapid assay to detect β-gal activity relies on the conversion of *o*-nitrophenol-β-D-galactoside (ONPG), a galactoside derivative, to yield galactose and the chromophore *o*-nitrophenol *(21).* *O*-nitrophenol can be detected by measuring absorbance at 420 nm using a spectrophotometer. The assay is sensitive and can be used when performing a quantitative determination of β-gal activity in cell extracts.

1.2. Fluorometric Assay Using MUG

The most simple and rapid assay to detect β-gal activity in cell extracts relies on the conversion of 4-methylumbelliferyl-β-D-galactoside (MUG), a nonfluorescent galactoside analog, to the highly fluorescent molecule 4-methylumbelliferone. The MUG product is measured using a fluorometer (excitation at 350 nm, and fluorescence emission read at 450 nm). The assay is extremely sensitive and is useful for quantitative measurements of β-gal levels in cell populations. Only a few thousand cells are required for accurate determinations. The assay is particularly useful for screening

Table 1
β-Galactosidase Assays

Substrate	K_m[a]	Instrument	Sensitivity[b]
Cell Extracts:			
MUG	170 μM	Fluorometer	10^6
ONPG	110 μM	Spectrophotometer	10^9
Intact Individual Cells:			
X-Gal		Microscope	10^3
FDG	17 μM	FACS	1–10

[a]Binding constant; references: MUG, M. Roederer, unpublished data; ONPG, (*32*); FDG, (*33*).
[b]Sensitivity is expressed as the minimum number of enzyme molecules required to obtain a measureable signal; thus, smaller numbers indicate greater sensitivity.

large numbers of populations by using conventional microtiter dish fluorescence readers, such as a Fluoroskan (Flow Laboratories). This assay has the widest dynamic range of the β-gal assays, allowing quantitation of activity in cell extracts having an average of 5 mol–10^6 mol of β-gal/cell.

1.3. Histochemical Assay Using X-Gal

Detection of β-gal activity *in situ* within cells in culture or in organs from transgenic animals can be performed using a histochemical stain (*22*) (*see* Figs. 1 and 2). This technique has been used to analyze cell lineages and patterns of gene expression within various tissues of eukaryotes during their development, e.g., rat nervous system (*23*), Drosophila embryos (*13–15*), murine embryos (*16–18*), and nematodes (*11*), and in cell-culture systems to study aspects of viral gene expression (*5,6,9,24–26*). In conjunction with plasmids that express β-gal in mammalian cells (*27*), this stain can also be used to assist in the identification of optimum conditions for DNA transfection or electroporation (*see* Fig. 1). The substrate, 5-bromo-4-chloro-3-indolyl-β-D-galactoside (X-gal), is hydrolyzed by β-galactosidases to generate galactose and soluble indoxyl molecules, which in turn are oxidized to insoluble indigo. The deep blue color generated by the hydrolysis of X-gal by β-gal facilitates subcellular localization of the β-gal activity.

Cells or tissues to be stained are first washed in phosphate-buffered saline (PBS) and fixed using an appropriate fixative (e.g., glutaraldehyde/paraformaldehyde). The components of the stain are

1. Sodium phosphate to buffer the pH of the system and to provide sodium ions, which activate the β-gal enzyme;
2. Magnesium ions, a cofactor for the enzyme;
3. Potassium ferrocyanide and potassium ferricyanide, which together act as an oxidation catalyst to increase the rate of conversion of the soluble

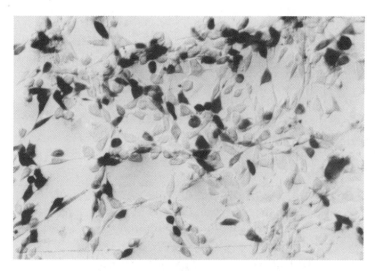

Fig. 1. GP +*env* AM12 cells expressing *E.coli* β-gal detected by X-gal histochemical stain. GP +*env* AM12 cells, a Moloney murine leukemia retroviral packaging cell line derived from NIH 3T3 cells, were electroporated with pCMVβ *(27)*, a vector that expresses *E.coli* β-gal under control of the human cytomegalovirus immediate early promoter. Forty-eight hours postelectroporation, cells were fixed and stained for β-gal activity with the X-gal stain as described in the text. Cells expressing β-gal at different levels can be seen as staining different shades of blue (gray). Cells not expressing β-gal, or expressing at a level below the sensitivity of the stain, appear clear. This illustrates one of the uses of this technique to assist in optimizing conditions for electroporation of different cell lines (*see* Chapter 5). Magnification 400×.

(and therefore diffusible) indoxyl molecules to the insoluble indigo form, thereby enhancing localization of the blue color; and
4. X-gal, the chromogenic indicator.

The stain is prepared and used to cover the fixed cells of whole or sectioned tissues. Following an incubation period, the indigo dye can be seen by eye or low-power microscopy. Further, the insoluble indigo dye precipitated in this manner is electron-dense, facilitating fine analysis of subcellular localization of β-gal fusion proteins by electron microscopy (*see* Notes). Although this technique for detection of β-gal activity is not as sensitive as an immunocytological method *(5)* or FACS-gal *(6)*, it has the advantage relative to the ONPG and MUG methods that it can detect a single cell expressing β-gal within a population of nonexpressing cells.

1.4. Analysis of β-Gal Expression in Viable Cells Using FACS-Gal

Of the four assays described here, the analysis of β-gal expression in cultured cells using fluorescein di-β-D-galactoside (FDG) and a FACS is the most powerful *(6,7)*. The assay relies on the hydrolysis of FDG by β-gal inside

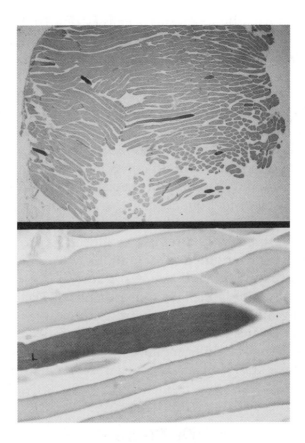

Fig. 2. Histochemical-based detection of *E.coli* β-gal in muscle of a transgenic mouse using X-gal stain. Leg muscle from an F2 transgenic mouse (G. R. MacGregor and P. A. Overbeek, unpublished observations), the transgene of which is composed of the Rous (avian) sarcoma virus long terminal repeat juxtaposed to the *E.coli* β-gal gene with RNA processing signals derived from SV40, fixed and stained for β-gal activity using X-gal as described in the text. Following staining, the tissue was embedded in plastic, sectioned, and counterstained with hematoxylin and eosin. Note the heterogeneity of β-gal expression as detected by the X-gal stain. It is probable that additional myofibers contain β-gal activity at levels below the sensitivity of detection afforded by this technique. Magnification (A) 40×, (B) 400×.

viable cells and the subsequent detection of the product, fluorescein, with the laser excitation and detection systems of the FACS. Cells to be analyzed are loaded with FDG by brief hypotonic shock at 37°C for 1 min. At the end of 1 min, the cells are returned to isotonic conditions by dilution into ice-cold medium. Although fluorescein passes through the cell membrane 200 times faster at 37°C than at 5°C, the V_{max} of β-gal is reduced only about tenfold by this temperature change. Thus, by lowering the temperature following loading of cells with FDG, β-gal activity proceeds without leakage of the fluorescein or FDG substrate from cells, thereby permitting discrimination between β-gal-positive and -negative subpopulations of cells (*see* Fig. 3). However, if the cells are allowed to warm to above 15°C, the fluorescein generated in β-gal-positive cells will leak through the cell membrane and be taken up by other cells, including β-gal⁻ cells, yielding a population that stains homogeneously positive for β-gal expression when analyzed by FACS.

The FACS-gal assay is unique in that cells can be analyzed, sorted, and cloned using the FACS on the basis of their level of β-gal activity and are viable throughout the process. Furthermore, it is both quantitative and extremely sensitive—under standard conditions, as few as 5 mol in a single cell can be detected. FACS-gal is more sensitive than immunocytochemical methods or the X-gal histochemical stain–for example, approx 1000 mol are necessary for a cell to be stained homogeneously blue by X-gal (Table 1). The fluorescence observed (fluorescein produced) is monotonically related to the number of β-gal tetramers present in the cell; calculations (MR, GPN, SF, and LAH, unpublished) indicate that fluorescence = (number of β-gal tetramers)$^{1.8}$ × constant × time. There exist many applications for this technique, including analysis of DNA transcription rates, studies of cellular epigenetic effects, transgene studies in immune lineage cells correlated to expression of cell-surface differentiation markers, and isolation of control elements for gene expression (e.g., using an "enhancer trap" system).

2. Materials

2.1. ONPG Analysis

1. PM-2 buffer (9): 23 mM NaH$_2$PO$_4$, 77 mM Na$_2$HPO$_4$, 0.1 mM MnCl$_2$, 2 mM MgSO$_4$, 40mM β-mercaptoethanol (stock is 14.2 M), pH 7.3. Filter the solution through a 0.45-μm disposable filter. It is stable at 4°C for up to 1 mo.
2. O-Nitrophenyl-β-D-galactopyranoside (ONPG, Sigma cat. no. N-1127). Dissolve at 4mg/mL in PM-2 buffer. Warm at 37°C, with vortexing, to form solution. Make fresh for each assay.
3. 1M Na$_2$CO$_3$.
4. Protein assay kit (BioRad cat. no. 500-0006 or equivalent).
5. Bovine serum albumin (50 mg/mL solution from BRL, cat. no. 5561UA, or equivalent).
6. Disposable plastic cuvets (1 mL) with 10-mm light path.
7. Phosphate-buffered saline (PBS): 15 mM sodium phosphate, pH7.3; 150 mM NaCl.

2.2. MUG Analysis

1. Z-buffer: 60 mM Na$_2$PO$_4$·7H$_2$O, 40 mM NaH$_2$PO$_4$·H$_2$O, 10 mM KCl, 1 mM MgSO$_4$·7H$_2$O. Adjust pH to 7.0 with NaOH or HCl.

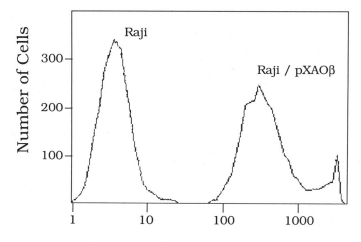

Relative Fluorescence Intensity

Fig. 3. Detection of human B lymphoblastoid cells expressing *E.coli* β-gal using FACS-FDG. Human Raji B lymphoblastoid cells were electroporated with an Epstein-Barr virus origin of replication episomal cDNA expression vector (G418 resistant) expressing the *E.coli* β-gal gene (pXAOβ, G. R. MacGregor, unpublished results) and a population of stable transfectants generated by selection with G418. This population was analyzed for expression of β-gal using the FACS-FDG method and chloroquine treatment as described in the text. The figure shows the result of an experiment in which equal numbers of parental Raji cells and the polyclonal Raji/pXAOβ population were mixed and analyzed for β-gal expression using FACS-FDG. Unelectroporated Raji cells can be distinguished with ease from the polyclonal population of Raji cells expressing the β-gal gene. Note the heterogeneity of expression revealed within the population by this method.

2. 1% TX-100: 1 mL Triton X-100 detergent in 100 mL (final vol) H_2O.
3. MUG stock: 3 m*M* methylumbelliferyl-β-D-galactoside (Sigma cat. no. M-1633) in Z-buffer. MUG at this concentration is not soluble at room temperature. To prepare the stock solution, add the appropriate amount of solid to Z-buffer and heat to boiling to form solution (should take 5–10 min). Aliquot into 1-mL tubes, and freeze until use. Just before starting the reaction, dissolve the stock by placing in boiling water (it should be completely in solution in 1–2 min at 80°C). Do not let the stock sit at room temperature for >10–15 min before using, since it may precipitate. If it does, simply reheat.
4. STOP buffer: 300 m*M* Glycine, 15 m*M* EDTA; adjust pH to 11.2 with NaOH. The pH of this solution is critical: Make sure that a 1:2 dilution of STOP with Z-buffer yields a pH of 10.5 or greater.

2.3. X-Gal-Based Histochemical Assay

1. Stock solutions of $1 M$ Na_2HPO_4, $1 M$ NaH_2PO_4 and $1 M$ $MgCl_2$: Prepare in double-distilled (dd) or Millipore milliQ-grade H_2O and store at room temperature.

2. Stock solutions of 50 mM potassium ferricyanide ($K_3Fe[CN]_6$) and 50 mM potassium ferrocyanide ($K_4Fe[CN]_6$): Prepare in ddH_2O and store in foil-wrapped glassware (in the dark) at 4°C, where they are stable for at least 3 mo.

3. X-Gal stock: Dissolve in *N,N*-dimethyl formamide at 20 mg/mL and store in a glass container (not polycarbonate or polystyrene) in the dark at −20°C.

4. 4% paraformaldehyde (Wear a mask and gloves when handling para-formaldehyde): In a fume hood, dissolve 8 g of powder in 150 mL of 0.1 M sodium phosphate, pH 7.3 (77 mM Na_2HPO_4, 23 mM NaH_2PO_4), stirring and heating to 60°C. Add 10N NaOH at a rate of 1 drop/min until the solution clears. Bring the vol to 200 mL with 0.1 M sodium phosphate, pH7.3. Store at 4°C for up to 1 mo.

5. Glutaraldehyde is purchased as a 25% solution.

6. To prepare the working fixative (2% paraformaldehyde/0.2% gluteral-dehyde), combine 50 mL of 4% paraformaldehyde with 49.2 mL of 0.1 M sodium phosphate, pH 7.3, and 0.8 mL of 25% glutaraldehyde. This can be stored at 4°C for up to 1 wk.

7. X-Gal stain: 100 mM sodium phosphate, pH 7.3 (77 mM Na_2HPO_4, 23 mM NaH_2PO_4), 1.3 mM $MgCl_2$, 3 mM $K_3Fe(CN)_6$, 3 mM $K_4Fe(CN)_6$, and 1mg/mL X-Gal. Filter through a 0.45-μm disposable filtration unit prior to use.

8. Phosphate-buffered saline (PBS): 15 mM sodium phosphate, pH 7.3; 150 mM NaCl.

2.4. FACS-Gal Analysis

1. Staining media: PBS (15 mM sodium phosphate, pH7.3; 150 mM NaCl) containing 10 mM HEPES, pH 7.3; 4% fetal calf serum.

2. Fluorescein-di-β-galactoside (FDG) was obtained from Molecular Probes, PO Box 22010, Eugene, OR 97402 (cat. no. F-1179). The FDG powder should be a very pale yellow. A dark yellow color indicates the presence of fluorescent contaminants. FDG powder is unstable and will hydrolyze spontaneously over a period of time even if dessicated and kept at −20°C. Therefore, prepare a stock solution as soon as it is received. As a solution, FDG is stable for many months. The 200 mM stock solution is made by dissolving 5 mg of FDG in 38 μL of 1:1 H_2O:DMSO. Mixing DMSO

and H_2O is exothermic, so it is necessary to cool the mixture before adding FDG. This stock should be yellow in color and will remain liquid at –20°C. To prepare a 2mM working solution, remove 10 µL and add to 990 µL of sterile water in a sterile clear tube. Since 2mM is near the maximum solubility for FDG, place the solution in a 37°C water bath for about 10 min to dissolve the FDG completely, ensuring that no precipitate remains. The solution should not be held at 37°C for extended periods of time, since this will enhance the rate of spontaneous hydrolysis of the FDG. This solution can be frozen and thawed as required and should be faint yellow in color. Alternatively, one can prepare many tubes of 2 mM FDG solution in aliquots of 1–2 mL and store them, frozen, until needed.

FDG solutions can be contaminated with minor quantities of fluorescent monogalactoside and/or fluorescein, both of which will contribute to background fluorescence. Although quality control ensures that the FDG prepared by Molecular Probes contains <10 ppm fluorescein-equivalent contaminants (an acceptable level for all FACS-related purposes), it is sometimes desirable to remove any background fluorescent components in the FDG stock solution prior to staining cells. This is achieved by photobleaching these fluorescent molecules by holding the Eppendorf tube containing the 2 mM solution directly in the path of the FACS 488-nm argon laser for 1 min or more (move the tube slowly to avoid melting the plastic). Hold the tube in such a manner that the laser strikes the solution at the miniscus. This will ensure optimal spread of the light throughout the solution. LASER GOGGLES MUST BE WORN DURING THIS PROCEDURE. After this treatment, the solution can be freeze-thawed without rebleaching.

3. Propidium iodide.
4. Nylon screen (optional): Cut 2-in.-square pieces of nylon screen. For sterile work, wrap these in aluminum foil and autoclave. Nitex monofilament screen cloth, cat. no. HD-3-85, was obtained from Fairmont Fabrics, PO Box 1515, Pacifica, CA 94044.

3. Methods

3.1. ONPG Analysis

1. Disperse the transfected cells by treatment with trypsin (if adherent) or centrifuge (if suspension) and wash once with PBS.
2. Resuspend pelleted cells in PM-2 buffer by vortexing. As a guide, we routinely resuspend 10^6 cells in 0.5–1 mL of PM-2. Transfer to a 1.5-mL Eppendorf tube.

3. Prepare cell extracts by 5 freeze-thaw cycles using liquid nitrogen (or dry ice/ethanol) and a 37°C water bath (*see* Note 3, Section 4.1.). Vortex samples briefly between each cycle. Following this treatment, spin the samples at 13,500g for 15 min at 4°C to pellet cellular debris.

4. Transfer the supernatant containing soluble protein to fresh Eppendorf tubes and place on ice.

5. Estimate the soluble protein concentration. A suggested technique is that of Bradford (*28, see also* Volume 3, this series), using a commercially available kit (BioRad). Values to generate a standard curve are obtained using BSA standards.

6. Dilute equal amounts of protein from cell extracts in PM-2 buffer to a final vol of 800 µL and place in disposable 1-mL plastic cuvets (*see* Note 1, Section 4.1.). Prepare two negative controls, one with BSA, the other with extract derived from untransfected cells.

7. Incubate the ONPG solution and the samples in the cuvets separately at 37°C for 15 min to allow temperature equilibration.

8. Initiate the reaction by the addition of 200 µL of prewarmed ONPG to each cuvet containing protein extracts. Cap the cuvets with parafilm and invert several times to ensure thorough mixing of the enzyme and substrate. Note the exact time of addition of ONPG. Perform enzyme incubations at 37°C.

9. Monitor the assays visually until a yellow color becomes apparent. For best results, this should give an absorbance at 420 nm of between 0.1 and 1.0.

10. Add 500 µL of 1 M Na_2CO_3 to each cuvet. This adjusts the pH of the reaction to approx 11, stopping further enzymatic conversion of ONPG. Note carefully the duration (in minutes and seconds) of each reaction (*see* Note 2, Section 4.1.).

11. Read the sample absorbance at 420 nm. Calculate β-gal activity as follows: U= ($380 \times A_{420}$) divided by time (in minutes), where 380 is a constant such that 1 U is equivalent to conversion of 1 nmol of ONPG/min at 37°C (*9*).

3.2. MUG Analysis

1. Resuspend the transfected cells to be assayed in Z-buffer. A reasonable starting concentration is about 5×10^5/mL. Deposit 105 µL of the cell suspension in a well of a microtiter dish (*see* Notes 1–6, Section 4.2.).

2. Add 15 µL of 1% TX-100 to each well (final concentration: 0.1%). Let these incubate for 5–10 min to solubilize the cells completely.

3. Add 30 µL of 3 mM MUG to each well. Time each reaction.

4. Add 75 µL of STOP to each well (1:2 dilution) after appropriate incubation time (*see* Note 7, Section 4.2.). The STOP solution not only stops

the reaction completely, but also increases the 4-methylumbelliferone fluorescence sixfold.

5. Measure the fluorescence of the reactions (excitation at 350 nm and fluorescence emission read at 450 nm).

3.3. X-Gal-Based Histochemical Assay

3.3.1. Adherent Cells

1. Aspirate media from the monolayers of cells to be assayed, and rinse gently but thoroughly twice with PBS.
2. Overlay the cells with fixative in a tissue-culture dish with fixative and incubate at 4°C for 5 min (*see* Note 7, Section 4.3.).
3. Aspirate the fixative and rinse gently, twice, with room temperature PBS.
4. Aspirate the PBS and overlay the fixed cells with X-gal stain.
5. *See* steps 5–6 of Section 3.3.2.

3.3.2. Suspension Cells

1. Spin down the cells (from 10^4–10^7). Wash once with 2 mL of PBS. Aspirate the PBS.
2. Agitate the tube to dissociate the pellet. Add 1 mL of fixative and incubate at 4°C for 5 min.
3. Spin down the cells and aspirate the fixative. Wash twice with 2 mL PBS. Aspirate the PBS.
4. Resuspend the fixed cells in 2 mL of X-gal stain. Transfer cells to 24-well culture dishes.
5. Replace the tissue-culture-dish lids and incubate in a humidified incubator at 37°C until a blue color develops (this may take anywhere from 30 min to overnight).
6. View the cells under a microscope. Cells expressing sufficient β-gal will appear blue (*see* Figs. 1 and 2).

3.4. FACS-Gal Analysis

3.4.1. Cell Preparation

1. Populations of cells expressing *E. coli* β-gal are harvested from exponentially growing cultures prior to staining (*see* Note 1, Section 4.4.). Trypsinize adherent cells or spin down suspension cells.
2. Resuspend the cells in staining medium and pipet to obtain a single-cell suspension. When working with FACS, cells must be in a single-cell suspension. If the cells are clumped as a result of inadequate trypsinization, cell death, or other reasons, clumps must be removed prior to running the analysis by passing the cells through a nylon screen.
3. Adjust the cell suspension to 10^7 cells/mL (*see* Note 2, Section 4.4.).
4. Aliquot 50 µL of cells into a 4-mL FACS tube (Becton Dickinson cat. no. 2058) and place cells on ice.

3.4.2. Staining for E.coli β-Gal Activity

1. Place the cells in the FACS tube in a 37°C water bath for 10 min.
2. Add to the cells 50 μL of 2 mM FDG in H_2O prewarmed to 37°C and mix rapidly and thoroughly (important). This part of the reaction can be scaled up or down without cause for concern. However, it is important that equal volumes of cells and 2 mM FDG in H_2O be used to generate the hypotonic shock.
3. Return the cells to a 37°C water bath for exactly 1 min. The staining procedure relies on an osmotic shock of the cells during the 1 min at 37°C; FDG is being taken up into the cells by passive osmotic loading.
4. Stop FDG loading at the end of 1 min by adding 2-mL of ICE-COLD staining media with 1 μg/mL propidium iodide. Use ice-cold pipets or tips to aliquot the staining media into the tube containing the cells. The uptake of FDG is stopped and the substrate and products locked in the cells by a rapid dilution into cold isotonic staining medium. This one step brings the cells back to isoosmotic conditions, stops the loading, and "freezes" the cell membrane, thereby locking the substrate and products inside the cell. Use propidium iodide to facilitate live/dead cell discrimination on FACS. It is necessary to gate out dead (propidium iodide bright) cells as these can interfere with the analysis.
5. Keep the cells on ice until ready to perform FACS analysis. The enzymatic conversion of FDG to fluorescein proceeds even though the cells are on ice. Any amount of enzyme will hydrolyze all of the available substrate, given enough time, yielding a homogeneous fluorescence distribution representing the amount of FDG loaded per cell. If one is interested only in qualitative discrimination of β-gal-expressing cells from nonexpressing cells, the above protocol is sufficient. For fluorescence-to-enzyme-content correlations, one must ensure that each sample is analyzed at the same time after loading and before the substrate levels are exhausted. Alternatively, one can use a competitive inhibitor of *E. coli* β-gal to stop or slow the reaction (*see* Section 4.4., Note 3).

3.4.3. Special FACS Requirements for FACS-Gal

1. Set up and calibrate the machine to detect fluorescein, propidium iodide, and forward scatter. Any FACS facility should be able to handle most requirements as outlined for FACS-Gal. A useful reference is Parks et al. *(30, see also* Chapter 29).
2. Using unstained cells identical to the type to be analyzed, set the autofluorescence compensation using the method of Alberti et al. *(31).* Cultured cells, adherent cells especially, and some cell types from isolated tissues have high levels of autofluorescence when excited at 488 nm. This auto-

fluorescence is caused primarily by cellular compounds (e.g., NADPH, complex hydrocarbons, and so on) that are excited at 488 nm and can emit across a broad range of wavelengths. It is essential, therefore, that autofluorescence compensation is set to perform accurate quantitation of β-gal activity. This is especially true when low levels of β-gal activity are being analyzed.

4. Notes

4.1. ONPG Analysis

1. To generate accurate readings for β-gal activity, it is important that the substrate should never be limiting during the reaction. To ensure that this is the case, duplicate reactions should be performed for each sample with two concentrations of protein extract. Absorbance values should be directly related to the concentration of cell extract used in each sample. For best results, the use of a spectrophotometer with a kinetics software accessory that permits the calculation of rates of substrate conversion is recommended (e.g., Beckman DU-60 series with Kinetics Soft-Pac™ module and thermostatted cuvet jacket).
2. At pH 11, β-gal activity continues, albeit extremely slowly. Samples should be read shortly after completing assays and not left for extended periods (e.g., overnight) before reading.
3. Repeated freeze-thawing can lead to inactivation of β-gal. It is also possible to lyse cells by an addition of Triton-X100, to a final concentration of 0.1% (*see* MUG procedure).

4.2. MUG Analysis

1. This protocol is designed for use with a fluorescence microtiter plate reader, although it can be easily adapted to be read by any fluorometer. The advantages of such a plate reader are many, including the ability to easily read 100- to 300-µL vols and to read 96 wells in 2–3 min. Thus, fluorescence microtiter plate readers are well-suited for performing large-scale screenings and/or quantitations of cell lines or reaction conditions. For use with a fluorometer, the reaction vol may be scaled up appropriately.
2. Cells also may be sorted directly from a FACS into wells. The advantage of this method is that a precise number of cells can be deposited, allowing extremely accurate quantitation. When using this method, deposit no more than 50 µL of cells in each well (generally about 20,000 cells, depending on the nozzle diameter), and dilute to 105 µL with Z-buffer. As a control well, deposit an equal vol of sheath fluid from the sorter and dilute with Z-buffer.

3. Include appropriate controls for MUG autohydrolysis. Although boiling the MUG does not result in significant hydrolysis, it can convert at a slow rate in Z-buffer during extended reactions.

4. The autofluorescence contribution of the lysed cells is negligible. However, autofluorescence can become significant with a large number of lysed cells/well (usually >200,000 cells/well). An appropriate control for all experiments is to deposit an equal number of parental (*LacZ⁻*) cells and measure their activity. This also controls for the contribution of the endogenous β-gal to the hydrolysis.

5. Because of inner-filter effect (quenching of fluorescence at high fluorescent product concentrations), it is important to standardize the measurements to ascertain that they are within a linear range. The reactions are easily standardized against dilutions of purified enzyme. Time-points (kinetics) should be chosen to ascertain the linearity of the reaction.

6. The reaction can be run at temperatures between 4 and 37°C. The hydrolysis rate is approx sixfold faster at room temperature than at 4°C, and again about fourfold faster at 37°C than at room temperature.

7. For 20,000 cells of a typical stably transfected cell line, a 1-h incubation at 37°C should be sufficient to obtain a reasonable fluorescence signal. The assay has been used successfully to quantitate β-gal activity in cells with an average of 5 mol of enzyme/cell, as well as in cells with over 800,000 mol of enzyme/cell. In the latter case, <100 cells/well were needed to quantitate the level of enzyme.

8. For transient assays, in which the number of transfected cells can be a small fraction of the total cell number, keep in mind that it is necessary to scale up the reaction to have sufficient activity for measurement.

4.3. X-Gal-Based Histochemical Assay

1. Often we have noted a heterogeneity of staining within cell populations, both clonal and polyclonal (*5;* Figs. 1 and 2, this Chapter). This is not a result of local variations in the permeability of cells for the stain, but reflects a true fluctuation in the level of β-gal activity on a per-cell basis. However, as quantitation of β-gal is relatively inaccurate using this technique, with cultured cells the investigator is advised to utilize the FACS-gal method for more accurate quantitation.

2. Fixation of whole tissues is performed essentially as described (*19*). Briefly, fixation is prolonged for 1–2 h, and sodium deoxycholate and NP-40 are added to the fixative, to final concentrations of 0.01 and 0.02%, respectively, to enhance permeability of the tissue. In addition, tissues are incubated with X-gal stain at room temperature (ca. 25–28°C) instead of

37°C in order to reduce background staining and minimize tissue damage. The sodium deoxycholate and NP-40 can be included in the stain without any harmful effects. Ater development of color, which may take anywhere from 1 to 24 h, tissues are rinsed thoroughly (twice in PBS with 3% DMSO, then three times in 70% ethanol) prior to storage in 70% ethanol. These rinses are necessary to prevent hydrolysis of residual X-gal. We have found that the indigo precipitate can be removed from tissue sections by exposure to xylene. For this reason, it is essential to prepare tissues for sectioning either by freezing or by embedding in plastic (NOT in paraffin). It is also important to have negative controls for each tissue examined.

3. With certain tissues we have encountered problems with a high background resulting from nonspecific hydrolysis of the substrate that leads to weak false positives. For example, with a transgenic line expressing β-gal under control of the Rous sarcoma virus promoter, although expression of the β-gal gene could be detected in the testes of transgenics by Northern analysis, no difference could be detected in the intensity of blue color observed between transgenic and nontransgenic littermates' testes (G.R. MacGregor and P.A. Overbeek, unpublished observations). Certain tissues, for example, kidney, testes, spleen, and pancreas of the mouse, appear to have higher backgrounds of β-galactosidase activity than others.

4. Commercially available antibodies (from Promega Biotech, Madison, WI) have been shown to have greater sensitivity in the detection of *E. coli* β-gal activity than the X-gal stain *(5)*. We have found that the antibody (a mouse monoclonal) works well for detection of β-gal within cultured cells *(5)*, but has failed to detect the enzyme in serial tissue sections from transgenics expressing β-gal, as shown by the histochemical (X-gal) method.

5. The indigo precipitate prepared by the above procedure is electron-dense and can be clearly revealed by transmission electron microscopy (EM) *(29)*. It is therefore possible to obtain precise subcellular localization of β-gal fusion proteins. To prepare cells for EM, stain for X-gal as above. Carry out standard cell preparation of EM. However, since the precipitated indigo dye is soluble in propylene oxide (a general reagent used in the preparation of sections for transmission EM), transfer cells from 100% ethanol directly to resin without propylene oxide treatment.

6. We have been unable to detect β-gal immunocytochemically following treatment of the cells with X-gal.

7. The fixative described here works well for NIH 3T3 cells (*see* Fig. 1). However, for other cell types, alternative fixatives may give better retention of cell morphology.

4.4. FACS-Gal Analysis

1. Keep cells as healthy as experimental conditions permit. We routinely maintain cells in a mid-log growth state for 1–2 d prior to analysis. Certain cell types, especially adherent cells, such as 293 or NIH 3T3, appear to have higher than usual endogenous β-D-galactosidase activity if they are abused or allowed to go to confluency. However, it is possible to reduce this background with a chloroquine treatment prior to analysis (*see* Note 4).

2. No dependency on the cell concentration has been found for staining patterns (using concentrations ranging from 10^5/mL to 10^7/mL).

3. Phenylethyl-β-D-thiogalactoside (PETG) (1 mM) has been found to be an ideal competitive reversible inhibitor of *E.coli* β-gal in viable mammalian cells *(7,8)*. It has a low K_i (ca. 1 μM); thus very little is required to inhibit the reaction. The thiol ester bond renders the reagent practically nonhydrolyzable by the enzyme, thereby simplifying its influence on the kinetics of the FDG-to-fluorescein conversion. Finally, it is hydrophobic and can cross the cell membrane readily, even at 4°C.

   Dissolve PETG (Sigma cat. no. P-4902 and Molecular Probes P-1692) in H_2O to give a 50 mM stock. Filter-sterilize and dispense into 500 μL aliquots. Store frozen at –20°C. Adding PETG to a final concentration of 1 mM stops conversion of FDG to fluorescein in live cells. After a predetermined period of incubation on ice of cells loaded with FDG (from 1 min to 2 h, depending on expected β-gal activity), add 40 μL of the 50 mM PETG and mix thoroughly (1 mM PETG can be used directly in the ice-cold isotonic loading termination solution to inhibit the reaction at the same time FDG loading is completed). The reaction is slowed to such an extent by 1 mM PETG that there is almost no conversion of FDG to fluorescein over a 3-h period.

4. Using the FACS-gal method, most cell lines examined have exhibited little or no background activity from endogenous β-galactosidases. These include several B and T lymphocyte lines; splenic, thymic, peripheral, or bone marrow lymphocytes; most fibroblasts; and embryo carcinoma cells. However, several mammalian cell types, including macrophages and adherent lines (such as 293 and NIH 3T3), have significant endogenous β-galactosidase activity. This activity stems from lysosomal β-galactosidases. Since these β-galactosidases are most active at an acidic pH, they can be partially inactivated by pretreating cells for 20 min prior to loading FDG with 300 μM chloroquine (a weak lysosomotropic base) *(34)*. Chloroquine is added (to a final concentration of 300 μM) to the ice-cold isotonic "stop-loading" medium. Otherwise, the protocol for FACS-gal analysis is identical. Alternatively, cells can be treated with 300 μM

chloroquine added directly to culture medium with actively dividing cells 2–3 h prior to performing the FACS-gal analysis, with essentially similar results.

5. Some cell types, bacteria and yeast, for instance, cannot be hypotonically loaded because the cell wall constrains hypotonic expansion. To overcome this difficulty, it is possible to pretreat the cells with a brief *hypertonic* shock (to shrink the cells within their cell walls) and then to load the FDG with a subsequent hypotonic treatment. Osmotic conditions should be varied depending on the organism's resilience; it is also necessary to carry out viability tests to ensure that your procedure does not harm the cells.

6. Molecular Probes makes available two kits (F-1180 and F-1181) containing premixed, quality-controlled reagents and a detailed protocol to carry out the FACS-gal procedure.

Acknowledgments

GRM was the recipient of an Arthritis Foundation postdoctoral fellowship. We thank Dorothy Lewis for assisting with the FACS analysis and Paul Overbeek for assisting in the generation and analysis of transgenic mice. We thank Gina Jager, Catherine Tarlinton, Jefferey Johnsen, Katrina Waymire, Gerri Hanten, and Mick Kovac for technical assistance. GRM is a research associate of the Howard Hughes Medical Institute.

References

1. Casadaban, M. J., Martinez-Arias, A., Shapira, S. K., and Chou, J. (1983) β-galactosidase gene fusions for analysing gene expression in *E. coli* and yeast. *Methods Enzymol.* **100**, 293–308.

2. An, G., Hidaka, K., and Siminovitch, L. (1982) Expression of bacterial β-galactosidase in animal cells. *Mol. Cell Biol.* **2**, 1628–1632.

3. Hall, C. V., Jacob, P. E., Ringold, G. M., and Lee, F. (1983) Expression and regulation of *E. coli lacZ* gene fusions in mammalian cells. *Mol. Appl. Genet.* **2**, 101–109.

4. Nielsen, D. A., Chou, J., MacKrell, A. J., Casadaban, M. J., and Steiner, D. F. (1983) Expression of a pre-proinsulin-β-galactosidase gene fusion in mammalian cells. *Proc. Natl. Acad. Sci. USA* **80**, 5198–5202.

5. MacGregor, G. R., Mogg, A. E., Burke, J. F., and Caskey, C. T. (1987) Histochemical staining of clonal mammalian cell lines expressing *E. coli* β-Galactosidase indicates heterogeneous expression of the bacterial gene. *Somat. Cell Mol. Genet.* **13**, 253–265.

6. Nolan, G. P., Fiering, S., Nicolas, J.-F., and Herzenberg, L. A. (1988) Fluorescence-activated cell analysis and sorting of viable mammalian cells based on β-D-galactosidase activity after transduction of *E. coli LacZ*. *Proc. Natl. Acad. Sci. USA* **85**, 2603–2607.

7. Nolan, G. P. (1989) Individual cell gene regulation studies and *in situ* detection of transcriptionally-active chromatin using Fluorescence Activated Cell sorting with a viable cell fluorogenic assay. PhD Dissertation, Stanford University, Stanford, CA.

8. Kerr, W. G., Nolan, G. P., and Herzenberg, L. A. (1989) *In situ* detection of transcriptionally-active chromatin and genetic regulatory elements in individual viable mammalian cells. *Immunology* (in press).

9. Norton, P. A. and Coffin, J. M. (1985) Bacterial β-galactosidase as a marker of Rous sarcoma virus gene expresion and replication. *Mol. Cell Biol.* **5,** 281–290.

10. Pennock, G. D., Shoemaker, C., and Miller, L. K. (1984) Strong and regulated expression of *E. coli* β-galactosidase in insect cells with a baculovirus vector. *Mol. Cell Biol.* **4,** 399–406.

11. Fire, A. (1986) Integrative transformation of *Caenorhabditis elegans*. *EMBO J.* **5,** 2673–2680.

12. Goring, D. R., Rossant, J., Clapoff, S., Breitman, M. L., and Tsui, L.-C. (1987) In situ detection of β-galactosidase in lenses of transgenic mice with a γ-crystallin/*lacZ* gene. *Science* **235,** 456–458.

13. O'Kane, C. J. and Gehring, W. J. (1987) Detection in situ of genomic regulatory elements in *Drosophila*. *Proc. Natl. Acad. Sci. USA* **84,** 9123–9127.

14. Ghysen, A. and O'Kane, C. (1989) Neural enhancer like elements as specific cell markers in Drosophila. *Development* **105,** 35–52.

15. Lis, J. T., Simon, J. A., and Sutton, C. A. (1983) New heat shock puffs and β-galactosidase activity resulting from transformation of Drosophila with an *hsp70-lacZ* hybrid gene. *Cell* **35,** 403–410.

16. Bonnerot, C., Rocancourt, D., Briand, P., Grimber, G., and Nicolas, J.-F. (1987) A β-galactosidase hybrid protein targeted to nuclei as a marker for developmental studies. *Proc. Natl. Acad. Sci. USA* **84,** 6795–6799.

17. Allen, N. D., Cran, D. G., Barton, S. C., Hettle, S., Reik, W., and Surani, M. A. (1988) Transgenes as probes for active chromosomal domains in mouse development. *Nature* **333,** 852–855.

18. Kothary, R., Clapoff, S., Brown, A., Campbell, R., Peterson, A., and Rossant, J. (1988) A transgene containing *lacZ* inserted into the dystonia locus is expressed in neural tube. *Nature* **335,** 435–437.

19. Sanes, J. R., Rubenstein, J. L. R., and Nicolas, J.-F. (1986) Use of recombinant retrovirus to study post-implantation cell lineage in mouse embryos. *EMBO. J.* **5,** 3133–3142.

20. Kalmins, A., Otto, K., Ruther, U., and Muller-Hill, B. (1983) Sequence of the *lacZ* gene of *E. coli*. *EMBO. J.* **2,** 593–597.

21. Miller, J. H. (1972) Assay of β-galactosidase, in *Experiments in Molecular Genetics*, (J. H. Miller, ed.) Cold Spring Harbor Laboratory, Cold Spring Harbor, NY, pp. 352–355.

22. Bondi, A., Chieregatti, G., Eusebi, V., Fulcheri, E., and Bussolati, G. (1982) The use of β-galactosidase as a tracer in immunocytochemistry. *Histochemistry* **76,** 153–158.

23. Price, J., Turner, D., and Cepko, C. (1987) Lineage analysis in the vertebrate nervous system by retrovirus-mediated gene transfer. *Proc. Natl. Acad. Sci. USA* **84,** 156–160.

24. Chakrabarti, S., Brechling, K., and Moss, B. (1985) Vaccinia virus expression vector: Co-expression of β-galactosidase provides visual screening of recombinant virus plaques. *Mol. Cell Biol.* **5,** 3403–3409.

25. Geller, A. I. and Breaksfield, X. O. (1988) A defective HSV-1 vector expresses *E. coli* β-galactosidase in cultured peripheral neurons. *Science* **241,** 1667–1669.

26. Huang, C. H., Samsonoff, W. A., and Grzelecki, A. (1988) Vaccinia virus recombinants expressing an 11-kilodalton β-galactosidase fusion protein incorporates active β-galactosidase in virus particles. *J. Virol.* **62,** 3855–3861.

27. MacGregor, G. R. and Caskey, C. T. (1989) Construction of plasmids that express *E. coli* β-galactosidase in mammalian cells. *Nucleic Acids Res.* **17,** 2365.

28. Bradford, M. M. (1976) A rapid and sensitive method for the quantitation of microgramme quantities of protein utilizing the principle of protein-dye binding. *Analyt. Biochem.* **72,** 248–254.

29. Bonnerot, C., Rocancourt, D., Briand, P., Grimber, G., and Nicolas, J. F. (1987) A β-galactosidase hybrid protein targeted to nuclei as a marker for developmental studies. *Proc. Natl. Acad. Sci. USA* **84,** 6795–6799.

30. Parks, D. R., Lanier, L. L., and Herzenberg, L. A. (1986) Flow cytometry and fluorescence activated cell sorting (FACS), in *The Handbook of Experimental Immunology*, 4th Ed. (Weir, D. M. and Herzenberg, L. A., eds.) Blackwell, Edinburgh, pp. 29.1–29.21.

31. Alberti, S., Parks, D. R., and Herzenberg, L. A. (1988) A single laser method for subtraction of cell autofluorescence in flow cytometry. *Cytometry* **8,** 114–119.

32. Wallenfels, K. and Weil, R. (1972) β-Galactosidase, in *The Enzymes*, vol. 7, 3rd Ed. (Boyer, P., ed.) Academic, New York, pp. 617–663.

33. Hofmann, J. and Sernetz, M. (1983) A kinetic study on the enzymatic hydrolysis of fluorescein di-acetate and fluorescein-di-β-D galactopyranoside. *Anal. Biochem.* **131,** 180–186.

34. Ohkuma, S. and Poole, B. (1978) Fluorescence probe measurement of the intralysosomal pH in living cells and the perturbation of pH by various agents. *Proc. Natl. Acad. Sci. USA* **75,** 3327–3331.

Chapter 18

Application of the Firefly Luciferase Reporter Gene

Vincent Giguère

1. Introduction

Reporter genes have become powerful tools to study regulation of gene expression in eukaryotes. In particular, chimeric transcription units generated by the fusion of the appropriate DNA regulatory sequences to reporter genes have led to the identification of a great number of DNA control elements that constitute eukaryotic promoters. Recently, transcription factors that interact with specific DNA control elements have been purified and the cDNAs encoding these DNA-binding proteins have been cloned. Among these factors, the steroid hormone receptors have been shown to belong to a superfamily of transcription factors that regulate gene expression in a ligand-dependent fashion (1). The cloning of their respective cDNAs provided the opportunity to identify the functional domains for hormone binding, DNA binding, and transactivation present in these proteins. To perform these studies, we developed a screening assay that uses cultured cells transfected with two expression vectors (2). The first vector directs the expression of the wild-type or in vitro mutagenized receptor, and the second contains a reporter gene linked to a hormone-responsive promoter. Application of the hormone or a related synthetic drug activates the reporter gene, and the effects of the mutations on the ability of hormone/receptor complex to acti-

From: *Methods in Molecular Biology, Vol. 7: Gene Transfer and Expression Protocols*
Edited by: E. J. Murray © 1991 The Humana Press Inc., Clifton, NJ

vate gene expression can be assessed. Because of the large number of experiments to be performed in these studies, the use of chloramphenicol acetyl transferase (CAT) (originally used in our cotransfection assay) as a reporter gene proved to be both laborious and onerous. In contrast, the luciferase gene possesses intrinsic qualities that most other reporter genes lack greater sensitivity, ease of use, instantaneous quantification, "environment friendliness" (no radiolabeled compound or organic solvent is used in this assay), and cost efficiency. Here, the properties of the luciferase system are briefly discussed and a simple and rapid protocol used in my laboratory to assay luciferase activity in extract obtained from cultured mammalian cells transfected with a luciferase reporter gene.

The luciferase enzyme catalyzes the bioluminescence in the firefly by oxidizing D(–)luciferin in the presence of ATP, Mg^{2+}, and O_2. The reaction produces oxyluciferin, CO_2, and a photon. The level of light emitted during the reaction is measured with a luminometer. In presence of an excess of ATP, light emission peaks at 0.3 s and, therefore, an integration over a 10-s period is sufficient. Because the luciferase enzyme has a specific requirement for ATP, the assay can be performed in the presence of other nucleosides without interference.

The firefly luciferase is composed of a single polypeptide, and the cDNA and gene encoding the protein have been cloned from the firefly *Photinus pyralis (3)*. Since the full-length cDNA was not cloned, de Wet and colleagues have created a hybrid luciferase gene by fusing part of the first exon obtained from a genomic clone to the remainder of the coding sequence from the cDNA. This hybrid luciferase gene can then be linked to the promoter of interest. A series of vectors that contain multiple cloning sites upstream of the luciferase gene has recently been engineered to facilitate the insertion of promoter sequences *(4)*. To date, the luciferase gene has proved to be functional in a variety of cell types derived from organisms ranging from yeast to humans *(5)*. The protocol described below has been optimized for the assay of luciferase activity in extracts prepared from mammalian cells.

2. Materials

1. PBS (phosphate-buffered saline, without Mg^{2+} or Ca^{2+}): 8.0 g NaCl, 0.2 g KCl, 5 g Na_2HPO_4, 0.2 g KH_2PO_4 per L of distilled H_2O.
2. Lysis buffer: 1% Triton X-100; 0.1 M KH_2PO_4, pH 7.8; 1 mM dithiothreitol (DTT).
3. 10 mM D(–)luciferin stock solution in 0.1M KH_2PO_4, pH 7.8. Keep in the dark at –20°C.

4. 1M K$_2$HPO$_4$, pH 7.8.
5. 0.1M ATP.
6. 0.1M MgCl$_2$.
7. Double-distilled H$_2$O (ddH$_2$O).
8. Luminometer.

3. Methods

1. Target cells (transfected using one of the techniques described in previous chapters) are washed twice with PBS (3 mL/60-mm tissue-culture dish). Cells grown in suspension, or that do not attached well to plastic, can be centrifuged and resuspended in PBS.
2. Add 1 mL PBS/dish and scrape the cells off the plate with a rubber policeman. Transfer the cells to an Eppendorf tube.
3. As soon as possible, centrifuge the cells for 15 s in a microcentrifuge, remove the supernatant, and resuspend the cell pellet in 100 µL of lysis buffer by pipeting up and down rapidly (*see* Note 1).
4. Spin for 5 min at 12,000g in a microcentrifuge at 4°C to pellet the cellular debris.
5. Transfer the supernatant to a new Eppendorf tube. The crude cell extract may be assayed immediately or stored at −20°C (*see* Note 2).
6. To perform the luciferase activity assay, the following reaction cocktail should be made fresh immediately before sampling analysis:

1M K$_2$HPO$_4$	5 µL
0.1M ATP	2.5 µL
0.1M MgCl$_2$	5 µL
ddH$_2$O	32.5 µL
total/sample	45 µL

7. Prepare a 1 mM D(−)luciferin solution in 0.1 M K$_2$HPO$_4$ from the stock solution described above, taking into account that 100 µL/sample is needed plus 1 mL (amount may vary depending on the make of the instrument) to preload the luminometer. The substrate should be kept in the dark until use (*see* Note 3).
8. Pipet 5 µL of crude cell extract into a test tube, add 45 µL of reaction cocktail, mix well, load into luminometer, inject 100 µL D(−)luciferin solution, and read the light emission. The assay is performed at room temperature, or around 25°C (*see* Notes 4–7).

4. Notes

1. The amount of cell extract used in the assay can be varied depending on the level of luciferase activity present. If needed, the extract can be diluted in lysis buffer or the quantity of H_2O in the cocktail in step 6 changed to accommodate more extract. However, the amount of lysis buffer in the reaction cocktail should be kept constant within a single experiment.

2. The luciferase enzyme activity present in cell extract decreases rapidly when stored at room temperature, but is stable for about a month at 4°C and for several weeks when frozen at –20°C or below. The enzyme is also unstable at extreme pH, therefore the assay should always be performed at a pH between 7.3 and 8.0 (pH 7.8 is optimal).

3. The substrate D(–)luciferin will not dissolve in water. Always prepare the stock solution of luciferin in the KH_2PO_4 buffer.

4. For cell lysis, has two advantages using Triton X-100 rather than the widely used freeze-thaw method: rapidity, since the cells lyse immediately upon addition of the lysis buffer, and enhanced light emission, since Triton X-100 increases the turnover of the enzyme-product complex *(6, 7)*.

5. It is possible to evaluate the absolute amount of enzyme being produced in the transfected cells by calibrating the luminometer periodically with a reliable source of purified luciferase of known specific activity.

6. To provide an internal control for transfection efficiency when comparing the efficacy of various expression vectors within an experiment, a second reporter gene under the control of a general promoter can be transfected along with the luciferase gene. We routinely use the *E. coli*, β-galactosidase gene (*see* Chapter 17) driven by the Rous Sarcoma virus-long terminal repeat. Transfected cell extracts assayed for both luciferase and β-galactosidase activity allows the derivation of a corrected value for each distinct construct.

7. Preferentially, the luminometer should be equipped with an automated injector to improve reproducibility of the assay and with an overload protector to prevent damage to the photomultiplier tube. Lists of commercial suppliers of available firefly luciferase reagents and luminometers have recently been compiled *(8, 9)*.

References

1. Evans, R. M. (1988) The steroid and thyroid hormone receptor superfamily. *Science* **240**, 889–895.
2. Giguère, V., Hollenberg, S. H., Rosenfeld, M. G., and Evans, R.M. (1986) Functional domains of the human glucocorticoid receptor. *Cell* **46**, 645–652.

3. de Wet, J.R., Wood, K. V., DeLuca, M., Helinski, D. R., and Subramani, S. (1987) Firefly luciferase gene: structure and expression in mammalian cells. *Mol. Cell. Biol.* **7**, 725–737.

4. Nordeen, K. (1988) Luciferase reporter gene vectors for analysis of promoters and enhancers. *BioTechniques* **6**, 454–456.

5. Subramani, S. and DeLuca, M. (1988) Applications of the firefly luciferase as a reporter gene. *Genetic Engineering* (Setlow, J. K., ed.), vol. 10, Plenum, New York, pp. 75–89.

6. Kricka, L. J. and DeLuca, M. A. (1982) Effects of solvents on catalytic activity of firefly luciferase. *Arch. Biochem. Biophys.* **217**, 674–681.

7. Williams, T. M., Burlein, J. E., Ogden, S., Kricka, L. J., and Kant, J. A. (1989) Advantages of firefly luciferase as a reporter gene: Application to the interleukin-2 gene promoter. *Anal. Biochem.* **176**, 26–32.

8. Van Dyke, K. (1985) *Bioluminescence and Chemiluminescence: Instruments and Applications* (Van Dike, K., ed.), vol. I, CRC, Boca Raton, FL, pp. 83–128.

9. Leach, F. R. and Webster, J. J. (1986) Commercially available firefly luciferase reagents, in *Bioluminescence and Chemiluminescence* (Part B) (DeLuca, M. and McElroy, W. D., eds.), *Methods in Enzymology*, vol. 133, Academic, Orlando, FL, pp. 51–70.

Section 4
Selection Techniques for Generating Stably Transfected Cell Lines

Use of Vectors to Confer Resistance to Antibiotics G418 and Hygromycin in Stably Transfected Cell Lines

Robert F. Santerre, Jenna D. Walls,
and Brian W. Grinnell

1. Introduction

The development of dominant selection markers to identify eukaryotic cells that have undergone a gene transformation event has greatly facilitated molecular genetic studies in higher eukaryotic cells. Selection schemes based on resistance to antibiotic cytotoxicity *(1,2)* will be described in this chapter. Other schemes—for example, based on resistance to inhibition of DNA synthesis by methotrexate *(3)* or mycophenolic acid *(4)*—are described in other chapters of this book. Prior to the development of dominant selection markers, the use of recessive markers, such as thymidine kinase *(TK)* or hypoxanthine-guanine phosphoribosyl transferase (HGPT) was limited to a handful of mutant cell lines that were *TK⁻* or HGPT⁻ *(5,6)*. If one wished to transfect a wild-type cell line, one had first to select a recessive mutant derivative cell line and characterize it before proceeding with the experiments of interest. Such restrictions posed a significant barrier to molecular genetic analyses in higher eukaryotic cells.

In microbial systems, genetic analysis has been greatly facilitated by the use of antibiotic resistance markers. Many of these markers were isolated

From: *Methods in Molecular Biology, Vol. 7: Gene Transfer and Expression Protocols*
Edited by: E. J. Murray © 1991 The Humana Press Inc., Clifton, NJ

from bacteria as autonomously replicating plasmid DNA molecules carrying genes for resistance to antibiotics, e.g., neomycin *(neo)* and kanamycin (Km) *(7)*. Resistance genes often code for enzymes that can chemically modify an antibiotic (e.g., by acetylation or phosphorylation), rendering it inactive. As an outgrowth of academic and industrial efforts to identify, characterize, and develop medically useful antibiotics (e.g., neomycin, gentamicin), a number of closely related derivatives with significant cytotoxicity in eukaryotes (e.g., G418) were identified *(8)*. Parallel work to clone the antibiotic resistance gene, Tn5, coding for neomycin phosphotransferase *(9)* and to clone and characterize the herpes simplex virus thymidine kinase gene *(10)* generated the necessary starting materials to enable construction of the first plasmid vector conferring antibiotic resistance to G418 in mammalian cell cultures *(1)*.

G418 and hygromycin B are aminoglycoside antibiotics produced by streptomycetes. The cytotoxicity of both antibiotics is based on inhibition of protein synthesis *(11,12)*. Hygromycin B has been shown to block translocation and stimulate misreading *(11)*. As stated above, G418 can be inactivated by phosphorylation. Hygromycin is similarly inactivated by phosphorylation *(2)*; however, the two phosphotransferase enzymes are quite specific and show no crossreactivity. Thus, it is possible to perform simultaneous or sequential drug selections employing both resistance markers. Both antibiotics exhibit broad specificity in prokaryotes and in eukaryotes as diverse as yeast and mammals. Although mammalian cells contain numerous phosphorylating activities, none are antibiotic-specific. In addition, antibiotic resistant mutants have not been identified in higher eukaryotic cells, although the level of drug tolerance can vary widely, presumably related to rates of metabolic turnover and drug transport.

The DNA transfection and antibiotic selection procedures described below are based on methods originally described by Graham and van der Eb *(13)*, Colbere-Garapin et al. *(1)* and Santerre et al. *(2)*.

2. Materials

2.1. Plasmid Vectors

Since the initial reports describing the use of these dominant antibiotic resistance selections in mammalian cells *(1,2)*, a variety of vectors employing different 5' and 3' regulatory elements have been constructed, many of which are now distributed to the scientific community by the American Type Culture Collection, Rockville, MD. Table 1 lists examples of some of these vectors and their important characteristics. Two vectors based on SV40 virus early promoter elements are shown in Fig. 1. The pSV2-*neo* vector has been described

Table 1
Examples of Plasmid and Viral Vectors
Utilizing Either G418 or Hygromycin Resistance as Selectable Markers

Vector	Type	Source
pRSV-*neo*	Integrative; Rous sarcoma virus promotor	ATCC[a]
pPB3	Integrative; SV*neo*, λ cos packaging sequences	ref. *16*
pDE104	Integrative; actin 15 promoter from Dictyostelium, *hyg*	ref. *17*
pMC1*Neo*	Integrative; polyoma enhancer, TK*neo*	ref. *18*
pTK-*hyg*	Integrative; *TK* promoter	ref. *19*
pRP-cneoX	Episomal, BK virus replicon; SV*neo.*	ref. *20*
p201	Episomal, Epstein-Barr virus replicon; TK*hyg*	ref. *21*
pTG4	Episomal, Bovine papilloma virus replicon; mouse metallothionein promoter, *hyg*	ref. *22*
pdBPV-MMT*neo*	Episomal, Bovine papilloma virus replicon; mouse metallothionein promotor, *neo*	ATCC
pSB302	Viral, M-MuLV, helper-free virus production in ψ-2 cells; polyoma promoter/origin, *neo*	ref. *23*
pJDT277	Viral, rescued with adeno-associated helper virus; *TKneo*	ref. *24*
pZIP-NeoSV(X)1	Viral, M-MuLV, helper-free virus production in ψ-2 cells; LTR promotor	ref. *25*
pLψPL-*neo*	Viral, Akv-MuLV, helper-free virus production in ψ-2 cells; LTR promoter	ref. *26*
MMCV-*neo*	Viral, M-MuLV, helper-free virus production in ψ-2 cells; *TKneo*	ref. *27*

[a]American Type Culture Collection, Rockville, MD.

(*14*). The pSV2-*hyg* vector was constructed by A. Smith (*15*) and can be obtained from P. Berg (Department of Biochemistry, Stanford University School of Medicine, Stanford, CA 94305-5425).

2.2. Cell Lines

Both the *hyg* and *neo* genes can be used as dominant selectable markers in a number of different cell lines. A partial list of cells that we have successfully transformed by this technique includes hamster cell lines (CHO, BHK-21), mouse cell lines (S180, Ltk⁻), monkey cell lines (CV-1, MK2) and human cell lines (HeLa, 293). Cells should be in exponential growth stage for selection (optimally, no more than 50% confluent [~1 × 10⁶ cells/100-mm plate] at the time of transfection).

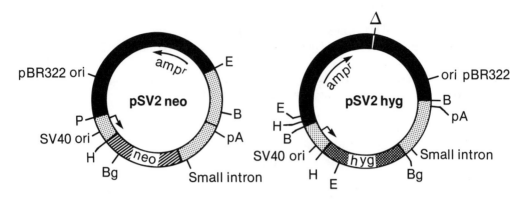

Fig. 1. Diagram of the general structure and gene components for pSV2*neo* and pSV2*hyg* plasmids. Both plasmids contain pBR322 sequences (filled segment) for a bacterial origin of replication (pBR322 ori) and an ampicillin resistance marker (*amp*) to enable propagation in *E. coli*. SV40 virus sequences (stippled segments) provide eukaryotic regulatory elements for transcription (⤻, early promoter), donor and acceptor sites for intron splicing (small intron), a poly A addition signal (pA), and an origin of replication (SV40 ori) requiring T-antigen for activity. Hatched segment, neomycin phosphotransferase *(neo)*; cross-hatched segment, hygromycin B phosphotransferase *(hyg)*; Δ, deletion of pBR322 nucleotides 1095–2485, creating the "poison sequence"-minus pML vector; B, BamHI; Bg, BglII; E, EcoRI; H, HindIII; P, PvuII.

2.3. Solutions and Reagents for DNA Transfection

1. 2× HEBS: 16.0 g NaCl, 0.74 g KCl, 0.19 g anhydrous Na_2HPO_4 (or 0.25 g $Na_2HPO_4 \cdot 2H_2O$), 10.0 g HEPES, distilled H_2O to 1 L. Adjust pH to 7.08 with $5M$ NaOH (1× will be 7.05). Filter-sterilize through a .22-µm membrane, aliquot, and store at –20°C.

2. $2M$ $CaCl_2$: 29.41 g $CaCl_2 \cdot H_2O$, distilled H_2O to 100 mL. Filter-sterilize as above, aliquot, and store at –20°C.

3. Plasmid DNA: CsCl-purified plasmid DNA precipitated in 70% ethanol (final concentration)/0.3M sodium acetate, dried and resuspended in sterile distilled H_2O.

4. Salmon-sperm or calf-thymus DNA resuspended in sterile dH_2O.

Avoid repeated freeze-thawing of solutions. Both 2× HEBS and $2M$ $CaCl_2$ will remain stable at 4°C for several months, but aliquots should be frozen for long term storage. DNA solutions may be stored at 4°C.

2.4. Drug Selection

1. G418 sulfate (Geneticin®) may be purchased from GIBCO Laboratories Life Technologies, Inc. (No. 860-1811). Hygromycin B may be purchased from Boehringer Mannheim Biochemicals (No. 843-555).

2. A 1000× hygromycin B stock solution (typically 200 mg/mL) may be made up in H_2O, filter-sterilized through a 0.22-μm membrane, and stored in aliquots at –20°C. Frozen stock solutions remain stable for several months. Stability in media stored at 4°C is at least equivalent to that of other labile media components (e.g., serum).

   CAUTION: Hygromycin B is toxic and can be absorbed into the body if contact is made with the eyes and/or skin. The compound can cause severe and permanent damage to the eyes, and moderate skin irritation. Wear impermeable gloves, skin covering, goggles, and an approved dust/mist respirator, especially when handling the powder.

3. G418 may be dissolved as a 100× stock in H_2O (typically 50 mg/mL), and sterilized by filtering through a 0.22-μm membrane. Because Geneticin® is supplied with approx 50% potency, the purity of the product must be taken into consideration when making stock solutions. Aliquots of stock solution may be stored at –20°C. G418 is stable in media stored at 4°C for 1–2 mo.

4. The addition of G418 to medium tends to lower the pH, whereas addition of hygromycin tends to raise the pH. Medium with sufficient buffering capacity should be used, or appropriate adjustment of the pH made with CO_2 or sodium bicarbonate.

2.5. Solutions and Reagents for Cell Culture

1. Medium requirements can vary from cell line to cell line, but this should not affect either the transfection or selection protocol. A formulation suitable for maintenance of the cell line of choice should be used. For the majority of cell lines we work with, we have used Dulbecco's Modified Eagle's Medium with high glucose (4500 mg/L) supplemented with 10% fetal calf serum and 50.0 μg/mL gentamicin.

2. 0.5% methylene blue: 0.5 g of powder dissolved in 100 mL of 50% methanol.

3. PBS: Dulbecco's phosphate-buffered saline, Ca^{2+}, Mg^{2+} free.

4. DMSO: Spectro-grade dimethyl sulfoxide sterilized by autoclaving for 20 min.

3. Methods

3.1. Determination of Drug Killing Curve

The amount of drug required for selection may vary with a number of factors, including cell type. The optimal concentration of drug required to select and maintain transformed cells must be determined for each cell type.

In practice, one needs only to determine the minimal concentration of drug required to kill all cells in the population. Generally, the effective concentration of both hygromycin and G418 is less in serum-free growth medium.

1. Prepare a single cell suspension at a concentration of 3.0×10^5 cells/mL in growth medium. Plate two 6-well (35-mm) tissue-culture plates containing 3 mL growth medium/well with 1 mL of cell suspension/well and incubate at 37°C overnight.

2. Prepare a series of twofold increasing concentrations of either hygromycin from 50 to 800 µg/mL, or G418 from 75 µg/mL to 1.2 mg/mL, in growth medium.

3. Aspirate medium from wells and add 4 mL of each concentration of selective medium/well in duplicate. Add growth medium without drug to one set of wells. Incubate at 37°C for colony formation.

4. When colonies have grown to approx 1–3 mm in diameter, aspirate medium, rinse wells with 2 mL of PBS/well, and stain colonies. Add 1 mL/well of 0.5% methylene blue for 20 min. Rinse with water to remove excess stain and air-dry.

The lowest drug concentration resulting in 100% kill is the dose required for selection. The drug concentrations used in this protocol may need to be adjusted for particularly sensitive or resistant cell lines.

3.2. DNA Transfection Protocol

1. One day prior to transfection, seed 100-mm tissue-culture plates with 1.0×10^6 cells/plate. If cells have a low plating efficiency, seeding an extra set of plates at a higher density (2.0×10^6) will help ensure a cell monolayer at the correct density for transfection. Likewise, if cells are particularly large in size or rapidly growing, plating a set at lower density (5.0×10^5) may be necessary to obtain the desired 50% confluency at time of transfection. Incubate the cells overnight.

2. A DNA/calcium phosphate coprecipitate is prepared using a modified version of the Wigler protocol (5) (*see also* Chapter 2, this vol). One milliliter of final precipitate will be required for each 100-mm plate. A mock precipitate with either salmon-sperm or calf-thymus DNA carrier or no DNA should be prepared as a control. Prepare one tube containing a 2× DNA/CaCl$_2$ solution by adding sterile distilled H$_2$O, plasmid DNA, or plasmid DNA plus carrier DNA (20–40 µg/mL final), and a 1:8 dilution of 2M CaCl$_2$ (250 mM final), in that order. Prepare a second tube containing an equal vol of 2× HEBS solution.

3. Insert a 1-mL sterile pipet (cotton-plugged) attached to an automated pipetor into the 2× HEBS solution and gently blow air bubbles through the solution while adding, drop by drop, the 2× DNA/CaCl$_2$ solution.
4. Let the solution stand 15–45 min at room temperature until a fine precipitate forms. Tubes should be of clear polystyrene to facilitate detection of precipitate formation. DNA concentration in the final mix is 10–20 µg/mL.
5. Mix precipitate gently with a pipet and add 1 mL of the suspension directly to each 100-mm plate containing 10 mL of growth medium covering the cell monolayer. Incubate at 37°C for 4 h, then aspirate medium and add 10 mL of fresh growth medium.

Critical aspects of this procedure, which should be followed explicitly, are the pH adjustment of the 2× HEBS solution and the time for formation of the precipitate. The DNA/calcium phosphate precipitate should appear as a slightly cloudy solution. Heavier precipitates with large visible particles can form with longer standing times. We have obtained lower transformation efficiencies with DNA mixtures containing heavy precipitates. A final concentration of 5–20 µg DNA/mL is required for optimal DNA precipitation. This concentration may be made up entirely of plasmid DNA or of plasmid plus carrier DNA if vector concentrations are low. Plasmid DNA concentration can also affect transformation efficiency. Optimal DNA concentration can be determined empirically for a specific plasmid vector and a specific cell line.

3.3. Drug Selection Protocol

1. Forty-eight to 72 hours after transfection, aspirate medium from plates and add 10 mL of growth medium containing the selective drug at a concentration determined by the killing curve. As indicated above, the cell monolayer should be subconfluent, i.e., in growth phase. Incubate and change medium every 2–3 d until the majority of the cell layer sloughs off. Continue feeding the plates once a week until colonies appear, and grow to 1–3 mm in diameter. This usually requires 2–3 wk with hygromycin selection and 3–4 wk with G418 selection.

   Selection with both G418 and hygromycin is most efficient when the cells are growing at their optimum. If, when adding selecting medium, the cell monolayer is confluent, it may be necessary to replate the cells at a lower density before adding the drug. This is particularly important when using G418 since nongrowing, e.g., contact-inhibited, cells are much more resistant to this drug than are actively growing cells. Because of its greater cytotoxicity, this is less of a problem with hygromycin selection. The decision to replate cells rather than apply selection to the original plate will depend on the growth characteristics of the cell line and its sensitivity to the selective drug. It should be kept in mind that, when cells are replated, the number of colonies eventually obtained will not represent independent transforming events, but will include a number of sister clones. Therefore, to minimize the number of sister colonies, it is desirable to replate cells directly in selecting medium within 24–48 h of transfection.

2. When colonies have reached the appropriate size (1–3 mm) they can be isolated and transferred to 24-well plates. With a black marker or grease pencil, draw a circle on the bottom of the tissue-culture plate around the clones to be transferred. Aspirate the colonies using a micropipet or a similar device set at 150 µL as follows: On a sterile surface, such as a plastic tissue-culture dish, bend the end of the pipet tip so that it forms an angle (~45°). While scraping the tip within the circled area, draw up the cells and medium, and transfer to a well containing 2 mL of selection medium. Continue picking clones in this manner, using a clean (and sterile) tip for each clone until a sufficient number have been collected. Clones also may be isolated using cloning rings as described (28).

Maintain cells on selection while subculturing and characterizing isolated transformants.

3.4. Storage of Drug-Resistant Lines

Drug-resistant cell lines can be stored in liquid nitrogen using the same standard protocols used to store the nontransfected parent line. Typically, we use a freeze medium containing 10% DMSO/90% fetal bovine serum, but no selective drug. When recovering cells from frozen storage, it is best to replate the thawed cells in medium without the selective drug for 24 h. Certain cells can be replated into selection medium immediately upon thawing, but we find that some cells require a short period of growth to allow for expression of the drug-resistance gene prior to the addition of drug.

4. Notes

1. Because the transcriptional efficiency of many eukaryotic promoters differs in different cell lines, the regulatory region chosen to drive the expression of the selectable marker can influence the transformation efficiency. For example, Thomas and Capecchi (18) have shown that the transformation efficiency with G418 selection in murine ES cells was 12–

16-fold greater if the *neo* gene was driven by the SV40 early promoter/ enhancer than if driven by the RSV LTR. Often, the efficiency of transformation is not critical if one simply wants to isolate a sufficient number of transformants to obtain a desired cell line. However, if high efficiency is required, the best promoter to drive expression of the selectable marker in a particular host cell can be determined using a reporter gene, as described in Section 3 of this vol.

2. To introduce a nonselectable gene into a host cell, the gene of interest can be introduced either by cotransfection with an independent vector containing the dominant selectable marker or by linking both genes on a multicistronic vector, i.e., one containing both the selectable and nonselectable genes or cDNAs, each with appropriate 5' and 3' regulatory signals. Although reasonably high frequencies of cointroduction of the nonselectable cistron(s) can be achieved by cotransfection of the selectable and nonselectable genes on separate plasmids (10–30%), a higher percentage of drug-resistant transformants, which also contain the nonselectable plasmid, can be obtained if the two plasmids are linearized by digestion with compatible restriction enzymes and ligated prior to transfection. We have found that ligation in a ratio of 1:5 or 1:10, selectable plasmid to plasmid with the nonselectable gene of interest results in cointroduction efficiencies as high as 90%. In most cells, the transformation efficiency is higher with linearized plasmids than with closed circular plasmids. Linking the gene of interest and the selectable marker, either through the construction of multicistronic plasmids or by simply ligating the two plasmids prior to a cotransfection, optimizes the retention of the gene of interest with the serial subculture of the drug-resistant line. This is especially true in heteroploid cells.

3. In the example above, we have used the calcium phosphate method for introducing the plasmid containing the selectable marker into the cell. As described in Section 1 of this vol, there are many techniques available for the introduction of genes into mammalian cells. Techniques such as electroporation, DEAE-dextran, microinjection, or liposome and protoplast fusion have been used successfully to introduce selectable markers into a variety of mammalian cells. In general, one should use the transfection technique that is most efficient for the host cell being used. Transformation efficiency can be enhanced in some cells by treatment with chloroquine or sodium butyrate, or by glycerol shock (also described in Section 1 of this vol; for example, Chapter 3).

4. To obtain optimal transformation efficiency, it is best to use DNA of high purity. We recommend using DNA that has been purified twice by

Table 2
Transformation Efficiencies Using Hygromcyin and G418 Selection
in the S180 Mouse Sarcoma Cell Line[a]

Plasmid	No. of cells/plate[b]	Drug colonies/ plate/10 µg DNA, mean (no. of dishes)	Transformation efficiency/ 10 µg DNA
pSV2-*neo*	7.3×10^5	210 (6)	2.9×10^{-4}
pSV2-*hyg*	7.3×10^5	4.1 (19)	5.6×10^{-6}
pTK-*hyg*	7.3×10^5	28.7 (20)	3.9×10^{-5}

[a]Cells were seeded at 5×10^5 cells/100-mm plate 16 h prior to transfection with the various plasmid DNAs. Drug selection was applied 24 h posttransfection (400 µg hygromycin/ mL or 500 µg G418/mL). The number of drug-resistant colonies was determined 19 d posttransfection.
[b]Average number of cells/plate at the time of plasmid DNA transfection.

CsCl-gradient ultracentrifugation. However, if high efficiency is not necessary, even relatively crude plasmid DNA can be used, such as that obtained from rapid-isolation techniques *(29)*.

5. Selection with G418 is more efficient than selection with hygromycin in all cells that we have examined. As an example, we have compared the transformation efficiencies using both G418 and hygromycin selection in the S180 mouse sarcoma cell line. With pSV2-*neo* and pSV2-*hyg,* both of which utilize the SV40 early promoter/enhancer, the transformation efficiency was 50-fold higher with G418 than with hygromycin selection (Table 2). However, the difference in efficiency between the two dominant selection markers is not this great in other cell lines, which show differences of approx five- to tenfold. Also in Table 2, we show that the transformation efficiency of pTK-*hyg,* which utilizes the herpes simplex virus *TK* promoter, was seven times higher than that of pSV2-*hyg.* These data emphasize the effect of choosing the optimal promoter for driving the expression of the selectable marker in a specific cell line. If efficiency is not critical, hygromycin selection has the advantage of killing cells more rapidly than G418. In addition, the drug is available in pure form.

6. If it is desirable to introduce multiple nonselectable genes into a cell by cotransfection with selectable markers, it is possible to use simultaneously selection with both hygromycin and G418. Alternatively, hygromycin clones can be isolated and used as host cells for sequential transformation and selection with plasmids conferring G418, or vice versa.

7. In general, stably transformed cells selected for either G418 or hygromycin resistance will maintain the plasmid sequences in the absence of drug

selection for as many as 50–75 cell doublings. This has been true even for extremely heteroploid cells, for example, the adenovirus-transformed human 293 cell line.

References

1. Colbere-Garapin, F., Horodniceanu, F., Kourilsky, P., and Garapin, A.-C. (1981) A new dominant hybrid selective marker for higher eukaryotic cells. *J. Mol. Biol.* **150,** 1–14.

2. Santerre, R. F., Allen, N. E., Hobbs, Jr., J. N., Rao, R. N., and Schmidt, R. J. (1984) Expression of prokaryotic genes for hygromycin B and G418 resistance as dominant-selection markers in mouse L cells. *Gene* **30,** 147–156.

3. Simonsen, C. C. and Levinson, A. D. (1983) Isolation and expression of an altered mouse dihydrofolate reductase cDNA. *Proc. Natl. Acad. Sci. USA* **80,** 2495–2499.

4. Mulligan, R. C. and Berg, P. (1981) Selection for animal cells that express the *Escherichia coli* gene coding for xanthine-guanine phosphoribosyltransferase. *Proc. Natl. Acad. Sci. USA* **78,** 2072–2076.

5. Wigler, M., Silverstein, S., Lee, L.-S., Pellicer, A., Cheng, Y.-C., and Axel, R. (1977) Transfer of purified herpes virus thymidine kinase gene to cultured mouse cells. *Cell* **11,** 223–232.

6. Graf, Jr., L. H., Urlaub, G., and Chasin, L. A. (1979) Transformation of the gene for hypoxanthine phosphoribosyltransferase. *Som. Cell Genet.* **5,** 1031–1044.

7. Davies, J. E. and Kagan, S. A. (1981) Aminoglycoside antibiotics: General aspects and resistance, in *New Trends in Antibiotic Research and Therapy* (Grassi, G. G. and Sabath, L. D., eds.), Elsevier/North Holland Biomedical, Amsterdam, pp. 83–94.

8. Daniels, P. J. L., Yehaskel, A. S., and Morton, J. B. (1973) The structure of antibiotic G-418. Abstr. 137, *13th Interscience Conference on Antimicrobial Agents and Chemotherapy*, Washington, DC.

9. Jorgensen, R. A., Rothstein, S. J., and Reznikoff, W. S. (1979) A restriction enzyme cleavage map of Tn 5 and location of a region encoding neomycin resistance. *Mol. Gen. Genet.* **177,** 65–72.

10. Colbere-Garapin, F., Chousterman, S., Horodniceanu, F., Kourilsky, P., and Garapin, A.-C. (1979) Cloning of the thymidine kinase gene of herpes simplex virus type 1 in *Escherichia coli* K-12. *Proc. Natl. Acad. Sci. USA* **76,** 3755–3759.

11. Gonzalez, A., Jimenez, A., Vazquez, D., Davies, J. E., and Schindler, D. (1978) Studies on the mode of action of hygromycin B, an inhibitor of translocation in eukaryotes. *Biochem. Biophys. Acta* **521,** 459–469.

12. Jimenez, A. and Davies, J. (1980) Expression of a transposable antibiotic resistance element in *Saccharomyces*. *Nature* **287,** 869–871.

13. Graham, F. L. and van der Eb, A. J. (1973) A new technique for the assay of infectivity of human adenovirus 5 DNA. *Virology* **52,** 456–467.

14. Southern, P. J. and Berg, P. (1982) Transformation of mammalian cells to antibiotic resistance with a bacterial gene under control of the SV40 early region promoter. *J. Mol. Appl. Genet.* **1,** 327–341.

15. Smith, A. and Berg, P. Personal communication.

16. Ghosh-Choudhury, G., Haj-Ahmad, Y., Brinkley, P., Rudy, J., and Graham, F. L. (1986) Human adenovirus cloning vectors based on infectious bacterial plasmids. *Gene* **50,** 161–171.

256 Santerre, Walls, and Grinnell

17. Egelhoff, T. T., Brown, S. S., Manstein, D. J., and Spudich, J. A. (1989) Hygromycin resistance as a selectable marker in *Dictyostelium discoideum*. *Mol. Cell. Biol.* **9,** 1965–1968.
18. Thomas, K. R. and Capecchi, M. R. (1987) Site-directed mutagenesis by gene targeting in mouse embryo-derived stem cells. *Cell* **51,** 503–512.
19. Santerre, R., unpublished results.
20. Grossi, M. P., Caputo, A., Rimessi, P., Chiccoli, L., Balboni, P. G., and Barbanti-Brodano, G. (1988) New BK virus episomal vector for complementary DNA expression in human cells. *Arch. Virol.* **102,** 275–283.
21. Yates, J. L., Warren, N., and Sudgen, B. (1985) Stable replication of plasmids derived from Epstein-Barr virus in various mammalian cells. *Nature* **313,** 812–815.
22. McAllister, W. T., SUNY Health Science Center, Brooklyn, NY (personal communication).
23. Berger, S. A. and Bernstein, A. (1985) Characterization of a retroviral shuttle vector capable of either proviral integration or extrachromosomal replication in mouse cells. *Mol. Cell. Biol.* **5,** 305–312.
24. Tratschin, J.-D., Miller, I. L., Smith, M. G., and Carter, B. J. (1985) Adeno-associated virus vector for high-frequency integration, expression, and rescue of genes in mammalian cells. *Mol. Cell. Biol.* **5,** 3251–3260.
25. Cepko, C. L., Roberts, B. E., and Mulligan, R. C. (1984) Construction and applications of a highly transmissible murine retrovirus shuttle vector. *Cell* **37,** 1053–1062.
26. Jensen, N. A., Jorgensen, P., Kjeldgaard, N. O., and Pedersen, F. S. (1986) Mammalian expression-and-transmission vector derived from Akv murine leukemia virus. *Gene* **41,** 59–65.
27. Stewart, C. L., Schuetze, S., Vanek, M., and Wagner, E. F. (1987) Expression of retroviral vectors in transgenic mice obtained by embryo infection. *EMBO J.* **6,** 383–388.
28. Merchant, D. J., Kahn, R. H., and Murphy, W. H. (1964) Cell culture techniques, in *Handbook of Cell and Organ Culture* (Burgess Publishing Co., Minneapolis, MN), pp. 52–58.
29. Birnboim, H. C. and Doly, J. (1979) A rapid alkaline extraction procedure for screening recombinant plasmid DNA. *Nucleic Acids Res.* **7,** 1513–1523.

CHAPTER 20

Selection of Cells Defective in Pyrimidine (TK⁻) and Purine (APRT⁻ and HPRT⁻) Salvage

Development of Host Strains Appropriate for Transfection

Mark Meuth and Janet Harwood

1. Introduction

The usefulness of the purine and pyrimidine salvage pathways in the study of the mechanisms of mutation and in the selection of cell lines stably transformed by vectors expressing these genes is well documented. Unfortunately, many investigators are deterred from selecting new host strains deficient in these enzymes because of the difficulties inherent in isolating recessive mutations of autosomal genes. Furthermore, considerable suspicion was cast over somatic cell genetics by the so-called epigenetic nature of some phenotypic changes (1). However, given the clear molecular basis of the vast majority of mutant phenotypes, such apprehensions are largely unwarranted, provided that careful, clean selections are employed (e.g., *see* ref. 2).

The three enzyme targets that have been used most frequently (Fig. 1) are thymidine kinase (TK), hypoxanthine-guanine phosphoribosyl transferase (HPRT), and adenine phosphoribosyl transferase (APRT). In cells, these enzymes salvage free bases and nucleosides from the culture medium for the synthesis of RNA and/or DNA. They are nonessential enzymes, be-

From: *Methods in Molecular Biology, Vol. 7: Gene Transfer and Expression Protocols*
Edited by: E. J. Murray © 1991 The Humana Press Inc., Clifton, NJ

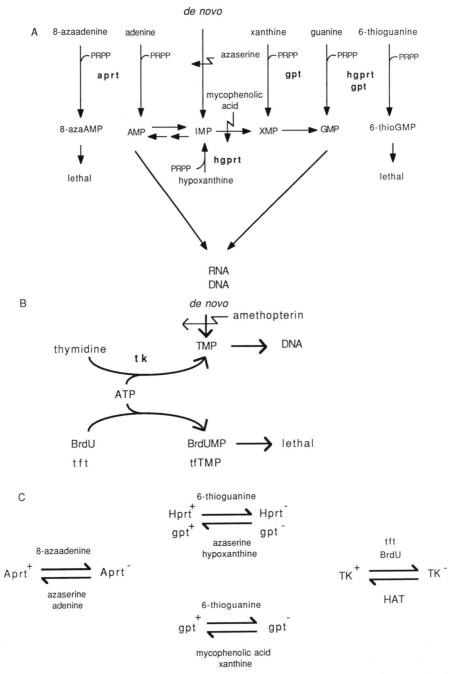

Fig. 1. Purine and pyrimidine salvage pathways. (A) Purine salvage pathways showing enzymes (**bold**) and inhibitors of interconversions. Metabolism of selective drugs is also indicated, and **gpt** refers to any transfected *E. Coli gpt* genes. In the absence of such an exogenously introduced gene, mammalian cells utilize xanthine poorly. (B) Role of thymidine kinase (**tk**) in pyrimidine salvage pathways. (C) Summary of selections for and against salvage enzyme activities.

cause deficient strains grow normally. On the other hand, these enzymes can be made essential by blocking *de novo* synthetic pathways, thus making the cells dependent on salvage for survival. This is the basis of the selections for stable transformants bearing vectors expressing such salvage enzymes. Cells can also use the bacterial equivalent of HPRT, xanthine-guanine phosphoribosyl transferase (GPT) for survival in the absence of HPRT. Alternatively, the ability of GPT to metabolize xanthine (in contrast to the cellular HPRT) can be used to select transfected cells in the presence of mycophenolic acid (Fig. 1 and ref. *3*).

The selection of enzyme-deficient cell lines is accomplished by supplying base or nucleoside analogs to cells so that metabolism of these drugs by the given salvage enzyme produces lethal metabolites (Fig. 1). The rare cells that survive are deficient in the salvage enzymes that metabolize the drugs to the toxic form. For an X-linked locus, such as HPRT, the protocol is simple, employing one-step selections for deficient phenotypes. Selections for recessive mutations in autosomal loci, however, are more complicated. The main difficulty is that all copies of the gene must be altered to obtain deficient strains. The approach usually taken to isolate such autosomal recessive mutations is stepwise selections, requiring the initial generation of hetero- or hemizygous strains by selection in intermediate drug concentrations followed by selection for completely deficient mutants (*4*). Figure 2A shows a schematic diagram of the survival of diploid, hemizygous, or heterozygous cell populations in a cytotoxic drug. The spontaneous frequency of each mutation in such selections is about 10^{-6}–10^{-7} in most cell lines. Thus, it is obvious that it is impractical to select the double mutant in a single step.

The selection of recessive autosomal mutations can be facilitated by the use of various mutagens (*see* Fig. 2B). Some mutagens (e.g., ethylmethanesulfonate [EMS]) cause limited chromosomal disruption and also may diminish the likelihood of epigenetic phenotypic changes (e.g., the loss of enzyme activity resulting from hypermethylation of the target gene). Frequencies of single-step recessive mutations can be increased as much as 1000-fold by EMS, making the selection of double recessive mutations more feasible. A potential disadvantage of mutagen treatment is the introduction of base substitutions into loci throughout the genome in the process of obtaining the mutation in the target gene. The well-defined stepwise selections are superior to serial selections (such as those employed to obtain amplified gene arrays), since these can lead to accumulation of chromosome abnormalities (from constant selection pressure) and epigenetic effects. This chapter describes approaches to the isolation and characterization of mutants deficient in these salvage enzymes.

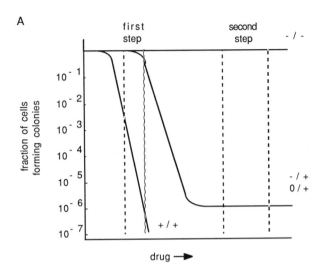

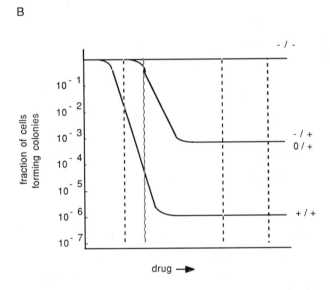

Fig. 2. Theory of the stepwise selection of recessive mutations of autosomal genes. Figures depict survival of cells (formation of colonies) in untreated (A) or mutagen-treated (B) cultures. Target concentration ranges for first- and second-step selections are indicated. Wild-type cells are represented as +/+, and hemi- or heterozygotes by o/+ or -/+, respectively. The survival of strains with mutations in both alleles is represented by -/-. The representative mutation frequencies presented are based on our studies with the autosomal *aprt* locus in hamster and human cell lines and may vary from cell line to cell line.

2. Materials

2.1. Generation of Purine/Pyrimidine Salvage Enzyme Mutations

1. Cell lines: Although the purpose of this chapter is to present some approaches for the isolation of mutants of any cell line, these approaches will be very tedious (if not futile) for strains that are grossly heteroploid for the chromosomes bearing the target genes. Thus, it is advisable to have some idea of the chromosome constitution of the starting cells and to use only lines that have limited changes in ploidy (*see also* Note 1).

2. Culture media: Ensure that no bases or nucleosides are present in the media used to grow your cell lines, since these are included in some formulations. For mutant selections and back selections, it is advisable to use dialyzed sera prepared by dialysis against four changes (~8 h/change) of a tenfold excess of phosphate-buffered saline solution (PBS). The dialyzed serum can be filtered through disposable 100-mL or 500 mL membrane filter assemblies (N®, *see* Note 2).

3. Base or nucleoside analogs: All drugs listed here are commercially available from a number of suppliers.

   a. 8-Azaadenine: 200× stock solution is 80 mM in water. Prepare by dissolving 200 mg in 15 mL of water and adding hydrochloric acid until it dissolves. Make the vol up to 20 mL. Filter-sterilize this solution and all others for cell culture. The solution is stable at 4°C. For mutant selection, use at a final concentration of 0.4 mM.

   b. 6-Thioguanine: Stock solution, 2 mM. Weigh 10 mg; dissolve in 20 mL of water. Add 1M NaOH dropwise until it dissolves. Adjust the pH to 9.5 using 1M acetic acid. Make the vol up to 30 mL and filter-sterilize. Store at –20°C. Most mutant selections use a final concentration of ~$10^{-5}M$.

   c. 5-Bromodeoxyuridine (BUdR): 50 mM stock solution in water. Dissolve 300 mg in water; make the vol up to 20 mL. The final concentration for selection is 0.5 mM.

   d. Triflurothymidine (TFT): 100× stock solution is 1 mM. Dissolve 6 mg in water and make the vol up to 20 mL. The final concentration for selection of TK-deficient mutants from hemizygous strains is usually 10 μM for CHO cells, 6 μM for human cell lines, and 13 μM for mouse cell lines. This analog is preferred by most laboratories for selection of TK⁻ strains because of more efficient killing of TK⁺ cells.

4. Ethylmethanesulfonate (EMS): Stock solution is 9.6M; dilute to a 0.8M working solution. A final concentration of 1.6 mM used to mutate CHO cells yields 60% survival, whereas for the human tumor cell line SW620, only 0.4 mM is required. Note that EMS is a suspected carcinogen, and care must be taken with handling and disposal.

2.2. Media for Back Selections

1. HAT medium: Stock solutions (1000×) are as follows:
   a. 50 mM hypoxanthine: Dissolve 680 mg in water adding a few drops of NaOH (to ph 9.0), and make up to 100 mL vol. Filter-sterilize and store at 4°C.
   b. 1 mM amethopterin: Dissolve 49 mg in water, add NaOH until it dissolves, and make up to 100 mL vol. Filter-sterilize, aliquot, and store at −20°C.
   c. 10 mM thymidine: Dissolve 240 mg in water, make up to 100 mL vol, and store at 4°C.
      Final concentrations for selection: 50 μM hypoxanthine, 1 μM amethopterin, and 10 μM thymidine.
2. Azaserine adenine (hypoxanthine): Stock solutions are as follows:
   a. 10 mM adenine: Dissolve 136 mg in water and make up to 100 mL vol. Store at 4°C.
   b. hypoxanthine solution as described above.
   c. 10 mM azaserine: Dissolve 173 mg in water and make up to 100 mL vol. Store at −20°C in aliquots.
      Final concentrations for selection: 10 μM adenine or 50 μM hypoxanthine, 20 μM azaserine, 10 μM thymidine (not essential).
3. Mycophenolic acid/xanthine: Stock solutions are as follows:
   a. 2.5 mg/mL mycophenolic acid: Dissolve in 0.1M NaOH, neutralize with 0.1M HCl, and store at −20°C.
   b. Xanthine: 25 mg/mL, store at 4°C.
      Final concentrations for selection: 25 μg/mL mycophenolic acid, 250 μg/mL xanthine. If background growth occurs, reduce xanthine to 25 μg/mL.

2.3. Generation of Cell Extracts
to Assay Salvage Enzyme Activity

1. Trypsin/EDTA: Available commercially from GIBCO as a 1× stock solution (catalog number 043-05300).

2. PBSA: Dissolve 10 g of NaCl, 0.25 g of KCl, 1.43 g of Na$_2$HPO$_4$, and 0.25 g of KH$_2$PO$_4$ in water, make the vol up to 1 L, and check that the pH is 7.2. Autoclave at 15 psi for 15 min. Store at room temperature.

3. 1 *M* Tris, pH 7.4: Dissolve 13.2 g of Tris-HCl and 1.94 g of Tris base in water. Make the vol up to 100 mL. Check the pH and adjust as necessary, using NaOH or hydrochloric acid.

4. Sonicator: MSE Soniprep 150.

5. Bio-Rad protein assay kit: Bio-Rad catalog number 500-0002.

6. 1 *M* MgCl$_2$: Dissolve 20.3 g of MgCl$_2$•6H$_2$O in water; make the vol up to 100mL.

7. Phospho-ribosyl pyrophosphate (PRPP): 12.5 m*M* PRPP stock solution (10×) is made by dissolving 4.8 mg in 1 mL water. Store at –20°C. PRPP should be made up fresh, we use a 10× stock solution for only 2 d.

8. DE81 filters: diameter 2.3 cm (Whatman).

9. 0.5 *M* EDTA, pH 8.0: Add 186.1 g of disodium ethylene diamine tetraacetic acid (dihydrate) to 800 mL of water. Adjust the pH to 8.0 by adding approx 20 g of NaOH pellets. Make the vol up to 1 L.

10. 10m*M* ammonium formate: dissolve 0.63 g in water; make the vol up to 1 L.

11. Toluene-based scintillation fluid. Permablend 3 (Packard): make up according to the manufacturer's instructions.

12. Radioactively labeled nucleoside: For HPRT activity, use 0.6 m*M* ^{14}C hypoxanthine (final SA 5 mCi/mmol). For APRT activity, use 0.3 m*M* ^{14}C adenine (final SA 5 mCi/mmol). For TK activity, use 50 µ*M* ^{3}H thymidine (final SA 20 mCi/mmol).

13. 1 *M* dithiothreitol: Prepare fresh prior to use. Dissolve 154 mg in water; make the vol up to 1mL. Aliquot and store at –20°C.

14. 0.1 *M* ATP: Dissolve 60 mg in water and adjust the pH to 7.0 using 1 *M* NaOH. Make the vol up to 1mL and store at –20°C.

15. Triton X-100, obtained from Sigma.

3. Methods

3.1. Generation of Mutant Pyrimidine/Purine Salvage Pathway Enzyme Cell Lines

3.1.1. By Spontaneous Mutation

1. Determine the sensitivity of the cell line to the given drug. Start by plating 100 or 1000 cells in each well of a 6-well dish in the presence of different drug concentrations: 8-azaadenine for APRT$^-$, 6-thioguanine for

HPRT$^-$, and bromodeoxyuridine for TK$^-$ (Fig. 1C). Once the concentration at which cell killing begins is known, increasing numbers of cells can be plated against increasing drug levels until a point is reached at which survival frequencies are <10^{-6} to 10^{-7} (*see* Note 3).

2. If survival at maximum drug concentrations is <10^{-7}, pick colonies from plates containing the highest drug concentration. Ideally the frequency of such colonies should be no more than 10^{-5}. Retest the sensitivity of these colonies to the full range of drug concentrations. If the colonies are true hetero- or hemizygotes, colonies should form at the highest drug concentrations, although at very low frequencies (i.e., 10^{-6}–10^{-7}, as represented in Fig. 2A). The colonies growing at these high drug concentrations should be resistant to the highest concentration of the drug, as determined by plating.

3.1.2. By EMS Mutagenesis

1. It is first necessary to check the sensitivity of cells to EMS, since this can vary greatly. Plate 100 or 1000 cells in increasing concentrations of EMS and incubate for 16 h. *See* Section 2.1., step 4 for examples.
2. Remove the medium, wash with PBSA, and return to normal growth medium.
3. After colonies form, stain the plates to determine the survival frequency. An adequate staining procedure using methylene blue is described in Chapter 19, Section 3.1.
4. To select for deficient strains, mutate cultures (~10^6 cells) as above for 16 h (*see* Note 4).
5. Then remove the EMS-containing medium, wash with PBS, and add back normal growth medium. Maintain the treated culture in this medium for 5–6 d (without selection) to allow the expression of the mutant phenotype.
6. Plate the mutated cultures in increasing concentrations of the selecting drug, as above. Double mutants may be obtained at low frequencies in a single step in such mutated cultures (Fig. 2B). If not, take colonies at intermediate drug concentrations (those at which survival is no more than 10^{-4}), remutate and replate at higher drug concentrations.
7. Colonies forming at highest drug concentrations should be picked and maintained in nonselective growth medium. They should be retested for drug resistance after a few weeks of growth. Any showing sensitivity to the drug should be discarded.

3.2. Back Selections

3.2.1. To Check Mutant Stability

1. Resistant strains should also be tested for in vivo salvage enzyme activity by plating on selective medium, making the cells dependent on the salvage enzyme for survival. This can be done by plating BUdR- or TFT-resistant cells (TK⁻) on HAT medium; 8-azaadenine resistant cells (APRT⁻) on azaserine adenine medium; and 6-thioguanine resistant cells (HPRT⁻) on azaserine hypoxanthine medium (Fig. 1C).
2. Survival of truly deficient mutants (i.e., the reversion frequency) should be $<10^{-7}$. *See* Note 5.

3.2.2. To Select for Cells Expressing Transfected Plasmids

1. These back-selection media are also used to obtain cells transfected with plasmids expressing salvage enzymes.
2. In addition to the combinations described above, mycophenolic acid/xanthine can be used as a dominant marker (in HPRT⁺ strains) to select for GPT expression, since mammalian cells normally utilize xanthine poorly.

3.3. Generation of Cell Extracts to Assay for Salvage Enzyme Activity

To examine in vitro salvage enzyme activities in the mutant lines, it is first essential to prepare cell-free extracts.

1. Grow $1-2 \times 10^7$ cells to 80% confluency.
2. Trypsinize to remove monolayers from plates, or pellet suspension cells by centrifugation.
3. Wash the cell pellets twice with PBS on ice.
4. Collect cells by centrifugation and resuspend the final pellet in 3 mL of $0.03 M$ Tris-HCl, pH 7.4, for APRT and HPRT assays, or in 100 µL 50 mM Tris-HCl, (pH 7.5), 1 mM EDTA, 0.2% Triton X-100, and 10 mM DTT for TK assays.
5. For APRT and HPRT assays, the cells can be disrupted either by sonication (four bursts of 5 s each, with 15-s cooling periods) or in a Dounce homogenizer. For TK assays, gently pipeting cells up and down in buffer that contains Triton X-100 is sufficient.
6. Spin the cell suspension at 12,000 rpm for 20 min at 4°C in a microfuge. Take the supernatant into a clean tube; this crude cell extract can be used directly in assays.

7. Determine the protein concentration using the Bio-Rad protein assay kit and bovine serum albumin as a standard.

3.3.1. Assay for APRT Activity

1. Reaction mix: 5 mM MgCl$_2$; 0.3 mM ^{14}C adenine (5 mCi/mmol); 30 mM Tris-HCl, pH 7.4; and 1.25 mM PRPP (Sigma).
2. Add cell extract to prewarmed reaction mixture at 37°C. For each assay, use between 10 and 50 µg of protein in a final reaction vol of 0.1 mL.
3. Incubate for 5–60 min (up to 120 min for low-activity extracts), taking 5-µL samples in duplicate at each time-point onto DE81 filters (Whatman). Dry the filters.
4. Wash the filters with 25 mL of 10 mM ammonium formate.
5. Dry under a heat lamp and count in toluene-based scintillation fluid.
6. Controls should include an assay run without PRPP to give background and with a filter spotted with 5 µL of the reaction, but not washed, to give the total counts per assay (*see* Note 6).

3.3.2. Assay for HPRT Activity

Reaction mixtures are identical to those for APRT assays, except for the substitution of 0.6 mM ^{14}C hypoxanthine for ^{14}C adenine.

3.3.3. Assay for TK Activity

1. Use 10–50 µg of protein from a freshly prepared cell extract.
2. Reaction mix: 100 mM Tris-HCl, pH 8.0; 2.5 mM MgCl$_2$; 5 mM DTT; 50 µM ^{3}H thymidine (20 mCi/mmol); and 5 mM ATP in a final vol of 100 µL.
3. Incubate cell extract and reaction mix at 37°C, spot 10-µL samples, taken in duplicate at various time-points, onto DE81 paper, and dry.
4. Wash the filters in 4 mM Tris-HCl, pH 8.0. Dry under a heat lamp.
5. Count the filters in toluene-based scintillation fluid. A blank control without extract should be run concurrently.

4. Notes

1. It is useful to optimize growth and plating conditions for a cell line before attempting selections or transfection experiments, since the plating efficiency of many cell lines is poor. Plating efficiency can be improved in some cases by adding a higher serum concentration or other nutrients to the medium. Many other details of cell-culture techniques and solutions are not included here. Please consult refs. 5 and 6 for further information.

2. If too much particulate materal is present to allow filtration, simply centrifuge the dialyzed serum (2000 rpm for 10 min) before filtering. Store sera at −20°C.

3. Plating densities are critical in such experiments, since cross-feeding effects can reduce the survival of mutants. Ideally, these effects should be determined by reconstruction experiments in which the plating efficiency of a known number of mutant cells is determined in the presence of the selecting drug concentration and increasing numbers of wild-type cells. When such an experiment is feasible, plate the maximum number of cells that do not affect the survival of the mutants. Unfortunately, you may not have the mutants necessary for the reconstruction, so, as a rough guide, plate no more than 500,000 cells/100-mm dish in selecting drug concentrations.

4. For the cell lines that we use, mutational frequencies reach a maximum when about 30–60% of cells survive. Additional mutagen does not increase frequencies further, but can have a number of undesirable side effects.

5. Some mutant strains with detectable base substitutions in the structural gene can still utilize the base, but not the analog, and therefore survive in the back-selection medium. These mutants are obviously not suitable hosts for use in transfection experiments.

6. Protein concentrations should be titrated to ensure that the amount of product formed is proportional to the amount of extract added.

References

1. Harris, M. (1982) Induction of thymidine kinase in enzyme deficient Chinese hamster cells. *Cell* **29**, 483–492.
2. Phear, G., Armstrong, W., and Meuth, M. (1989) Molecular basis of spontaneous mutation at the *APRT* locus of hamster cells. *J. Mol. Biol.* **209**, 577–582.
3. Mulligan, R. C. and Berg, P. (1981) Selection for animal cells that express the *Escherichia coli* gene coding for xanthine-guanine phosphoribosyltransferase. *Proc. Natl. Acad. Sci. USA* **78**, 2072–2076.
4. Jones, G. E. and Sargent, P. A. (1974) Mutants of cultured cells deficient in adenine phosphoribosyl transferase. *Cell* **2**, 43–54.
5. Jacoby, W. B. and Pastan, I. H., eds. (1979) *Methods in Enzymology*, vol. LVIII: *Cell Culture* (Academic, New York).
6. Cole, J. and Arlett, C. F. (1984) The detection of gene mutations in cultured mammalian cells, in *Mutagenicity Testing: A Practical Approach* (Venitt, S. and Parry, J. M., eds.), IRL, Oxford, pp. 233–273.

SECTION 5
ANALYSIS OF STEADY-STATE-LEVEL TRANSCRIPTION IN TRANSFECTED CELL LINES

CHAPTER 21

Quantitative and Qualitative Analysis of Exogenous Gene Expression by the S1 Nuclease Protection Assay

Maggie E. Walmsley and Roger K. Patient

1. Introduction

The S1 nuclease protection procedure allows the precise definition of the beginning and end of gene transcripts as well as the position of intron/exon boundaries in a gene. Alternatively, when these parameters are already known, the technique can be used to quantify transcript levels in a variety of expression systems.

In the standard procedure developed by Weaver and Weissmann *(1)*, a ^{32}P end-labeled DNA probe (*see* Note 1) is hybridized to total cytoplasmic or polyA$^+$ RNA. Subsequent treatment of the RNA–DNA hybrid with S1 nuclease (*see* Note 2), which shows a high specificity for single-stranded RNA or DNA, removes those single-stranded sequences that lie outside the RNA–DNA hybrid. The size of the DNA fragment protected from nuclease digestion by mRNA is then determined by polyacrylamide gel electrophoresis (*see* Note 3).

1.1. Probe Strategies

The choice of DNA probe is tailored to the individual experiment and the information being sought. Single- or double-stranded DNA probes may be used. Probes labeled at the 5' end by polynucleotide kinase *(2)* are used to detect the 5' start of a transcript or the 5' end of an exon at an intron/exon

From: *Methods in Molecular Biology, Vol. 7: Gene Transfer and Expression Protocols*
Edited by: E. J. Murray © 1991 The Humana Press Inc., Clifton, NJ

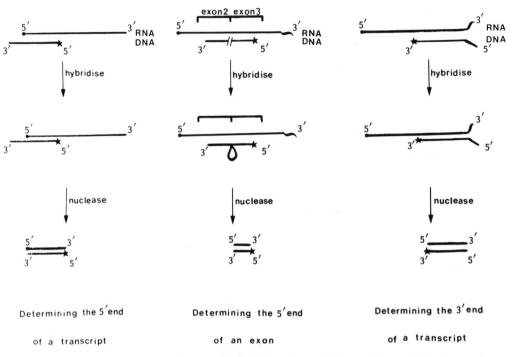

Fig. 1. Determining the ends of an RNA transcript and the positions of the intron/exon boundaries by S1 nuclease mapping. The end-labeled DNA probe is hybridized to the RNA transcript. RNA sequences not protected by the probe (at either end of the probe) or intron sequences in the DNA not present in the mRNA transcript are removed by the single-strand-specific S1 nuclease. The length of resultant hybrid is determined by polyacrylamide gel electrophoresis. The scheme for determining only the 5' end of an exon is shown. The procedure for determining the 3' end of an exon is similar, except that a 3' end-labeled probe is used.

junction (Fig. 1). Probes labeled at the 3' end by the Klenow fragment of DNA polymerase I (2) are used to detect the 3' end of a transcript or the 3' end of an exon (Fig. 1). The restriction sites used for isolating a probe should be chosen such that the protected fragment is at least 10% shorter in length than the full-length probe and can be easily distinguished from it on polyacrylamide gels. This is necessary because probes are normally in excess of RNA transcripts and, when double-stranded DNA probes are used, a certain proportion of probe renaturation occurs and is seen as a full-length probe band. Even single-stranded probes are usually contaminated with a small amount of the complementary strand that will protect full-length probe from nuclease attack. For determining the 5' end of a transcript or exon, restriction sites should be selected that will yield a probe that can be 5' end-labeled in the strand complementary to the mRNA and that spans the cap site or intron/exon boundary. Similarly, to determine the 3' end of a transcript or exon, choose restriction sites that yield a DNA fragment that can be 3' end-labeled in the strand complementary to the mRNA and that spans the end of the transcript or the exon/intron junction (Fig. 1). Single-stranded, end-labeled probes are separated from the cold complementary strand on a denaturing polyacrylamide gel *(2)*. When planning a single-stranded probe, restriction sites should be chosen to maximize the size difference between the labeled strand and the cold complementary strand in order to facilitate separation of the strands on polyacrylamide gels. For example, 5' end-labeling at an NcoI site followed by a recut with PstI will result in an eight-nucleotide difference in length between the labeled and cold strands. Furthermore, to avoid a lengthy run on the strand-separation gel, a probe fragment of no longer than 250 bases should be planned.

1.2. Hybridization Conditions

When double-stranded probes are used, hybridization in the presence of formamide is essential in order that formation of RNA–DNA hybrids is favored over DNA–DNA probe renaturation (*see* Note 4). In the case of single-stranded probes, hybridization may be carried out either in aqueous, high-salt conditions (which maximize stability and rate of duplex formation) or in the presence of formamide. Although formamide conditions result in suboptimal hybrid formation, probe and RNA degradation (and therefore background) are significantly reduced, since formamide decreases the melting temperature (T_m) of a hybrid such that the hybridization can be carried out at lower temperatures (*see* Note 4).

1.3. Choosing a DNA Probe

The double-stranded probe method is less sensitive, as a result of probe renaturation. Formamide reduces this, but renders hybrid formation suboptimal. However, if transcript levels are high, ease of probe preparation may make this the method of choice. Single-stranded, end-labeled probes are at least an order of magnitude more sensitive, since the contribution of probe renaturation is low and hybridization can occur in highly favorable aqueous conditions. However, probe preparation is lengthier. Single-stranded, uniformly labeled probes are yet more sensitive, but require cloning of the appropriate DNA fragment into M13, and can only be used when the precise boundaries of the transcript are already known. Such boundaries can be mapped only with uniquely end-labeled probes because, when the radioactive label is distributed throughout the length of the probe, spurious bands caused by probe degradation can be seen. Uniformly labeled probes are, therefore, most useful for detection of very low levels of transcripts that have been characterized previously.

2. Materials

All buffers or solutions must be treated with diethylpyrocarbonate (DEPC). Add DEPC to solutions at a concentration of 0.1%, shake vigorously for 1 min and then incubate overnight at 37°C. Finally, autoclave for 15 min to eliminate the DEPC. Centrifuge tubes and pipet tips must also be autoclaved. Whenever possible, use sterile plasticware instead of glass. Wear gloves at all times. Wash down the bench, microfuge, and automatic pipets with 10% SDS at the start of the experiment. These precautions should minimize loss of RNA resulting from RNase contamination.

1. Deionized formamide: Use the highest quality formamide available. Deionize by stirring for 30 min at room temperature with AG501-X8 mixed bed resin (Bio-Rad; approx 1 g resin/100 mL formamide) using a fresh glass bottle and magnetic stirring bar that have been treated with 0.1% DEPC and then autoclaved. Pour the supernatant into a fresh DEPC-treated bottle, add more resin, and repeat stirring for 30 min. Pass the formamide through a sterile filter, and store frozen and protected from light.

2. 10× NaCl/PIPES/EDTA: $4 M$ NaCl; $0.4 M$ PIPES, pH 6.5; 10 mM EDTA; made up with DEPC H_2O.

3. Formamide buffer: 80% formamide; $0.4 M$ NaCl; 40 mM PIPES, pH 6.5; 1 mM EDTA. Combine 500 µL deionized formamide with 62.5 µL 10× NaCl/PIPES/EDTA and 62.5 µL DEPC H_2O.

4. S1 buffer: $0.25 M$ NaCl; $0.03 M$ NaOAc, pH 4.6; 1mM ZnSO$_4$; 20 µg/mL denatured salmon-sperm DNA. Phenol-extract DNA twice, precipitate with ethanol, and resuspend at 1 mg/mL. Boil for 5–10 min and transfer to ice. Add DNA to the other S1 buffer ingredients at a final concentration of 20 µg/mL and store at –20°C. Before use, redenature S1 buffer for 10 min at 90°C and transfer immediately to ice. When cold, add nuclease S1 (BCL, London) to a concentration of 1500U/mL.

5. Formamide dyes: 90% formamide, 10 mM NaOH, 10 mM EDTA, 0.1% (w/v) bromphenol blue, 0.1% (w/v) xylene cyanole.

6. TE: 10 mM Tris-HCl, pH 8.0; 1 mM EDTA.

7. 70% EtOH/DEPC H_2O: 70 mL absolute ethanol, 30 mL DEPC-treated water.

8. Yeast tRNA: Make up to 25 mg/mL with DEPC H_2O in the maker's bottle to avoid RNase contamination during weighing. Filter-sterilize and store in sterile plastic tubes at –20°C.

9. 10× Klenow buffer: $0.5 M$ Tris-HCl, pH 7.2; $0.1 M$ MgSO$_4$; 1 mM DTT. Filter-sterilize.

10. 10× CAP buffer: $0.5M$ Tris-HCl, pH 9.0; 10 mM MgCl$_2$, 1 mM ZnCl$_2$, 10 mM spermidine.
11. 10× STE: 100 mM Tris-HCl, pH 8.0; $1M$ NaCl; 10 mM EDTA.
12. 10× kinase buffer: $0.5M$ Tris-HCl, pH 7.6; $0.1M$ MgCl$_2$, 50 mM DTT; 1 mM spermidine; 1 mM EDTA.
13. $3M$ sodium acetate (NaOAc): Brought to pH 5.4 with glacial acetic acid, DEPC-treated, and autoclaved for 15 min.
14. G50 Sephadex: Suspend Sephadex in approx 50 vol of TE. Autoclave for 15 min (Sephadex will swell) and allow to cool to room temperature. Store at 4°C in a capped bottle.

3. Methods

3.1. Preparation of RNA

Any of the standard published methods of RNA isolation are suitable for analysis by the S1 nuclease protection assay (*see also* Chapters 24,32). Rigorous precautions must be taken to avoid RNAse contamination (*see* Section 2.). No shortcuts should be contemplated. The most sensitive DNA probe is of no value if RNA samples are degraded. For an excellent review of the RNA isolation procedures available and required precautions, *see* ref. *(3)*.

3.2. Probe Preparation

3.2.1. Double-Stranded End-Labeled Probes

Probes are labeled with ^{32}P at their 3' ends using the Klenow fragment of DNA polymerase I. The 5' termini are labeled using the enzyme polynucleotide kinase (PNK) following the removal of the 5' end phosphates by the action of calf alkaline phosphatase (CAP). PNK then replaces these phosphates with the terminal γ–phosphate of the substrate γ-^{32}P-ATP.

1. For 3' end-labeling, in a plastic Eppendorf tube, combine 1 pmol of 3' ends of plasmid DNA restricted with an appropriate restriction enzyme (*see* Note 5), 5 μL 10× Klenow buffer, 2 μL (20 μCi, α-^{32}P-dNTP SA >400 Ci/mmol), 2 μL each of 2 mM solutions of the other three unlabeled dNTPs, 5 μL 1 mg/mL BSA, 2 U Klenow, and DEPC H$_2$O to 50 μL.
2. Incubate at room temperature for 30 min.
3. Heat-kill the enzyme at 65°C for 10 min.
4. Separate labeled DNA from unincorporated ^{32}P-dNTP by spinning through a Sephadex G50 column equilibrated with TE (*see* Note 6).
5. For 5' end-labeling, dephosphorylate appropriately restricted plasmid DNA by combining, in a plastic Eppendorf tube, 1 pmol 5'ends, 5 μL 10× CAP buffer, 0.1 U CAP, and DEPC H$_2$O to 50 μL.

6. Incubate for 1 h at 37°C for protruding 5' ends or 56°C for blunt ends.

7. Add a further 0.1 U CAP and continue incubation for a further hour.

8. Stop the reaction by the addition of 10 μL 10× STE, 5 μL 10% SDS, and DEPC H$_2$O to 100 μL.

9. Heat at 65°C for 15 min.

10. Extract once with phenol and once with chloroform; then ethanol-precipitate by adding 2.5 vol cold 100% ethanol.

11. Wash the pellet with 70% EtOH/DEPC H$_2$O), dry under vacuum, and resuspend the pellet in DEPC H$_2$O at a concentration of 1 pmol 5'ends/5 μL (*see* Note 7). Store at –20°C.

12. To 5' end-label the dephosphorylated DNA, in a plastic Eppendorf tube, combine 1 pmol 5' ends, 2 μL 10× kinase buffer, 7 μL α-^{32}P-ATP (70 μCi, SA 3000 Ci/mmol), 15–20 U PNK, and DEPC H$_2$O to 20 μL.

13. Incubate for 30 min at 37°C.

14. Add 5 μL 3 *M* NaOAc and 25 μL DEPC H$_2$O.

15. Extract once with phenol and once with phenol:chloroform.

16. Transfer the aqueous layer to a G50 Sephadex column (*see* Note 6).

17. For both 3' and 5' end-labeled probes, precipitate labeled DNA in the column eluate with 2 vol of ethanol in the presence of 0.3 *M* NaOAc. Wash the pellet with 70% EtOH/DEPC H$_2$O, dry under vacuum, and resuspend the pellet in formamide buffer at approx 10^4 cpm/μL. Store at –20°C.

18. When a second restriction enzyme cut is necessary (*see* Note 5), extract the G50 eluate with phenol followed by chloroform. Ethanol-precipitate in the presence of 0.3 *M* NaOAc as above; dry and resuspend the pellet in TE. Recut with the appropriate restriction enzyme.

19. Separate the labeled probe fragment from the rest of the digest on low-gelling-temperature agarose and recover by phenol extraction of the excised gel slice *(2)*. For an alternative probe purification using nondenaturing polyacrylamide gel electrophoresis *(2)*, *see* Note 8.

20. Concentrate the eluted probe to 200 μL vol with butanol, extract once with phenol:chloroform and twice with chloroform, and precipitate with ethanol in the presence of 0.3 *M* NaOAc. Wash the pellet with 70% EtOH/DEPC H$_2$O, dry under vacuum, and resuspend the probe in formamide buffer or DEPC H$_2$O at approx 10^4 cpm/μL. Store the probe at –20°C until use.

3.2.2. Single-Stranded End-Labeled Probes

1. End-label and recut 1–5 pmol of 5' or 3' ends of plasmid DNA as in Section 3.2.1.

2. Ethanol-precipitate the restriction enzyme digest in the presence of 0.3*M* NaOAc as above; wash the pellet with 70% EtOH/DEPC H$_2$O, dry, and resuspend in 20 µL of formamide dyes.

3. Denature at 90°C for 3 min, transfer to ice, and load on a 5% denaturing polyacrylamide gel, along with a labeled DNA mol wt size marker (*see* Note 9). Load approx 10^4–10^5 cpm of the labeled marker so that it can be seen easily after a 10-min exposure at room temperature. Run the gel for the appropriate length of time.

4. Remove the top glass plate from the gel, cover with plastic wrap, and expose the gel to autoradiographic film for 10 min at room temperature in an autoradiography casset in the dark.

5. Develop the film and cut out a window in the film where the probe band appears. Align the film with the gel (use the radioactivity trapped in the gel slots for alignment) and cut out a slice of acrylamide containing the labeled probe (*see* Note 10).

6. Extract the probe from the polyacrylamide slice (*see* Note 8).

7. Perform step 20 of Section 3.2.1.

3.2.3. Uniformly-Labeled Single-Stranded Probes (See Note 1)

For a detailed description of the cloning and synthesis of these probes in M13, *see* Volume 2, this series.

3.3. S1 Nuclease Protection Assays

3.3.1. Formamide Method

1. Combine RNA and excess labeled probe (*see* Note 11).

2. Add 1/10 vol 3*M* sodium acetate (pH 5.4), and then add 2.5 vol of ethanol. Mix well and precipitate nucleic acid by centrifuging for 15 min in a microfuge.

3. Remove supernatant (check that all counts have been precipitated on a Geiger-Muller counter) and wash the pellet with 0.5 mL of 70% ethanol/DEPC H$_2$O.

4. Dry the pellet under vacuum and suspend it thoroughly in 20 µL formamide buffer (*see* Note 12).

5. Denature samples at 90°C for 3 min and transfer immediately to hybridization temperature (*see* Note 4).

6. Hybridize overnight (*see* Note 13).

7. To each sample, add 200 µL of ice-cold S1 buffer containing 200–600 U, freshly added, of S1 nuclease (BCL). Vortex briefly and transfer to a water bath at the temperature that is optimal for the S1 reaction. Incubate for the empirically determined optimal time (*see* Note 14).

8. Add 10 µg of carrier tRNA and 2.5 vol of ethanol. Mix well and centrifuge for 15 min in a microfuge (*see* Note 15).

9. Wash the pellet with 0.5 mL of 70% ethanol/DEPC H_2O, dry, and resuspend in 5–10 µL of formamide dyes.

10. Denature samples for 3 min at 90°C, and transfer at once to ice.

11. Load the samples on a denaturing polyacrylamide gel.

12. Electrophorese and autoradiograph.

3.3.2. Aqueous Method

1. Perform steps 1–3 as in Section 3.3.1. above.

2. Resuspend the pellet in 30 µL of 0.05M HEPES, pH 7.0; 1mM EDTA, 0.75M NaCl (*see* Note 16).

3. Vortex, spin down solution briefly, and incubate at 68°C for 10 min.

4. Transfer to 43°C water bath for 6 h or overnight (*see* Note 17).

5. Proceed through steps 7–12 of Section 3.3.1. above.

4. Notes

1. A more sensitive alternative to end-labeled probes are uniformly labeled, single-stranded DNA probes, which can be prepared if the appropriate DNA fragment is cloned into Ml3. Using single-stranded Ml3 DNA, a universal oligonucleotide sequencing primer, ^{32}P labeled dNTPs, and the Klenow fragment of DNA polymerase I, a single-stranded probe of very high specific activity can be produced (*see* Volume 2, this series) (4).

2. Mung bean nuclease (5) or *E. coli* exonuclease VII (6,7) have been used as alternatives to S1 nuclease.

3. The size of the protected fragment can be determined to within a nucleotide by coelectrophoresis of a Maxam and Gilbert sequencing ladder (8) of the end-labeled probe.

4. In 80% formamide, a narrow temperature range can be found in which RNA–DNA hybrids are greatly favored over DNA–DNA hybrids; thus, probe renaturation is greatly diminished. In aqueous solvents containing 0.4M NaCl, RNA–DNA hybrids of average G+C content are 5–10°C more stable than corresponding DNA–DNA hybrids. The presence of formamide increases this temperature difference between homo- and heteroduplexes by differentially lowering the T_m of the two types of duplex. However, since T_m depends on base composition and probe length, and since the relationship between T_m depression and formamide concentration is not linear for RNA–DNA hybrids, the optimal temperature for RNA–DNA hybridization in the presence of formamide must be

empirically determined for each new DNA probe. A first approximation of the temperature optimum can be calculated as follows:

In aqueous solutions containing 0.4M NaCl (the salt concentration used here), $T_m = 0.41$ (% G+C) + 74.9 for DNA duplexes.

Assume a reduction in T_m of 0.62°C/% formamide used. Thus, for example, for a probe with a G+C content of 50%, a reasonable estimate for the temperature of hybridization in 80% formamide would be 0.41 (50) + 74.9–80(0.62) = 45.8°C.

Since this represents the T_m for DNA–DNA hybrids, these would be unstable at this temperature, whereas RNA–DNA hybrids would be relatively favored. A range of temperatures above and below this calculated figure should be tested. For double-stranded DNA probes 80% formamide is essential; however, for single-stranded probes, 50% formamide, 0.4M NaCl, 40 mM PIPES (pH 6.5, and 1mM EDTA compose a commonly used solvent.

5. One mole of 5' or 3' ends equals the number of base pairs of plasmid DNA × 660 g/number of ends. Whenever possible, choose a unique restriction site in the plasmid DNA for labeling. Alternatively, make certain that the other labeled fragments in the digest will not hybridize to the RNA transcript. No purification is then required. If neither of these alternatives are possible, recut the labeled digest with a second restriction enzyme that will generate a small probe fragment (100–300 bp) that can, on an agarose or polyacrylamide gel, easily be separated from the larger, labeled fragments.

6. Prepare G50 Sephadex columns as follows: Plug the nipple of a 2-mL sterile plastic syringe with polymer wool and fill the syringe with a concentrated slurry of Sephadex. Suspend the syringe over a sterile plastic centrifuge tube and spin at 1500 rpm in a swing out rotor for 5 min. Discard the centrifuge tube and buffer contents, and transfer the syringe to a fresh tube. Load the labeled DNA onto the top of the column, and thoroughly wash out the Eppendorf tube with 50 µL of TE to ensure transfer of all the label to the column. Spin at 1500 rpm for 5 min. Labeled DNA will be found in the eluate; unincorporated label will be located at the top of the column. A successfully labeled DNA probe should register full scale on a Geiger counter. If this does not happen, try washing the column with a further 50–100 µL of TE. If the eluate still fails to register full scale on the counter, your labeling has been unsuccessful. Remove 1 µL of the probe and determine the specific activity by Cerenkov counting. The specific activity should be in the region of 2–5 × 10^6 dpm/pmol 5' or 3' ends.

7. It is useful to dephosphorylate 10–20 pmol of 5' ends of restricted plasmid. This can then be used as a stock for future end labelings.

8. Incubate the excised polyacrylamide slice containing the labeled probe in 0.5 mL TE containing 10 µg carrier tRNA at 55°C for 1 h or overnight. Remove the polyacrylamide slice.

9. For a 200-nucleotide fragment, approx 3.5 h is needed for the electrophoretic run.

10. Avoid cutting out too wide a slice, since this leads to contamination with the cold complementary strand.

11. Probe should be in an approx fivefold molar excess. Larger excesses of probe will increase background. Usually, a minimum of 1 pg of target RNA must be used to detect a signal. When target RNA concentrations are unknown, serial dilutions of a known source of target RNA should be included in control samples to ensure that probe is in excess for test samples. If probe is in excess over the whole (or part of the) dilution range and test samples fall within this range, then the assay is quantitative for the test samples. The amount of RNA used in nuclease protection assays in general should not exceed 20 µg to avoid the use of excessive amounts of nuclease for complete digestion and overloading of polyacrylamide gels. A control reaction containing an equal amount of an RNA not complementary to the probe (e.g., yeast tRNA) should be included in each assay to control for bands produced from probe, which do not represent hybridization to target RNA. All samples should be brought to the same concentration of RNA by addition of carrier tRNA.

12. At this point, it is common to transfer samples to siliconized, DEPC-treated capillaries in order to avoid evaporation of samples. We have found that, if tight-fitting or screw-capped Eppendorf tubes are used and if the tubes are well submerged in a well-filled water bath with a tight-fitting lid, then condensation is minimized and transfer to capillaries is not necessary. Wrapping Parafilm™ around the top of the Eppendorf tube ensures no leakage of water into the reaction mix. This holds true for temperatures in the range of 42–52°C. At higher temperatures, capillaries may be needed.

13. When there are large amounts of target RNA present, hybridization times can be reduced to 6 h, particularly when quantitative results are not required.

14. S1 conditions: To obtain the cleanest results, a range of temperatures (13–37°C), a range of S1 concentrations (1000–3000 U/mL), and incubation for 0.5–2.5 h should be investigated. At higher temperatures and nuclease concentrations, AT-rich sequences and mismatched bases will

breathe and provide regions for nuclease attack, producing bands smaller than the true signal. At lower temperatures or suboptimal nuclease concentrations, larger bands will appear in addition to the real signal because of incomplete digestion.

15. Many authors recommend a clean-up step with phenol and chloroform following the S1 reaction. We find that this step can be omitted.

16. If pellets prove difficult to resuspend in this high-salt buffer, try the following: Take up pellets in 20 µL of 0.075 M HEPES (pH 7.0) and 1.5m M EDTA. When dissolved completely, add 10 µL 2.25 M NaCl.

17. Hybridization occurs more rapidly in aqueous conditions. Also, since the temperature range for aqueous hybridization is greater than that for formamide conditions, most probes will work at approx 43°C. However, stronger and cleaner results may be achieved by determining the optimum hybridization temperature for each probe.

References

1. Weaver, R. F. and Weissmann, C. (1979) Mapping of RNA by a modification of the Berk-Sharp procedure: The 5' termini of 15S β-globin mRNA precursor and mature 10S β-globin mRNA have identical map coordinates. *Nucleic Acids Res.* **7**, 1175–1193.

2. Maniatis, T., Fritsch, E. F., and Sambrook, J. (1982) in *Molecular Cloning: A Laboratory Manual* (Cold Spring Harbor Laboratory, Cold Spring Harbor, NY).

3. Berger, S. L. (Chs. 19,21), McDonald, R. J., Swift, G. H., Przybyla, A. E., and Chirgwin, J. M. (Ch. 20); Nevins, J .R. (Ch. 22); and Mechler, B. M. (Ch. 23) (1987) All in *Guide to Molecular Cloning Techniques*, sections VII, VIII, Preparation and Characterization of RNA (Berger, S. L. and Kimmel, A. R., eds.), Academic, San Diego, pp. 215–248.

4. Calzone, F. J., Britten, R. J., and Davidson, E. H. (1987) Mapping of gene transcripts by nuclease protection assays and cDNA primer extension, in *Guide to Molecular Cloning Techniques* (Berger, S. L. and Kimmel, A. R., eds.), Academic, San Diego, pp. 616–619.

5. Kowalski, D., Kroeker, W. D., and Laskowski, M. Sr. (1976) Mung bean nuclease I. Physical, chemical and catalytic properties. *Biochemistry* **15**, 4457–4463.

6. Chase, J. W. and Richardson, C. C. (1974) Exonuclease VII of *Escherichia coli.* Purification and properties. *J. Biol. Chem.* **249**, 4545–4552.

7. Chase, J. W. and Richardson, C. C. (1974) Exonuclease VII of *Escherichia coli.* Mechanism of action. *J. Biol. Chem.* **249**, 4553–4561.

8. Maxam, A. M. and Gilbert, W. (1977) A new method for sequencing DNA. *Proc. Natl. Acad. Sci. USA* **74**, 560–564.

CHAPTER 22

The RNase Protection Assay

Mitchell H. Finer

1. Introduction

A sensitive method for quantitation of mRNA in gene transfer studies is mRNA protection using end-labeled DNA probes. In addition, this technique also provides structural information about the transcript under study *(1)*. In vitro labeled antisense RNA can be used as an alternative to end-labeled DNA probes *(2,3)*. RNA probes have attained wide popularity because of the ease of synthesis and high yield of probe in a labeling reaction. This has been made possible by the recent characterization of single subunit bacteriophage RNA polymerases and their promoters *(4,5)*. Currently, three different bacteriophage RNA polymerase/promoter combinations are in use. They are derived from bacteriophage SP6 of *Salmonella typhimurium (3)*, bacteriophage T3 of *E. coli (6)*, and bacteriophage T7 of *E. coli (6)*. These RNA polymerases are ideal for in vitro synthesis of labeled transcripts because of their ease of purification, stability, high rate of polymerization (10 times faster than *E. coli*), and their high specificity resulting from the recognition of large promoter sequences.

The strategy for mRNA protection using labeled RNA probes can be divided into three steps. First, the probe fragment is cloned in reverse orientation into a plasmid vector, downstream from the bacteriophage RNA polymerase promoter (Fig. 1). Second, the plasmid is linearized downstream of the probe fragment and transcribed in vitro with labeled nucleotides (Fig. 2). The runoff transcripts initiate at the phage promoter and terminate

From: *Methods in Molecular Biology, Vol. 7: Gene Transfer and Expression Protocols*
Edited by: E. J. Murray © 1991 The Humana Press Inc., Clifton, NJ

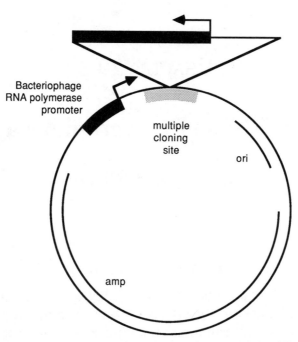

Fig. 1. Construction of a template for in vitro RNA synthesis. The probe fragment is cloned in reverse orientation downstream of a bacterial RNA polymerase promoter in the multiple cloning site. For 5' end mapping, the probe fragment overlaps the transcription initiation site.

at the end of the linear template. The template is removed by DNase treatment and the probe used directly, or the probe can be gel-purified. The latter method removes the template as well as enriching for full-length probe. Third, the probe is hybridized to mRNA, followed by digestion with a combination of RNase A (C- and A-specific) and RNase T1 (G-specific). Double-stranded RNA/RNA hybrids are protected from digestion. Single-stranded material, corresponding to nontranscribed sequences within the probe, is digested. The digestion products are fractionated on denaturing polyacrylamide gels. Only double-stranded RNA, corresponding to transcribed regions, gives rise to the protected fragments seen on the gel (Fig. 2).

Probes synthesized by in vitro transcription have several advantages over end-labeled DNA probes.

1. In vitro transcription with one out of the four nucleotides labeled results in a uniformly labeled probe. This yields greater specific activity and results in increased sensitivity compared to end-labeled DNA probes. The specific activity of the probe is constant (provided the labeled nucleotide has the same specific activity) whenever the probe is synthe-

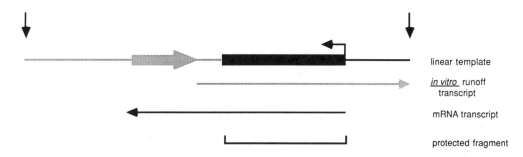

Fig. 2. Messenger RNA protection with in vitro labeled RNA. The template is linearized with a restriction enzyme that cuts downstream of the probe fragment. Transcription of the template generates a uniformly labeled antisense RNA probe. The probe is hybridized to mRNA followed by digestion with ribonuclease A and T1 and fractionation on a denaturing polyacrylamide gel. Only double-stranded RNA, corresponding to transcribed regions, gives rise to the protected fragments seen on the gel.

sized, and the counts incorporated reflect the total amount of probe synthesized. Therefore, once the mass of probe (in cpm) to achieve probe excess has been determined, this number of counts always reflects the same mass of probe. In addition, probes for different mRNAs transcribed simultaneously have the same specific activity. This allows direct comparison between the signals for two different protected fragments run on the same gel, normalizing for the length difference between the protected fragments. In contrast, end-labeled probes differ in specific activity from labeling to labeling. Comparison of different end-labeled probes on the same gel is not possible in consequence of differential labeling efficiency of fragments generated by restriction enzymes.

2. Separation of in vitro labeled RNA probes from the transcription template is simple and rapid. Digestion with RNase-free DNase removes the template. The probe can then be ethanol-precipitated and used directly. Even though some RNA probes must be gel-purified, the size differential between the template and the probe precludes contamination. In contrast, DNA probes must be strand-separated for optimal performance. Poor strand separation results in hybridization of the probe to the complementary strand, thereby reducing the amount of probe available for hybridization.

3. Quantities of probe RNA, sufficient for 200 hybridizations (3) can be synthesized in a single reaction. In order to prepare a similar amount of end-labeled probe, large quantities of plasmid must be digested and the resulting fragment labeled in multiple labeling reactions.

4. The sensitivity obtained using RNA probes is further enhanced by virtue of the greater stability of RNA/RNA hybrids in comparison to DNA/

RNA hybrids *(7)*. This allows the use of more stringent hybridization conditions.

2. Materials

Store all buffers at room temperature unless indicated.

2.1. Probe Synthesis and DNase Treatment

Store buffers 1–5 and 12 in aliquots at –20° C. Freeze and thaw an aliquot not more than five times.

1. 10× Transcription buffer: 400 mM Tris-HCl, pH 7.5; 60 mM MgCl$_2$; 20 mM Spermidine.
2. 20× dithiothreitol: 200 mM.
3. 10× Bovine serum albumin (BSA): 1 mg/mL.
4. 10× XTPs: 5 mM of each of the three unlabeled nucleotides: GTP, ATP, and CTP for use with α-^{32}P UTP; ATP, CTP, and UTP for use with α-^{32}P GTP.
5. 10× DNase Buffer (10× TM): 100 mM Tris-HCl, pH 7.5; 100 mM MgCl$_2$.
6. α-^{32}P GTP or UTP.
7. Human placental ribonuclease inhibitor. Store at –20°C.
8. SP6, T7, or T3 RNA polymerase. Store at –20°C.
9. RNase-free DNase, 1 mg/mL. Store at –20°C.
10. 5M Ammonium acetate (NH$_4$Ac).
11. Ethanol, absolute. Store at –20°C.
12. 5 mg/mL transfer RNA, ribonuclease free.
13. Phenol, saturated with 10 mM Tris-HCl, pH 7.5, 1 mM EDTA.
14. Chloroform.
15. Elution buffer: 1% w/v sodium dodecyl sulfate; 0.5M ammonium acetate; 5 mM EDTA, pH 7.5.
16. 2 mM EDTA, pH 7.5.
17. 10 mM Tris-HCl pH 7.5, 1 mM EDTA pH 7.5.
18. 70% ethanol.
19. DEPC-treated water *(see* Section 4.1., Note 1).

2.2. Hybridization

1. 10× Hybridization buffer: 4M NaCl; 100 mM PIPES, pH 6.4; 10 mM EDTA.
2. 3× Recrystalized formamide.

2.3. RNase Digestion and Gel Electrophoresis

1. RNase buffer: 300 mM NaCl; 10 mM Tris-HCl, pH 7.5; 5 mM EDTA, pH 7.5.

2. 5 mg/mL transfer RNA. Keep this separate from the tRNA used for probe synthesis.
3. RNase A: 10 mg/mL. Store frozen in aliquots at –20°C.
4. RNase T1: 1 mg/mL. Store at 4°C.
5. Sodium dodecyl sulfate (SDS): 20% w/v.
6. Proteinase K: 10 mg/mL, in 50 % glycerol. Store at –20°C.
7. Sample loading buffer: 80% v/v formamide; 0.1%w/v xylene cyanol; 0.1% w/v bromophenol blue; 1 m*M*EDTA, pH 7.5.
8. 5× TBE: 450 m*M*Tris-HCl, pH 8.3; 450 m*M*boric acid; 5 m*M*EDTA.
9. Acrylamide solutions: 20% acrylamide (29:1 acrylamide:bisacrylamide), 8.3*M*urea, 1×TBE; 8% acrylamide (19:1 acrylamide:bisacrylamide), 8.3 *M*urea, 1×TBE.
10. 1× TBE, 8.3*M*urea acrylamide dilution buffer.
11. 10% ammonium persulfate in water.
12. TEMED.

3. Methods

3.1. Preparation of the Labeled Probe

1. Linearize the template with the appropriate restriction enzyme that cuts downstream from the insert. Avoid enzymes that generate 3' overhangs. Linearize sufficient template for a large number of transcription reactions (50 μg for 50 reactions) *(see* Section 4.3., Notes 1,2).
2. Extract the digest once with an equal vol of TE-saturated phenol and once with an equal vol of chloroform. Add 0.1 vol of 3*M* sodium acetate and precipitate with 2 vol of ethanol. Recover the DNA by centrifugation.
3. Wash the DNA pellet by adding 100 μL of 70% ethanol, followed by a 2-min spin at full speed in an Eppendorf centrifuge. Discard the 70% ethanol and lyophilize the DNA pellet. Resuspend in RNase-free TE at a concentration of 1 μg/μL.
4. Add the components to the transcription reaction in the following order at room temperature:

> 2 μL 10× transcription buffer *(see* Note 3, Section 4.3.).
> 2 μL 10× XTP mix for use with labeled UTP or labeled GTP.
> 1 μL 20× DTT.
> 2 μL 10× BSA.
> 10 μL α-^{32}P-UTP or GTP.
> 1 μL linear template DNA, 1 μg/μL.
> 1 μL 5 U/μL human placental RNase inhibitor.
> 1 μL bacteriophage RNA polymerase (3–10 U/μL).

Incubate at 40°C for 30 min for SP6 RNA polymerase, 37°C for 30 min for T3 and T7 RNA polymerase. If the probe is to be gel-purified, omit steps 5–7 and continue with gel purification as described below.

5. For DNase digestion of the template, add the following:

   4 μL human placental RNase inhibitor (5 U/μL).

   65 μL DEPC H_2O.

   10 μL of 10× TM.

   1 μL of 1 μg/μL RNase free DNase.

   Incubate at 37°C for 10 min.

6. Add 100 μL of DEPC H_2O and 1 μL of 5 μg/μL RNase-free tRNA. Extract the probe once with an equal vol of TE saturated phenol and once with an equal vol of chloroform. Add 200 μL of 5 *M* ammonium acetate and 800 μL of ethanol. Precipitate by chilling in a dry ice/ethanol bath for 15 min. Spin for 15 min in an Eppendorf centrifuge cooled to 4°C. Remove the supernatant, wash with 70% ethanol as described above, and lyophilize to dryness.

7. Resuspend in 200 μL of 2 m*M* EDTA, pH 7.5. Reprecipitate as described in step 6. Resuspend in 150 μL of 2 m*M* EDTA, pH 7.5. Count 3 μL in a scintillation counter to determine net synthesis (*see* Section 4.3., Note 4).

3.2. Gel Purification of Labeled Probe

1. Pour a small (17 cm × 17 cm) 4% denaturing polyacrylamide/8.3 *M* urea gel for probe purification. Use the thin spacers identical to those found in DNA sequencing gels (0.3 mm). Mix 20 mL 8% acrylamide, 8.3 *M* urea with 20 mL 1× TBE, 8.3 *M* urea. Degas in a heavy-walled vacuum flask using a water aspirator for 10 min. Add 20 μL TEMED, 200 μL 10% ammonium persulfate, mix, and pour. Polymerize for 1 h. Prerun gel for 1 h in 0.5× TBE at 500–1000 V. Check the temperature of the gel plates to prevent them from cracking.

2. Follow steps 1–4 of probe synthesis. Omit step 5 and go directly to step 6. After lyophilization to dryness, resuspend the probe in 10 μL of sample loading buffer. Vortex vigorously to resuspend the probe. Load and run at 500–1000 V. It is useful to determine how each probe runs with respect to the tracking dyes on an analytical gel prior to running the preparative gel.

3. Separate the gel plates and cover the gel with Saran wrap™. CAUTION: Because 50–80% of the labeled nucleotide is incorporated into the probe, the gel is highly radioactive. Use appropriate safety measures. In a darkroom, tape a piece of X-ray film to the gel. Using a 18-gage needle, poke holes through the film into the gel for registration marks. Expose for 1–2 min.

4. Develop and dry the film. Line up the registration marks and retape the film to the gel. Cut out the appropriate band by cutting through the film into the gel. Separate the film and the Saran wrap™ from the gel slice. Place the gel slice in an Eppendorf tube. Crush the gel slice with a sealed, siliconized Pasteur pipet. Add 0.5 mL of elution buffer. Mix on a shaker for 1–2 h at 37°C.

5. Remove the acrylamide by pelleting the acrylamide in the Eppendorf centrifuge. One microliter of RNase-free tRNA (5 μg/μL) is added to the probe containing supernatant. The probe is then extracted once with an equal vol of TE saturated phenol and once with an equal vol of chloroform, and precipitated by the addition of 1.0 mL of ethanol. No salt is necessary because of the ammonium acetate in the elution buffer. The probe is resuspended in 100 μL of 2 m*M*EDTA, pH 7.5. Count 3 μL in a scintillation counter to determine net synthesis.

3.3. Hybridization, RNase Digestion, and Gel Fractionation

1. Prepare sufficient hybridization cocktail for the number of reactions that will be set up. Hybridization cocktail contains the following for each reaction:

    24 μL 3× recrystalized formamide (*see* Section 4.4., Note 1).
    3 μL 10× hybridization buffer.
    3 μL labeled probe.

2. To prepare RNA for hybridization, ethanol-precipitate RNA samples (*see* Section 4.4., Note 2). Wash the pellet in 70% ethanol and lyophilize to dryness. Resuspend each sample in 30 μL of hybridization cocktail by vortexing vigorously. Heat to 85°C for 10 min. Hybridize at 45–55°C overnight (>12 h) (*see* Section 4.4., Notes 3–5).

3. After hybridization is complete, add 350 μL of RNase buffer to each sample. Using tRNA, adjust all samples to 10 mg/sample of RNA. This is necessary only if small amounts of RNA are used in the protection reaction (<1 mg). This normalizes the digestion conditions for all samples. Add RNase A to 40 μg/μL and RNase T1 to 2 μg/μL. Digest at 30°C for 30 min (*see* Section 4.4., Note 6).

4. Remove the RNase by addition of 10 μL of 20% SDS and 5 μL 10-mg/mL proteinase K, followed by digestion for 15 min at 37°C. Add 1 μL of 5 μg/μL tRNA to each reaction. The samples are extracted with an equal vol of phenol and an equal vol of chloroform. The protected fragments are then recovered by addition of 800 μL of ethanol, chilled in dry ice/ethanol for 15 min, and spun in the Eppendorf centrifuge for 15 min. The supernatant is discarded and the the pellet is lyophilized to dryness. Resuspend each sample in 2 μL of loading dye, boil for 2 min, and then quickly chill on ice.

5. Fractionate digested products on a denaturing polyacrylamide/8.3M urea DNA sequencing gel. Pour and prerun the gel as described above for the gel used in the isolation of the probe. The gel used here is usually longer (40 cm) and has a higher percentage of acrylamide (6–12%). The percentage of acrylamide used depends upon the size of the protected fragment. The range of protected fragment sizes and the suggested percentages of acrylamide gels are as follows:

acrylamide concentration	protected fragment size range
6%	150–400 nucleotides
8%	100–250 nucleotides
10%	20–150 nucleotides
12%	10–100 nucleotides

The 6% acrylamide is made by diluting the 8% stock with 1× TBE, 8.3M urea. The 10 and 12% acrylamide is made by diluting the 20% stock with 1× TBE, 8.3M urea (*see* Section 4.4., Note 7).

4. Notes

4.1. Precautions for Working with RNA

Because of the ubiquitous presence of RNase, appropriate precautions must be taken for the preparation of reagents to be used in this work. All water used for the preparation of solutions should be of the highest possible purity, such as that provided by Millipore Corporation's Milli-Q purification system. Next, the water used to prepare solutions should be treated with diethylpyrocarbonate (DEPC) to inactivate any ribonuclease. DEPC is added, to a final concentration of 0.1%, followed by autoclaving for 30 min to inactivate any remaining DEPC. CAUTION: DEPC is a suspected carcinogen and should be handled only in a chemical fume hood. All solutions should be made up and stored in tissue-culture plastic ware. These materials have been sterilized by ethylene oxide or γ-irradiation and have been found by the author to be RNase-free. Furthermore, because copious amounts of RNase are used to digest the RNA/RNA hybrids, a set of "RNase pipetmen" should be used for the RNase digestion and be kept separate from the ones used for probe synthesis and hybridization. If possible, a separate lab bench should be used for the RNase digestions.

4.2. Plasmid Vectors Used for In Vitro Transcription

1. The first step in a mRNA protection assay is the selection of the probe fragment. Several alternatives are shown in Fig. 3. Probe fragments that overlap the transcription initiation site, the polyadenlyation site, splice donors, and splice acceptors can be chosen. For optimal synthesis of

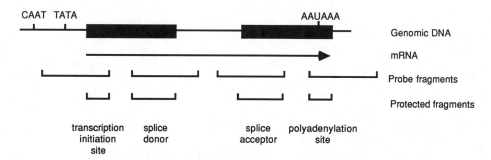

Fig. 3. Probes for mRNA protection. Genomic DNA fragments that contain both transcribed and nontranscribed sequences can be used for 5' and 3' end probes. Fragments that contain both intron and exon sequences can be used to map splice donors and acceptors.

labeled probe, the probe fragment should not be greater than 500 nucleotides *(8)*, and the protected fragment should be no greater than 400 nucleotides *(8)*. These limits can be exceeded with less than optimal results.

2. After a probe fragment has been selected, the fragment is cloned into a plasmid vector containing a bacteriophage RNA polymerase promoter. Many different plasmids are available for this purpose; some of them are listed in Table 1. All of the plasmids contain the ampicillin-resistance gene and the origin of replication of pBR322. Another common feature of these plasmids is a multiple cloning site (MCS). This has been derived from the MCS found in pUC12,13,18, or 19 *(9)*. Promega Biotec has added new MCSs with up to 15 unique restriction sites. In addition, Promega Biotec (Madison, WI) has introduced a polylinker that lacks restriction sites that generate 3' overhangs. The reason for this is discussed below. For each plasmid, both orientations of the MCS with respect to the RNA polymerase promoter are available. A few of the plasmids contain the a complementation fragment of β-galactosidase. These plasmids offer the ability of blue/white X-gal selection for recombinants *(10)*. This list excludes bacteriophage λ cloning vectors that have bacteriophage RNA polymerase promoters flanking an MCS and plasmids containing single strand bacteriophage origins of replication (phagemids). Plasmid vectors containing a single RNA polymerase promoter or RNA polymerase promoters flanking the polylinker are available. Multiple promoters allow synthesis of both sense and antisense transcripts. For the purposes discussed here, only the antisense transcript is necessary. However, if the sense strand may be of use at some future time, then these plasmids should be utilized.

3. Of the three RNA polymerases, one is not more efficient for probe syn-

Table 1
Survey of Bacteriophage Promoter-Containing Plasmids

Plasmid selection	Vendor	Promoter/Multiple Cloning Site[a]	*lac* z
SP64	Boehringer Mannheim	SP6: HindIII...EcoRI (pUC12/13)	−
SP64	Promega Biotec		−
SP18	Bethesda Research Laboratories	SP6: HindIII...EcoRI (pUC18/19)	−
SP65	Boehringer Mannheim	SP6: EcoRI...HindIII (pUC12/13)	−
SP65	Promega Biotec		−
SP19	Bethesda Research Laboratories	SP6: EcoRI...HindIII (pUC18/19)	−
T3T7lac	Boehringer Mannheim	T7: EcoRI...HindIII: T3 (pUC18/19)	+
T3T7-18	Bethesda Research Laboratories		
T3T7-19	Bethesda Research Laboratories	T3: EcoRI...HindIII: T7 (pUC18/19)	−
pT71	Boehringer Mannheim	T7: EcoRI...HindIII (pUC12/13)	−
pT71	US Biochemicals		
pT713	Bethesda Research Laboratories		−
pT72	Boehringer Mannheim	T7: HindIII...EcoRI (pUC12/13)	−
pT72	US Biochemicals		−
pT712	Bethesda Research Laboratories		−
pGem 1	Promega Biotec	T7: EcoRI...HindIII: SP6 (pUC12/13)	−
DP1	New England Nuclear		−
pGem 2	Promega Biotec	SP6: EcoRI...HindIII: T7 (pUC12/13)	−
DP2	New England Nuclear		−
pGem 3	Promega Biotec	T7: EcoRI...HindIII: SP6 (pUC18/19)	−
pGem -3z	Promega Biotec		+
SPT18	Pharmacia		−
SPT18	Boehringer Mannheim		−
pGem 4	Promega Biotec	SP6: EcoRI...HindIII: T7 (pUC18/19)	−
pGem-4z	Promega Biotec		+
SPT19	Pharmacia		−
SPT19	Boehringer Mannheim		−
SP6/ T7-19	Bethesda Research Laboratories		+
SP70	Promega Biotec	SP6: XhoI, Pvu II, HindIII, EcoRI, ClaI, Eco RV, Bgl II:T7[b]	−
SP71	Promega Biotec	T7: XhoI, Pvu II, HindIII, EcoRI, ClaI, Eco RV, Bgl II:SP6[b]	−

(continued)

Table 1 *(continued)*

Plasmid selection	Vendor	Promoter/Multiple Cloning Site[a]	*lac* z
SP72	Promega Biotec	SP6: Xho I...pUC18/19...Bgl II: T7[c]	–
SP73	Promega Biotec	T7: Xho I...pUC18/19...Bgl II: SP6[c]	–
pBS	Stratagene	T7: EcoRI...SphI: T3[d]	–
SP6/T3	Bethesda Research Laboratories	T3: EcoRI...HindIII: SP6	–

[a] The restriction sites found in pUC12 are EcoRI, SacI , SmaI, BamHI, XbaI, SalI, PstI, and HindIII. The restriction sites found in pUC18 are EcoRI, SacI, KpnI, SmaI, BamHI, XbaI, SalI, PstI, SphI, and HindIII. The multiple cloning site (MCS) of pUC13 and pUC19 is in the opposite orientations of that in pUC12 and 18, respectively.

[b] These MCSs lack sites for enzymes that generate 3' overhangs.

[c] These MCSs contain the restriction sites found in SP70 and SP71 with a pUC18/19 polylinker inserted between the EcoRI and HindIII sites. This yields a polylinker with 15 unique sites.

[d] This MCS is derived from the pUC18 MCS with the HindIII site deleted.

thesis than the others *(6)*. However, different enzymes do transcribe different templates with varying efficiencies *(8)*. If a particular polymerase shows a strong stop within a particular probe fragment, switch to a different promoter/polymerase combination.

4. T3 and T7 RNA polymerase are approx fivefold less expensive per unit than SP6 RNA polymerase.

5. The stability of the coliphage RNA polymerases in the hands of the author are greater than that of SP6 RNA polymerase. However, if the SP6 enzyme is divided into small aliquots, and if one minimizes the time the enzyme spends outside of –20°C, its stability is just as great as the coliphage RNA polymerases.

4.3. Template Preparation, Transcription, and Purification

1. The template must be linearized prior to transcription. Digestion with restriction enzymes that generate a 3' overhang should be avoided in view of the possibility of "end artifacts" *(8)*. Some examples of "end artifacts" are the presence of full-length protected probe. Digestion of the template with an enzyme that generates a 5' overhang usually eliminates this problem.

2. When linearizing the probe, it is essential that it is 100% cut. Incomplete digestion of the template results in background bands in the final acrylamide gel. One alternative is to digest the template with a restriction enzyme that cuts the template many times. Another is to use a single cutter and purify the linear template by one of the numerous

methods available.

3. The buffer described in the materials is the one originally described for transcription by SP6 polymerase *(3)*. This buffer can be used for transcription with T3 and T7 RNA polymerases as well. This is also the buffer recommended for transcription with the latter enzymes by at least one supplier of these enzymes.

4. Following transcription and digestion of the template with DNase, the labeled probe can be purified by precipitation with ammonium acetate and ethanol. Some probes provide excellent results when prepared in this fashion. However, others yield significant background bands. For some probes, this can be eliminated by gel purification of the labeled probe prior to hybridization. The purification protocol described in the Methods Section results in high yields of full-length probe. Although time-consuming, the improvement in the signal-to-noise ratio is significant enough in some cases to make it worthwhile.

4.4. Hybridization, RNase Digestion, and Gel Fractionation

1. The formamide used in these hybridizations is 3× recrystalized, as suggested by Casey and Davidson *(7)*. To recrystalize formamide, place a stir bar into a 1-L bottle of formamide and close the lid tightly. Place the bottle in an ice bucket filled with ice, and place the bucket on a stirring motor in a cold room. Stir overnight. Formamide will crystalize on the sides of the bottle. Decant unrecrystalized formamide, thaw the crystals at room temperature, and recrystalize twice more. One liter of formamide yields 200 mL of 3× recrystalized formamide.

2. The amount of RNA added to the hybridization can vary over a wide range. The abundance of the mRNA under study and the yield of RNA from a particular cell or tissue type govern the limits. As little as 10 ng of total RNA from adult human blood gives a signal within an hour when probed for β-globin *(11)*. The maximum amount of RNA that can be added to a hybridization has not been determined. In practice, the range of RNA is 2–20 μg/reaction. As much as 50 μg can be used (M. Finer, unpublished observations). When using very small amounts (<2 μg), tRNA can be added as carrier for the RNase digestion in order to avoid overdigestion.

3. The temperature for hybridization must be empirically determined for each probe. A suggested starting range is between 45 and 55°C.

4. To ensure that the hybridization is quantitative, a probe excess determination must be carried out. This can be carried out in either of two ways. First, a RNA source is selected that is highly enriched in the RNA under study. A maximum amount (20 μg) of RNA is hybridized to increasing

amounts of probe, in twofold increments. When probe excess is achieved, no further increase in signal will be detectable. This amount of probe is used for all subsequent hybridizations. In the second approach, a fixed amount of probe (10^6 cpm) is hybridized in twofold increments to increasing amounts of RNA derived from a tissue that is highly enriched for the RNA under study. The relationship between RNA input and signal from the protected fragment should be linear when in probe excess. This will determine the maximum amount of RNA put into the hybridization.

5. A necessary control to include in each assay is the hybridization of the probe to a nonspecific RNA (i.e., yeast RNA). This identifies RNase-resistant fragments from the probe itself. In some cases, these will be the same size as the protected fragment, and a new probe will have to be selected. In practice, two different plasmids should be constructed for each desired probe. This ensures that at least one will be useful.

6. In the work of Melton et al. *(3,8)*, the suggested conditions for RNase digestion are reported to be 40 µg/mL RNase A and 2 µg/mL RNase T1. These are good starting concentrations. The exact concentration depends on specific activity of the RNase preparations. For both RNases, titration on both sides of these concentrations is essential. A recommended titration for RNase A is 20, 40, 60, and 80 µg/mL. RNase A should be stored in aliquots frozen at –20°C. RNase T1 must also be titrated over the range of 1–4 µg/mL. It is difficult to obtain RNase T1 as a lyophilized powder. Most preparations come as an ammonium sulfate suspension. Prior to use, the suspension must be spun in an Eppendorf centrifuge at full speed for 15 min, the supernatant vol determined and the supernatant discarded, and the pellet resuspended in a vol of TE equivalent to the original vol of the supernatant. Failure to do so results in a large ammonium sulfate precipitate when the protected fragments are recovered by ethanol precipitation. This precipitate will redissolve in sample buffer. However, the samples will take a long period of time to run into the gel, and the gel will run poorly. RNase T1 can be stored at 4°C for up to 6 mo.

7. Single-stranded RNA probes possess one potentially major drawback. Some probes generate numerous background bands, in addition to the protected fragment, even though the probe hybridized to itself or to nonspecific RNA is free of background bands. This is most prevalent when highly homologous RNAs are also present within the same RNA population, or in gene transfer studies in which the exogenous and endogenous transcripts are from closely related species. Short regions of homology will be protected from digestion and appear on the gel because the probe is uniformly labeled. With an end-labeled probe,

unless these short duplexes include the end where the probe is labeled, they will not be seen on the gel. Careful selection of the sequence to be used for a probe, or testing two or more probes for a specific mRNA, can reduce or eliminate this problem.

References

1. Berk, A. and Sharp, P. (1977) Sizing and mapping of early adenovirus mRNAs by gel electrophoresis of S1 endonuclease-digested hybrids. *Cell* **12**, 721–732.
2. Zinn, K., DiMaio, D., and Maniatis, T. (1983) Identification of two distinct regulatory regions adjacent to the human β-interferon gene. *Cell* **34**, 865–879.
3. Melton, D., Krieg, P., Rebagliati, M., Maniatis, T., Zinn, K., and Green, M. (1984) Efficient synthesis of biologically active RNA and RNA hybridization probes from plasmids containing a bacteriophage SP6 promoter. *Nucleic Acids Res.* **7**, 1175–1193.
4. Butler, E. and Chamberlin, M. (1982) Bacteriophage SP6 specific RNA polymerase. I. isolation and characterization of the enzyme. *J. Biol. Chem.* **257**, 5772–5778.
5. Kassavetis, G., Butler, E., Roulland, D., and Chamberlin, M. (1982) Bacteriophage SP6 specific RNA polymerase. II. Mapping of SP6 DNA and selective *in vitro* transcription. *J. Biol. Chem.* **257**, 5779–5787.
6. Chamberlin, M., Kingston, R., Gilman, M., Wiggs, J., and DeVera, A. (1983) Isolation of bacterial and bacteriophage RNA polymerases and their use in synthesis of RNA *in vitro*. *Methods Enzymol.* **101**, 540–568.
7. Casey, J. and Davidson, N. (1977) Rates of formation and thermal stabilities of RNA:DNA and DNA:DNA duplexes at high concentrations of formamide. *Nucleic Acids Res.* **4**, 1539–1552.
8. Krieg, P. and Melton, D. (1987) In vitro RNA synthesis with SP6 RNA polymerase. *Methods Enzymol.* **155**, 397–415.
9. Yanisch-Perron, C., Vieria, J., and Messing, J. (1985) Improved M13 phage cloning vectors and host strains: Nucleotide sequence of M13mp18 and pUC19 vectors. *Gene* **33**, 103–119.
10. Messing, J. (1983) New M13 Vectors for Cloning. *Methods Enzymol.* **101**, 20–77.
11. Dzierzak, E., Papayannopoulou, T., and Mulligan, H. (1988) Lineage-specific expression of a human β-globin gene in murine bone marrow transplant recipients reconstituted with retrovirus-transduced stem cells. *Nature* **331**, 35–41.

CHAPTER 23

Primer Extension Analysis of mRNA Isolated from Transfected Cell Lines

Mark W. Leonard and Roger K. Patient

1. Introduction

Primer extension is a relatively quick and convenient means by which transcription from a gene transfected into tissue-culture cells can be monitored. The technique can be used to accurately determine the site of transcription initiation or to quantify the amount of cap-site-specific message produced.

The principle of this technique is shown in Fig. 1. In brief, a radiolabeled probe fragment (preferably single-stranded) is hybridized to its complementary sequence near the mRNA 5' terminus. This primer is then extended by the enzyme reverse transcriptase back to the initiation point of the message. The products of the reaction are run on a denaturing polyacrylamide gel and exposed to autoradiography.

The major advantage of primer extension for mRNA analysis is its convenience (compared to S1 mapping or RNase mapping). The technique enables precise determination of the start point of transcription. Also, because very clean results can be obtained, more than one mRNA can be quantitatively analyzed in a single reaction. For example, the transcripts from a transfected marked gene can be distinguished from the cell's endogenous gene products, or, by judicious choice of primers, transcription from a test gene and a cotransfected (internal standard) control gene can be monitored in

From: *Methods in Molecular Biology, Vol. 7: Gene Transfer and Expression Protocols*
Edited by: E. J. Murray © 1991 The Humana Press Inc., Clifton, NJ

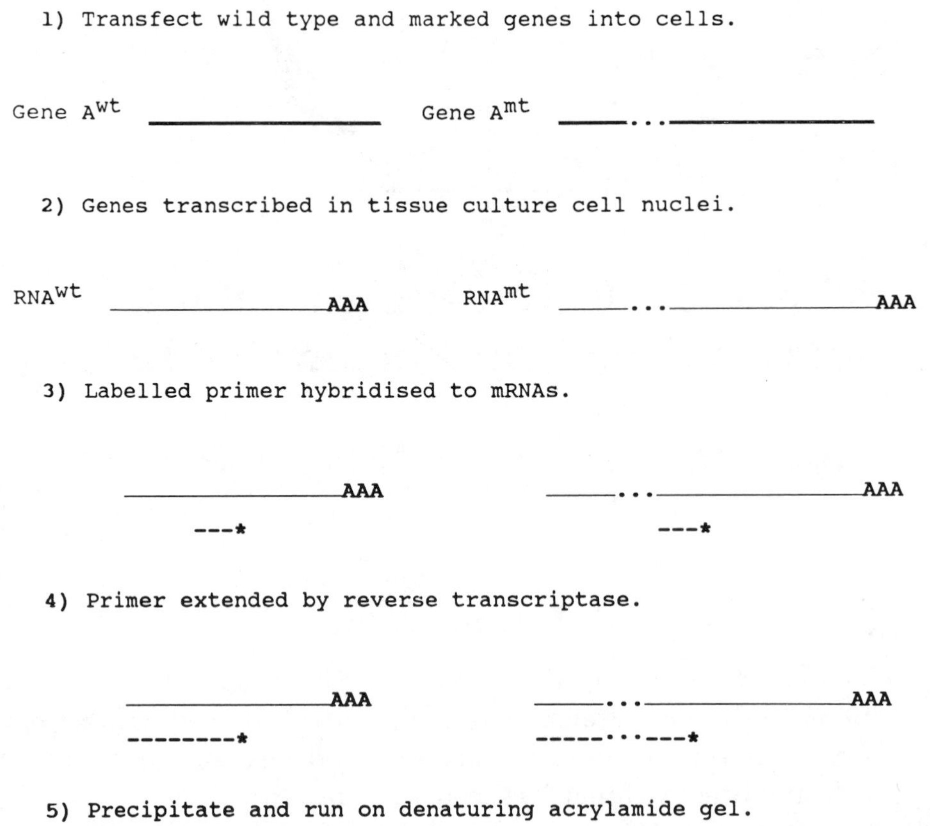

1) Transfect wild type and marked genes into cells.

Gene A^{wt} _____   Gene A^{mt} _____..._____

2) Genes transcribed in tissue culture cell nuclei.

RNA^{wt} _____**AAA**   RNA^{mt} _____..._____**AAA**

3) Labelled primer hybridised to mRNAs.

_____**AAA**   _____..._____**AAA**
          ---*   ---*

4) Primer extended by reverse transcriptase.

_____**AAA**   _____..._____**AAA**
    ---------*   -----··-·---*

5) Precipitate and run on denaturing acrylamide gel.

Fig. 1. Distinguishing transcripts from wild type and marked copies of the *X. laevis* β-globin gene by primer extension: Schematic representation of the primer extension reaction.

the same reaction (*see* Fig. 2). Finally, in genes with multiple cap sites, the amount of transcription from each site can be distinguished in a single reaction.

Many of the above considerations apply equally to the analysis of mRNA by S1 or RNase mapping (*see* Chapters 21 and 22, this vol). Although these latter techniques are usually more sensitive, the convenience of primer extension means that it is often the method of choice for RNA analysis.

2. Materials

As with all procedures involving RNA, extreme care must be taken to avoid RNase contamination and degradation of samples (*1*). Work surfaces should be clean, and gloves should be worn at all times. Stock solutions and glassware should be treated with the RNase inhibitor diethylpyrocarbonate (DEPC) (0.1% for 30 min or longer at 37°C). DEPC cannot be used to treat

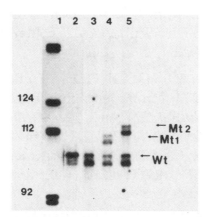

Fig. 2. An example of a primer extension reaction: Total cytoplasmic RNA from cultured cells containing Xenopus β-globin gene constructs, analyzed using a single 5'-labeled oligo primer. Lane 3, wild-type, β-globin gene introduced alone; Lanes 4 and 5, wild-type gene plus genes marked by insertion of different-sized oligonucleotides into the first exon. Samples are run alongside a labeled DNA size marker (Lane 1) and total cytoplasmic RNA (50 ng) from *X. laevis* erythroblasts (Lane 2) to show the cap site used in vivo.

solutions containing Tris, since it is unstable in the presence of this buffer. Tris buffers should be made with DEPC-treated autoclaved water and then reautoclaved. It is important to remove all traces of DEPC (by autoclaving) prior to use to prevent carboxymethylation of RNA and proteins. Sterile disposable plasticware can be treated in the same way, but is usually sufficiently RNase-free that pretreatment is not required. Separate stocks of plasticware and reagents should be maintained solely for RNA work.

Glass capillaries for the hybridization reaction should be siliconized (optional for plasticware). Items for siliconization are rinsed in a 5% solution of dichlorodimethyl silane in chloroform in a fume hood (this solution is toxic and highly volatile). Siliconized items should be rinsed several times with DEPC-treated water and baked (100°C, 2h) before being DEPC-treated themselves.

The most convenient source of single-strand primer is a chemically synthesized short oligonucleotide (*see* Note 1). This should be 18 nucleotides or longer, and should ideally be located within 100 bases of the mRNA cap site. Care should be taken to ensure that the chosen oligomer does not contain repeats capable of inter- or intraprobe hybridization, since this will reduce the efficiency of annealing to mRNA.

Usually, the primer is 5' end-labeled *(2–4)* (*see* Note 2), particularly if the sequence of the extension products is to be determined by the method of Maxam and Gilbert *(3,5)*. The specific activity of the primer should be determined by Cerenkov counting after removal of unincorporated nucleotide (by centrifugation through a Sephadex G25 column). Primers should have a SA of $>5 \times 10^5$ dpm/pmol.

1. 10× Kinase buffer: 500 mM Tris-HCl (pH 7.6), 100 mM MgCl$_2$, 50 mM dithiothreitol (DTT), 1 mM spermidine, 1 mM EDTA.
2. 5× Hybridization buffer: 2M NaCl, 50mM PIPES (pH 6.4).
3. 1× Extension buffer: 5 µL of 1M Tris-HCl (pH 8.3) 5 µL of 200 mM DTT, 5 µL of 120 mM MgCl$_2$, 2.5 µL of 1 mg/mL actinomycin D, 5 µL each of 10 mM dATP, dCTP, dGTP, dTTP, 1 µL (approx 40 U) RNasin *(see below)*, and DEPC water to 89 µL.
4. Formamide loading dye: 80% deionized formamide, 45 mM Tris-HCl borate, 45 mM boric acid, 1.25 mM EDTA, 0.02% xylene cyanole.
5. G25 Sephadex: Suspend Sephadex in approx 50 vol of TE (10 mM Tris-HCl, pH 7.5; 1 mM EDTA). Autoclave for 15 min (Sephadex will swell) and allow to cool to room temperature. Store at 4°C in a capped bottle.
6. Carrier (yeast) tRNA: Make up to 25 mg/mL with DEPC H$_2$O. Use the maker's bottle to avoid RNase contamination during weighing. Store in sterile plastic tubes at –20°C.
7. 3M sodium acetate (NaOAc), brought to pH 5.4 with glacial acetic acid, DEP-treated, and autoclaved for 15 min.
8. 70% EtOH/DEPC H$_2$O: 70 mL absolute ethanol, 30 mL DEPC-treated water.

The NaCl, MgCl$_2$, EDTA, and PIPES should be DEPC-treated as described above. The remaining buffer components should be made up in DEPC-treated autoclaved water, but not treated this way themselves. Actinomycin D is light-sensitive and toxic, and should not be autoclaved. DTT is thermally unstable and cannot be autoclaved (stock 1M DTT should be made up in DEPC-treated 10 mM NaOAc, filter-sterilized, and aliquoted at –20°C). Stocks of dNTPs should be filter-sterilized.

These buffers can be aliquoted and stored at –20°C. If the RNase inhibitor RNasin is to be present, it should be added fresh to the extension buffer on the day it is to be used. Reverse transcriptase (stored in aliquots at –70°C) should, similarly, be added fresh to the extension mix immediately prior to use.

3. Methods

Protocols for the labeling, hybridization, and extension reactions are given below. The hybridization reaction is frequently carried out in sealed capillaries as described; however, the protocol is greatly simplified by using the modification given in Note 3.

3.1. Kinasing Primer

1. In a plastic microfuge tube, mix
   1–50 pmol oligonucleotide 5' (unphosphorylated) ends,
   2 μL 10× kinase buffer,
   70 μCi aqueous gamma ^{32}P-ATP (3000 Ci/mmol),
   10–20 U T4 polynucleotide kinase, and
   DEPC water to 20 μL.
2. Incubate at 37°C for 30 min.
3. Add 4 μL of 250 mM EDTA.
4. Remove unincorporated labeled nucleotide by centrifugation down a Sephadex G-25 column (*see* Note 4).
5. Extract with phenol:chloroform:isoamyl alcohol (25:24:1) (v/v).
6. Add 10 μg tRNA (carrier for the precipitation).
7. Add 1/10 vol 3M NaOAc, ethanol-precipitate by adding 2 vol 100% ethanol and pelleting in a microfuge for 15 min. Wash the pellet in 70% ethanol and dry under vacuum.
8. Resuspend (0.25–2.5 fmol/μL) in DEPC water.

3.2. Hybridization Reaction

1. In a plastic microcentrifuge tube (siliconization is not essential), mix
   2 μL (0.5–5 fmol) labeled primer (*see* Note 5),
   2 μL 5× hybridization buffer,
   0.1–1 fmol target mRNA (up to 20 μg total RNA), and
   DEPC water to 10 μL.
2. Take the mixture up in a siliconized glass capillary (*see* Note 3).
3. Seal both ends of the capillary in a Bunsen flame and label the sample with indelible marker (on water-proof tape if necessary).
4. Heat the sample to 70°C by submerging in a water bath for 3 min (*see* Note 6).
5. Hybridize for 3–6 h, submerged in a water bath at the optimum temperature (*see* Notes 7–11).

3.3. Extension Reaction

1. Dry the capillaries and remove the ends with a glass cutter.
2. Remove both ends of the capillary, connect to a pipet and expel the hybridization mix into 89 μL of extension buffer in a microfuge tube (including 1 μL [approx 40 U] RNasin if desired; *see* Note 12).
3. Add 1 μL (approx 20 U) AMV reverse transcriptase per sample.
4. Incubate the extension mix at 42°C for 1 h (*see* Note 13).
5. Add 11 μL of 3M NaOAc, ethanol-precipitate total nucleic acid as in step 7, Section 3.1., wash with 70% ethanol, and vacuum dry.

6. Take the pellet up in 5–10 μL of formamide loading dye.
7. Heat-denature at 90°C for 3 min; chill on ice.
8. Electrophorese on an appropriate percentage of denaturing polyacrylamide gel, along with suitable size markers or DNA sequencing ladders.

The labeled extension products are run on a standard denaturing urea–acrylamide gel of suitable percentage (dependent on the distance of the primer from the 5' end of the message) to enable good resolution of cap site length transcripts. This is particularly important when the site of transcription initiation is to be determined, but is also important for quantification experiments if multiple start sites exist in the gene of interest (*see* Notes 14–16).

4. Notes

1. A single-stranded (5' unphosphorylated) oligonucleotide is the most convenient source of primer. Alternatively, the primer can be generated by restriction enzyme digestion of the cloned gene under study. A pair of infrequently cut restriction sites with cohesive ends of different lengths, separated by approx 20–100 bp, are cleaved so as to produce coding and noncoding strands of different lengths. A radiolabeling step between the first and second cleavages yields a uniquely end-labeled fragment that can be separated from the noncoding strand by denaturing acrylamide gel electrophoresis (*3*) and autoradiography (*6*) (*see* Chapter 21). The greater the difference in size between the two strands, and the smaller the restriction fragment, the better the probe separation. It is possible to use a uniquely end-labeled double-stranded primer, since RNA–DNA hybrids are more stable than the corresponding DNA–DNA hybrids (by approx 5°C). However, the use of a double-stranded primer requires precise determination of the hybridization temperature and reduces the efficiency of the technique.
2. Ideally, the primer should be 5' end-labeled. The 5' terminal phosphate groups of restriction fragments must be removed by treatment with alkaline phosphatase (*4*) prior to kinasing; oligomers should be obtained without a terminal phosphate to preclude this step. Such 5' end-labeling is particularly important if the sequence of the extension products is to be determined by the method of Maxam and Gilbert. However, if the objective is merely to quantitate the amount of a particular message, then a 3' labeled primer can be used (*4,7*). Practically, this may be simpler in some instances in which restriction-enzyme-generated probes are to be used (for example, labeling may be important in generating strands

of different sizes). The sensitivity of the primer extension analysis can be improved by using a uniformly labeled (M13 vector-generated) probe *(4,7)*.

3. The hybridization reaction is frequently performed in siliconized capillaries but the protocol can be greatly simplified by carrying out this step directly in plastic microfuge tubes. It is important to completely submerge the microfuge tubes in the water bath to prevent evaporation, since this will alter the salt concentration of the reaction and affect the hybridization. Care must be taken to ensure the tubes are adequately sealed; screw-capped microfuge tubes are best for this purpose. The extension reaction can then be carried out in the same tubes.

4. Prepare G25 Sephadex columns as follows: Plug the nipple of a 2-mL sterile plastic syringe with polymer wool and fill the syringe with a concentrated slurry of Sephadex. Suspend the syringe over a sterile plastic centrifuge tube and spin at 1500 rpm in a swing-out rotor for 5 min. Discard the centrifuge tube and buffer contents, and transfer the syringe to a fresh tube. Load the labeled primer on to the top of the column, rinsing out the tube with 50 μL of TE to ensure transfer of all the label to the column. Spin at 1500 rpm for 5 min. Labeled primer will be found in the eluate, unincorporated label will be located at the top of the column. A successfully labeled probe should register full-scale deflection on a Geiger counter. If this does not happen, rewash the column with a further 50–100 μL of TE. Remove 1 μL of the probe and determine the SA by Cerenkov counting. Probes should not be used with SA <2–5×10^6 dpm/pmol.

5. It may be more convenient to mix the labeled primer with the RNA that is to be analyzed while preparing the RNA. The primer and the RNA can then be coprecipitated, after which the pellet can be taken up in DEPC-treated water and the remaining components of the hybridization reaction added directly to the resuspended pellet.

6. The primer and RNA for analysis are mixed with hybridization buffer, briefly heated to 70°C to remove any RNA (or primer) secondary structure, and then allowed to anneal.

7. The hybridization is carried out with the primer in approx 10-fold molar excess over the target complementary RNA; too great an excess (particularly at suboptimal hybridization stringency) can result in nonspecific priming.

8. The optimum temperature for the hybridization will depend on the length of primer and its base composition. Formulae for the estimation of RNA–DNA hybrid melting temperatures *(8, 9)* are not accurate for short

DNA primers. For most probes, the value is in the range 45–65°C in the buffer given, but pilot experiments should be carried out over this range of temperatures to determine the optimum hybridization temperature for the specific primer–mRNA combination being used.

9. A simple way to monitor the hybridization efficiency is to perform a modified S1 nuclease mapping reaction on the RNA–primer hybrids (*see* Chapter 21, this vol). Briefly, the oligomer and RNA under analysis are hybridized (3–6 h) at a range of temperatures, the hybrids digested with S1 nuclease and the amount of protected (hybridized) oligomer determined by denaturing acrylamide electrophoresis. The temperature at which the maximum amount of S1 nuclease resistant labeled primer occurs should be used for subsequent hybridization reactions.

10. It may also be necessary to optimize the amount of target mRNA present in a typical reaction by carrying out hybridizations with varying amounts of the RNA preparation. Total cytoplasmic RNA can be used in the reaction, although greater sensitivity (and cleaner results) may be achieved using poly A⁺ RNA.

11. The hybridization is carried out for 3–6 h. RNA is susceptible to thermal degradation at elevated temperatures (although this effect is reduced at the acid pH used here), so primers with high optimum hybridization temperatures should be annealed for as short a time as possible.

12. The ribonuclease inhibitor RNasin can be included in the extension reaction (1 μL, approx 40 U) but is less effective in the hybridization reaction. This is because the 70°C incubation to remove secondary structure and the high temperatures required in the annealing reaction are likely to cause denaturation of the RNasin protein. Additionally, the activity of RNasin is critically dependent on the presence of a minimum amount of 1 mM dithiotreitol, which is also unstable at elevated temperatures. Ribonucleoside–vanadyl complex RNase inhibitors can reduce the efficiency of extension under certain conditions (>2 mM inhibitor in the presence of low [1 mM] concentrations of dNTPs).

13. The elongation reaction is carried out at 42°C to reduce the amount of mRNA secondary structure, which can cause premature termination of the reverse transcriptase.

14. The further the primer is located from the cap site, the greater the likelihood of premature termination by the reverse transcriptase at sites of RNA secondary structure or RNA cleavage (e.g., by RNase). The presence of the resulting discrete "drop off" bands will cause a reduced cap-site signal. Changing the position of the primer to a site 5' to strong secondary structure extension barriers will improve the yield of cap-site product.

15. The extension reaction often generates more than one band in the vicinity of the cap-site (*see* Fig. 2). These may represent genuine multiple start sites of transcription. Additionally, it is thought that methylation of the mRNA at the cap-site, or adjacent nucleotide, causes premature termination of the reverse transcriptase enzyme in a portion of the molecules. Such effects should be taken into account when determining the precise point of transcription initiation. The ratio of the cap-site bands can vary between different transfected cell types, but is constant for a given source of mRNA.

16. Additional bands may be produced as a result of fold-back cDNA synthesis by reverse transcriptase, although the incorporation of actinomycin D in the extension buffer should reduce this activity. Sodium pyrophosphate (80 mM) appears to be even more effective in this function, but may be inhibitory to reverse transcriptase from some sources. Spurious bands occasionally may arise by cross hybridization of the primer to either endogenous tissue-culture-cell RNA or carrier tRNA. Such bands can be identified by performing a control primer extension reaction on RNA isolated from nontransfected culture cells.

Further Reading

Maniatis, T., Fritsch, E. F., and Sambrook, J. (1982) *Molecular Cloning: A Laboratory Manual* Cold Spring Harbor Laboratory, Cold Spring Harbor, New York.

Williams, J. G. and Mason, P. J. (1985) Hybridization and analysis of RNA, in *Nucleic Acid Hybridization—A Practical Approach* (Hames, B. D. and Higgins, S. J., eds.), IRL, Oxford, Washington, DC, pp. 139–160.

Krug, M. S. and Berger, S. L. (1987) First strand cDNA synthesis primed with oligo dT, in *Methods in Enzymology*, vol. 152 (Berger, S. L. and Kimmel, A. R., eds.), Academic, London, New York, pp. 316–325.

Calzone, F. J., Britten, R., and Davidson, E. H. (1987) Mapping gene transcripts by nuclease protection assays and cDNA primer extension, in *Methods in Enzymology*, vol. 152 (Berger, S. L. and Kimmel, A. R., eds.), Academic, London, New York, pp. 611–632.

References

1. Blumberg, D. (1987) Creating a ribonuclease-free environment, in *Methods in Enzymology*, vol. 152 (Berger, S. L. and Kimmel, A. R., eds.), Academic, London, New York, pp. 20–24.

2. Richardson, C. C. (1965) Phosphorylation of nucleic acid by an enzyme from T4 bacteriophage infected *E. coli. Proc. Natl. Acad. Sci. USA* **54,** 158–165.

3. Maxam, A. M. and Gilbert, W. (1980) Sequencing end-labeled DNA with base specific chemical cleavages, in *Methods in Enzymology*, vol. 65 (Grossman, L. and Moldave, K., eds.), Academic, London, New York, pp. 499–560.

4. Arrand, J. E. (1985) Preparation of nucleic acid probes, in *Nucleic Acid Hybridisation—A Practical Approach* (Hames, B. D. and Higgins, S. J.), IRL, Oxford, Washington, DC, pp. 139–160.
5. Maxam, A. M. and Gilbert, W. (1977) A new method for sequencing DNA, *Proc. Natl. Acad. Sci. USA* **74,** 560–564.
6. Boffey, S. (1987) Autoradiography and fluorography, in *Techniques in Molecular Biology,* vol. 2 (Walker, J. M. and Gaastra, W., eds.), Croom and Helm, London, Sydney, pp. 288–295.
7. Tsang, A. S., Mahbubani, H., and Williams, J. G. (1982) Cell-type-specific actin mRNA populations in dictyostelium discoideum. *Cell* **31,** 375–382.
8. Schildkraut, C. and Lifson, S. (1965) Dependence of the melting temperature of DNA upon salt concentration. *Biopolymers* **3,** 195–208.
9. Britten, R. J. and Davidson, E. H. (1985) Hybridisation strategy, in *Nucleic Acid Hybridisation—A Practical Approach* (Hames, B. D. and Higgins, S. J., eds.), IRL, Oxford, Washington, DC, pp. 3–15.

CHAPTER 24

Northern Blot Analysis
of Gene Expression

Robb Krumlauf

1. Introduction

In the analysis of gene expression, the steady-state level of RNA transcripts is one of the most convenient parameters used to monitor the activity of an endogenous or introduced gene in cell lines and tissues. A variety of methods, such as S1 hybridization (Chapter 21, this vol), RNase protection (Chapter 22), and Northern blotting, can be used to measure RNA levels. Which assay system is best depends largely on the type of information required, levels of sensitivity, and limitations of the particular in vivo system being examined. This chapter details the method for analyzing RNA by Northern blotting, which basically involves the isolation of RNA, its size fractionation by electrophoresis, transfer to a membrane, and detection by nucleic acid hybridization and autoradiography.

There are several advantages to Northern blotting analysis. Transcription patterns of genes are often complex, and multiple RNA species can be generated from the same gene. Northern analysis provides information on the relative number, size, and abundance of RNAs derived from a gene, which cannot be obtained by the alternative methods. This technique also generates a record of the RNA that is stored on a membrane that can be used many times. Therefore, the expression of several genes can be analyzed on the same RNA samples by using multiple probes to rehybridize the filter. There are two disadvantages often associated with this technique. The RNA isolated

From: *Methods in Molecular Biology, Vol. 7: Gene Transfer and Expression Protocols*
Edited by: E. J. Murray © 1991 The Humana Press Inc., Clifton, NJ

from cells or tissues must be of high quality, not degraded, which can be difficult in some tissues or for inexperienced workers. This is not a problem for the alternative S1 nuclease protection or RNase protection methods, since enzymes are used to degrade the RNA as part of these assays. The Northern assay is also generally considered to be less sensitive, and it involves more steps than the alternatives. Therefore, it requires larger amounts of RNA or starting material and more time to obtain the results.

Many of the problems associated with the Northern blotting method can be eliminated by optimizing the transfer and coupling of RNA to membrane supports and utilizing more sensitive single-stranded probes. Nylon membranes, such as GeneScreen® supplied by Du Pont, Wilmington, DE), are flexible, tear-resistant supports to which the RNA can be permanently coupled by UV-crosslinking. One of the main advantages of performing filter hybridization to UV-crosslinked RNA is that very-high-stringency conditions can be used, which improves sensitivity, reduces background, and enables convenient multiple reuse of the filters. In many cases, when the concentration of the desired RNA species is high or large amounts of sample are available, these may not be critical parameters. However, RNA samples frequently need to be isolated from small amounts of tissues or from cells that are very hard to obtain (transgenic mice, clinical samples or embryonic material). In transfection experiments, it is desirable to minimize the amount of RNA needed for analysis to enable more DNA constructs to be examined and reduce the amount of cell culturing required. In these cases optimal conditions are essential. Sensitivity is greatly enhanced by using single-stranded RNA probes, but these often generate very high backgrounds by nonspecific hybridization to rRNA species, especially when total RNA is being used. It is therefore beneficial to isolate poly A$^+$ RNA, even if the amount of total RNA in the sample is very small. Analyzing only poly A$^+$ RNA will improve the signal-to-noise ratio and avoid RNA overloading, which can result in incomplete coupling of the RNA to the filter.

RNA:RNA hybrids are very stable and often the proper stringency conditions for hybridization are not used, resulting in high background or crosshybridization to other RNA species. By increasing the stringency of both the hybridization and washing conditions, the nonspecific signals are greatly reduced or eliminated; however, if the RNA has not been UV-crosslinked to the filter, these conditions can remove much of the sample, resulting in loss of signal. The conditions can also be severe that nitrocellulose membrane supports become brittle and break apart, which is why nylon membranes (GeneScreen®) are essential in obtaining optimal reproducible results.The choice of hybridization buffers is not critical, but minimizing the temperature of hybridization and washing can reduce the degree of RNA degradation and extend the reusable life of the filter. This can be accomplished by using formamide in the buffers to control the stringency and reduce the melting temperatures of the hybrids.

Utilizing these modifications to the Northern blotting method to optimize the conditions, the assay is as sensitive as RNase protection or S1 analysis and provides a convenient long-term record of important samples that may be repeatedly analyzed. This chapter describes in detail the protocols for carrying out high-sensitivity Northern blots that have successfully been used in the laboratory to examine genes that are expressed at very low levels in small amounts of early embryonic tissues and in transgenic mice *(1–3)*. Generally, the protocol is not drastically different from existing Northern methods and requires no specialized equipment except a UV light source. The method depends on an easy means of isolating high-quality poly A⁺ mRNA, UV-crosslinking on the RNA to nylon membranes, and hybridization to single-stranded RNA probes. However, it is equally applicable to Northern analysis of all types, and alternative RNA isolation procedures or hybridization methods may be substituted into the protocol with little change in efficiency or results. DNA probes may also be used in most cases, but they will be less sensitive than the single-stranded RNA probes.

2. Materials

Methods for RNA isolation require pure reagents and care in preparation to avoid RNA degradation. It is advisable to wear gloves at all times. Heavy metals or other contaminants can result in chemical cleavage of RNA, thus deionized distilled water and high-grade analytical reagents should be used. Autoclaving buffers alone is not sufficient to inactivate any contaminating RNases, since renaturation may follow heat denaturation. The chemical diethylpyrocarbonate (DEPC) binds to RNase, irreversibly inactivating it, and is the most convenient means of producing RNase-free solutions (CAUTION: DEPC is a carcinogen—use gloves).

2.1. Isolation of RNA

2.1.1. LiCl–Urea Method

1. DEPC water: Add 1–2 drops of diethylpyrocarbonate/L glass-distilled deionized water and autoclave to sterilize. This removes the DEPC, which breaks down to ethanol, CO_2, and water.
2. Homogenization buffer: $3M$ LiCL, $6M$ urea. Dissolve 126 g LiCl and 360 g urea in 1 L of sterile DEPC water and filter through a 0.2 μm filter.
3. $2M$ Tris-HCl, pH 7.6: Make buffer in DEPC water and adjust to pH 7.6. Place in a glass bottle, add 1–2 drops of DEPC, and autoclave *immediately*. DEPC can destroy Tris, so check the pH of the buffer after autoclaving, and never autoclave dilute Tris buffers.

4. $0.5M$ EDTA: Make the EDTA stock, and add 1–2 drops of DEPC, and autoclave.
5. 10% SDS: Make the SDS stock, add 1–2 drops of DEPC, and incubate at 68°C overnight. Do not autoclave.
6. $3.0M$ sodium acetate, pH 5.2: Adjust the acetate stock to the appropriate pH with acetic acid and add 1–2 drops of DEPC. Autoclave.
7. 95% ethanol.
8. Phenol—redistilled: Melt at 65°C, saturate with an equal vol of TES, and let set overnight. Add 5mL m-Cresol, 0.2 mL 2-mercaptoethanol, and 0.1 g of 8-hydroxy quinoline per 100 mL of phenol. Mix until dissolved; then remove as much of the aqueous layer as possible.
9. Phenol:chloroform:isoamyl alcohol(24:24:1): Use treated phenol (step 8) and AR-grade chloroform and isoamyl alcohol. Keep the mixture in the dark and do not store for long periods.
10. TES: 10 mM Tris-HCl, pH 7.6; 1 mM EDTA; 0.5% SDS. Make in DEPC water.
11. TE: 10 mM Tris-HCl, pH 7.6; 1 mM EDTA; make in DEPC water.
12. Sterile disposable RNase-free centrifuge tubes: Standard 1.5-mL Eppendorf microfuge tubes work for small preparations. They can be used directly from the box if handled with gloves. Falcon also supplies 5-mL (#2063), 15-mL (#2059), and 50-mL (#2070) sterile polypropylene tubes.

2.1.2. Hot Phenol Method

1. 50 mM sodium acetate, pH 5.2: Add 1–2 drops of DEPC and autoclave.
2. Lysis buffer: 50 mM sodium acetate, pH 5.2; 1% SDS; 3.5M NaCl. Make with DEPC water and autoclave.
3. 5M NaCl: Make buffer, treat with DEPC, and autoclave.
4. 95% ethanol.
5. Saturated phenol: Melt redistilled phenol and add 1/4 vol of 50 mM sodium acetate, pH 5.2, and mix. Let stand until the phases separate, and remove as much of the aqueous layer as possible. Store the phenol in small aliquots at –20°C until needed. Refreeze any unused phenol after RNA isolation.
6. NaCl/ice slurry: Add NaCl to ice and mix until the temperature reaches –10 to –13°C.

2.2. Isolation of Poly A⁺ RNA

1. Oligo dT cellulose, T3 grade.
2. 0.1N NaOH: Dilute Analar-grade 10N NaOH stock.
3. 10% SDS: Prepare as in Section 2.1.1., step 5.
4. 6M LiCl: 252 g LiCl/L treated with 1–2 drops of DEPC and autoclaved.
5. 2M Tris-HCl, pH 7.6: Prepare as above.

6. 0.5*M* EDTA: Prepare as above.
7. Binding buffer: 20 m*M* Tris-HCl, pH 7.6; 0.6*M* LiCl; 1 m*M* EDTA; 0.2% SDS made from RNase-free stocks and DEPC water.
8. Low-salt binding buffer: 20 m*M* Tris-HCl, pH 7.6; 0.1*M* LiCl; 1 m*M* EDTA; 0.2% SDS made from RNase-free stocks and DEPC water.
9. Elution buffer: 10 m*M* Tris-HCl, pH 7.6; 1 m*M* EDTA; 0.1% SDS made from RNase free stocks and DEPC water.
10. 95% ethanol.
11. 3*M* sodium acetate, pH 5.2: Prepare as above.
12. Plastic oligo dT columns, top and bottom closures, and rack for 20 columns—Isolabs, Cleveland, Ohio (Quicksep #QS-P) or Advanced Labs Techniques (Tunbridge Wells, Kent, UK).

2.3. Electrophoresis, Transfer, and Crosslinking

1. DEPC water: As above.
2. 20× MOPS stock: 0.1*M* sodium acetate, 0.4*M* MOPS, and 20 m*M* EDTA. Make in DEPC water.
3. Agarose: SeaKeem.
4. Formamide: There is no need for deionization.
5. 37% formaldehyde supplied as a liquid stock.
6. Blue juice dye: 0.1% xylene cyanol, 0.1% bromophenol blue, 1× MOPS, 50% glycerol. Make with DEPC water and autoclaved glycerol.
7. 0.1*M* ammonium acetate.
8. Ethidium bromide: 10 mg/mL in water. CAUTION! This is a potential carcinogen!
9. 20× SSC: 3*M* NaCl, 0.3*M* sodium citrate. To make 6× SSC and 2× SSC, dilute with autoclaved distilled water.
10. Denaturing buffer: 50 m*M* NaOH, 0.1*M* NaCl.
11. Neutralizing buffer: 100 m*M* Tris-HCl, pH7.6, diluted in DEPC water.
12. Nylon membrane: 200 × 200 mm GeneScreen® squares (Du Pont).
13. Whatman 3MM filter paper.
14. Paper towels (flat).
15. Plastic wrap (Saran Wrap™ or Clingfilm™).

2.4. Hybridization

1. 5× Denhardt's solution: 0.05% (w/v) BSA, 0.05% (w/v) polyvinyl pyrrolidone, 0.05% Ficoll 400.
2. Prehybridization buffer: 50–60% formamide, 5× SSC, 5× Denhardt's solution, 50 m*M* sodium phosphate buffer, pH 6.8; 250 µg/mL sheared denatured salmon-sperm DNA; 100 µg/mL yeast tRNA; and 1% SDS. All stocks should be made in DEPC water.
3. Hybridization buffer: 50–60% formamide; 5× SSC, 1× Denhardt's 20 m*M*

sodium phosphate buffer, pH 6.8, 100 µg/mL sheared denatured salmon-sperm DNA; 100 µg/mL yeast tRNA, 1% SDS, and 10% dextran sulfate.

4. 20× SSC: Prepare as above.
5. 10% SDS.
6. RNase A: 10 mg/mL stock in 10 mM Tris-HCl, pH 7.6.
7. Formamide: Fluka high grade.
8. All dilutions for washing buffers are done in DEPC water from the RNase-free stocks, as detailed above.

3. Methods

3.1. Isolation of Total RNA

3.1.1. LiCl-Urea Method

This method works for large and small amounts of fresh or frozen tissue, and may also be used for cultured cells. It is efficient at inhibiting nucleases in order to produce high-quality biologically active RNA and is based on the method of Auffray and Rougenon *(4)*. No ultracentrifugation steps are required, and the entire method can be performed using a refrigerated benchtop centrifuge with a swing-out rotor capable of handling standard sterile disposable plastic centrifuge tubes (1.5- to 50-mL vol). This eliminates the need for specially treated glassware, and the method can be used to isolate RNA from large numbers of samples at the same time.

1. Weigh the fresh or frozen tissue and place in a plastic disposable centrifuge tube of appropriate size.
2. Add LiCl-urea homogenization buffer in a ratio of 5–10 mL of buffer to 1 g of starting material.
3. Homogenize the sample for 2 min at 0°C (on ice) using a Polyton, Ultraturrax, or similar motor-driven homogenizer (*see* Note 1).
4. To complete the DNA shearing, sonicate the sample on ice for 1–2 min. A microtip should be used on small samples placed in 1.5-mL Eppendorf microcentrifuge tubes.
5. Spin the sample at low speed (1000 rpm) for 3–5 min at 0°C in a benchtop centrifuge to pellet any nonhomogenized material and membrane debris.
6. Pour the supernatant into a new centrifuge tube and store overnight at 0–4°C (*see* Note 2).
7. The DNA remains in solution and the RNA is harvested by centrifugation. Depending on the sample size and type of tube, centrifugation is done either in a Sorvall HB-4 rotor at 9000 rpm for 10 min at 0°C or in a refrigerated benchtop centrifuge at 3000–4000 rpm (max rated speed) for 30 min at 0°C.

8. Pour off the supernatant and discard. Then add 0.5 vol of LiCl-urea homogenization buffer (4°C), vortex or mix the sample, and leave on ice for 30 min.

9. Recentrifuge the sample to pellet RNA and discard the supernatant (*see* Note 3).

10. Dissolve the pellet in TES using 5 mL/g of original tissue or 0.5 vol of original homogenization buffer. The sample should be mixed well to dissolve the RNA pellet.

11. Add an equal vol of phenol:chloroform:isoamyl alcohol (24:24:1) and extract the sample for 5–10 min with vigorous shaking (*see* Note 4).

12. To separate the phases, spin at 3000–4000 rpm (max rated speed or *g* force) in a benchtop centrifuge at room temperature.

13. Carefully remove the top aqueous phase and place in a new tube. If the interface is very thick, reextract the organic phase by adding 0.5 vol of TES and recentrifuging.

14. Combine the aqueous phases and reextract a second time with an equal vol of phenol:chloroform:isoamyl alcohol.

15. Spin at 3000–4000 rpm in a benchtop centrifuge to separate the phases, and carefully remove the top aqueous layer to a new tube. Repeat the extraction procedure until the interface is clear.

16. Add 1/10 vol of 3*M* sodium acetate, pH 5.2, and 2 vol of 95% ethanol. Mix and store at –20°C. The RNA is stable indefinitely at this stage.

17. Harvest the RNA by centrifugation in a benchtop or Sorvall centrifuge (as in step 5) and discard the supernatant. Rinse the pellet by adding an equal vol of 70% ethanol and recentrifuging.

18. Dissolve the RNA in TE and measure the absorbance at 260 nm (40 µg/ mL = 1 A_{260} unit) (*see* Notes 5 and 6).

3.1.2. Hot Phenol Method

This method is a fast protocol for isolating RNA from tissue-culture cells. It is very useful for extracting RNA from large numbers of different samples generated in transfection experiments. The DNA is removed because it is soluble in 60°C phenol at pH 5.2.

1. Trypsinize cells from 3–9 90-mm tissue-culture plates, and pellet by centrifugation in 50-mL plastic tubes. Resuspend in PBS and repellet. Repeat the PBS wash. This removes all traces of serum.

2. Resuspend the cell pellet in 1 mL of 50 m*M* sodium acetate, pH 5.2, by vortexing. Make sure all cell clumps are dispersed.

3. Add 10 mL of 50 m*M* sodium acetate, pH 5.2, and 1% SDS and mix by inversion to lyse the cells.

4. Add an equal vol (11 mL) of phenol, saturated with 50 mM sodium acetate, pH 5.2, and prewarmed to 60°C.

5. Mix by vortexing and place the tube in a 60°C bath for 15 min. During the incubation, frequently remove the tube and revortex for a few seconds.

6. Remove the tubes from the bath and immerse in an NaCl/ice slurry for 5 min.

7. Spin at 3000 rpm for 10 min at 2°C in a refrigerated benchtop centrifuge. Insert a pipet and remove the bottom phenol layer leaving the interface.

8. Add 10 mL of 60°C saturated phenol and vortex. Incubate the sample for 15 min at 60°C with repeated vortexing.

9. Remove from the bath and incubate in NaCl/ice slurry for 5 min.

10. Spin at 3000 rpm for 10 min at 2°C.

11. Carefully remove the top aqueous layer and add 1/10 vol of 5M NaCl and 2 vol of 95% ethanol. Store at –20°C.

12. Pellet total RNA at 9000 rpm for 10 min at 4°C in a Sorvall HB-4 swing-out rotor and pour off the supernatant. Rinse with 70% ethanol and repellet.

13. Redissolve the RNA in TE and read the A_{260} to measure concentration. Store frozen at –20°C.

3.2. Isolation of Poly A⁺ RNA

The isolation of poly A⁺ RNA can be done by chromatograghy on oligo dT cellulose in batch operation, using centrifuge tubes, or in sterile RNAse-free plastic columns, often used for radioimmune assays. It works for large or small amounts of total RNA, as long as the binding capacity of the oligo dT cellulose is not exceeded. When the amount of total RNA is very small, carrier RNA is added to the sample to reduce background losses. In this way poly A⁺ RNA can be easily isolated from as little as 10–100 µg of total RNA *(5)*. This method is based on the method of Aviv and Leder *(6)*.

1. Oligo dT cellulose is suspended in water and allowed to swell for several hours.

2. Gently mix the cellulose and allow the material to settle for 20 min. Pour off fines, add sterile water, and resuspend the cellulose. Repeat these steps to remove any fine particles that may clog the column.

3. Resuspend the oligo dT cellulose in 0.1 N NaOH and pour the slurry into a plastic column (10 mm diameter). Allow the liquid to flow through until a packed vol of 5–7 mm of cellulose forms at the bottom.

4. Rinse the cellulose by carefully pipeting 5 mL of binding buffer onto the column, and allow it to flow through. Repeat three times to remove all

traces of NaOH by checking eluant with pH paper. Columns are now ready for samples (*see* Note 7).

5. Dissolve total RNA in TES, usually 1–2 mL for small samples and 5–10 mL for large samples (5–10 mg RNA). In the case of very small samples (<100 µg RNA), add 5µL of a 100µg/mL poly A stock to the sample to act as carrier.

6. Heat the RNA at 60°C for 10 min in a water bath, remove, and adjust the salt to 0.6 *M* LiCl by adding 1/10 vol of 6 *M* stock.

7. Vortex and immediately pour the sample carefully onto the oligo dT column to minimize disturbing the bottom cellulose layer.

8. Collect the run-through and reapply it to the column to ensure complete binding of poly A$^+$ RNA.

9. Collect the run-through again and save as poly A$^-$ RNA.

10. Add 5 mL of binding buffer, being careful to minimize disturbance of the bottom cellulose layer.

11. Allow the binding buffer rinse to flow through and repeat three times with 5 mL of binding buffer.

12. Rinse three times with 5 mL of low-salt binding buffers which further removes traces of ribosomal RNA on the column.

13. Allow the column to run dry and elute the poly A$^+$ RNA with TES. If large amounts of RNA were bound to the column, use 5–10 successive 1 mL rinses with TES collected in sterile 1.5 mL microfuge tubes. Read the A_{260} of each fraction blanked against TES to determine which fractions contain RNA (usually the first 3–4).

14. To elute small samples of RNA, add 75 µL of TES and allow it to drip through. Place a 1.5-mL microfuge tube under the column and elute the RNA with four 150-µL washes with TES. Allow 1–2 min between each rinse.

17. Collect another set of four 150-µL TES washes into a second tube. Usually all of the poly A$^+$ RNA is in the first tube.

18. The RNA is precipitated by adding 1/10 vol of 3 *M* sodium acetate, pH 5.2, and 2 vol 95% ethanol, and storing at –20°C.

19. Spin the sample for 15–20 min in a microfuge at 4°C or in a Sorvall HB-4 rotor at 9000 rpm at 4°C for 10 min. Discard the supernatant and wash the sample by adding an equal vol of 70% ethanol, and then respin. Dissolve the RNA in TE and store at –20°C (*see* Note 8).

3.3. Gel Electrophoresis, Transfer, and UV-Crosslinking

The methods for electrophoresis and transfer of nucleic acids by capillary action have been described in detail in many methods books; the protocols below represent slightly modified versions of the standard techniques (6–8). The UV-crosslinking method is based on tests designed to optimize the permanent binding of RNA to GeneScreen® membranes (9).

3.3.1. Electrophoresis

1. Carefully clean the gel box, casting tray (plates), and combs with mild detergent, and rinse with clean distilled water, giving a final rinse with sterile distilled water. Use gloves in all steps to avoid contamination with RNase.

2. Set up the casting tray and comb in a fumehood, since the formaldehyde vapors given off during the pouring and setting of the gel are strong and irritating to the eyes.

3. For a 200-mL gel, dissolve 2.89 g agarose in 156-mL sterile distilled water in a 500-mL flask by boiling (*see* Note 9).

4. Remove from heat; cool in a 60°C water bath.

5. When the sample is cooled to 60°C, add 10 mL of 20× MOPS stock and 34 mL of 37% formaldehyde. Mix briefly by stirring or gentle swirling and pour the gel immediately. Avoid creating air bubbles on the surface of the gel. If they form, they can be removed by touching with a sterile syringe needle.

6. Allow the gel to set for 30 min and gently remove the comb. Gels with formaldehyde have less tensile strength than normal agarose gels and tear easily. Use care in handling.

7. RNA samples are placed in a 1.5 mL-microfuge tube with a dye-denaturation cocktail as follows: Mix 1 μL 20× MOPS, 10 μL 100% formamide, 3.5μL 37% formaldehyde, 2 μL blue juice dye, and 5 μL RNA in TE. Usually 1–2 μg of poly A$^+$ is sufficient. If the RNA is too dilute, it can be dried down and resuspended in 5 μL of TE. Samples in the cocktail can be prepared ahead of time and then stored at 4°C for a few hours or overnight.

8. Heat shock the samples to denature the RNA at 60°C for 10–15 min in a water bath and cool on ice. Load the gel immediately.

9. Gel-running buffer is 1× MOPS with no formaldehyde. Gel is run for 5–7 h at 60–70 V (*see* Notes 10 and 11).

10. Stop electrophoresis and cut off the mol wt marker lanes to be stained. Staining can prevent efficient transfer of the RNA to the membrane, so do not stain the part of gel that is to be used for hybridization. Useful markers are poly A$^-$ RNA or commercial RNA-size ladders.

11. To stain the marker strip, rinse twice for 20 min in distilled water, and twice for 20 min in 0.1M ammonium acetate. These rinsing steps are necessary to remove the formaldehyde, which binds ethidium bromide. Then incubate for 15 min in 0.1M ammonium acetate with 0.1 μg/mL ethidium bromide.

13. Destain the gel twice, for 25 min each time, in 0.1M ammonium acetate. If background is still high, the gel can be destained for several hours or overnight at 4°C in 0.1M ammonium acetate without the RNA bands diffusing. A picture can be taken on a standard UV transilluminator setup.

3.3.2. Transfer

1. GeneScreen® nylon membranes (cut to approx gel size) are prepared for transfer by being floated onto distilled water until they are completely wet; then they are immersed in the water. After 10 min they are transfered to 2× SSC and stored until transfer.
2. Soak the gel in 50 mM NaOH, 0.1M NaCl for 20 min with gentle shaking. This partially cleaves the RNA and aids the transfer of large species. Do not leave longer than 20 min, and use DEPC-treated water at this step if transferring RNA <800 bases.
3. Neutralize the gel by incubating in 0.1M TrisHCl, pH 7.6, for 20 min followed by 2× SSC for 20 min with gently shaking.
4. Capillary transfer in 20× SSC is used to transfer the RNA from the gel in a standard manner. Sheets of Whatmann 3MM paper are soaked in 20× SSC and placed on a glass plate over a reservoir of 20× SSC. The ends are immersed in the reservoir to act as a wick for the SSC buffer.
5. The gel is placed on the wet 3MM with the comb side down to provide a smooth even surface for contact with the membrane.
6. Surround the gel with strips of parafilm on the exposed areas of the 3MM wick to allow flow of 20 × SSC through the gel only .
7. Wet the surface of the gel with 20× SSC and carefully lay the wet GeneScreen® membrane on top of the cell. Be careful to avoid trapping air bubbles between the gel and membrane.
8. Place three layers of 3MM cut to the exact size of the gel (prewet in 20× SSC) on top of the GeneScreen® membrane. Be careful again to avoid trapping air bubbles.
9. Place several inches of paper towels on the 3MM filter papers, and cover with a glass plate and a lead weight. Replace the towels if they become completely wet.
10. Following overnight transfer, the toweling is removed and the position of the lanes and the orientation of the gel is marked on the membrane with a pen.
11. Trim the edges of the membrane with a razor and peel the filter from the gel. Immerse the membrane in 6× SSC for 1–2 min.

3.3.3. UV-Crosslinking

1. Place a large piece of Saran Wrap™ or Clingfilm™ plastic wrap on the benchtop and pipet 2–4 mL of 6× SSC onto the middle of the plastic.
2. Remove the membrane from the 6× SSC and carefully place it on the plastic film such that the side that was in direct contact with the gel during transfer is facing down. Avoid air bubbles between the membrane and the plastic.

3. Fold over the excess plastic wrap to completely enclose the membrane and place on a glass plate. The side of the membrane in contact with the gel should be facing up.

4. Place the filter on the plate under a UV source that delivers 600 μW/cm² at a wavelength of 254 nm (*see* Notes 14–19).

5. Expose the filter to UV light for 5 min, remove from the source, and take the filter out of the plastic wrap.

6. Place the filter between two sheets of 3MM paper and bake at 80°C for 60 min.

7. The filter is now ready for hybridization.

3.4. Filter Hybridization

A large variety of hybridization buffers or systems are available and can be used with equal success in the filter hybridizations. This method is based on Wahl et al. *(10)*. Regardless of the protocols, high backgrounds can be a problem when using nylon membranes. This can usually be avoided by including high concentrations of SDS in both the hybridization and the washing steps. The UV-crosslinking prevents the high levels of SDS from eluting the RNA from the membrane. This protocol works for crosslinking DNA, as well as RNA, to the nylon membrane. A typical example of a final Northern result is shown in Fig. 1. The figure also illustrates how special RNase wash treatments can be useful.

1. Place the membrane in a plastic bag sealed on three sides. Pour in prehybridization buffer and seal the remaining side with a bag seal (*see* Notes 12,13).

2. Place the bag in a water bath at the hybridization temperature determined by the type of probe being used (*see* Table 1). For single-stranded RNA probes this temperature is 60–65°C.

3. Prehybridize for 2–4 h; then remove the bag, cut a corner, and pour out the prehybridization buffer.

4. Generate a single-stranded ³²P-labeled RNA probe by in vitro transcription as described in Chapter 22. A typical transcription will produce 1×10^8 cpm.

5. Place the probe in 10–15 mL of hybridization buffer and prewarm at the hybridization temperature for 20 min.

6. Carefully pour the hybridization buffer with probe into the plastic bag and reseal, avoiding, as much as possible, the formation of air bubbles.

7. Hybridize the filter overnight (12–24 h).

8. Cut open the bag and remove the hybridization buffer.

9. Remove the filter and rinse 3 × with 500 mL of 2× SSC at room temperature to rinse out most of the nonhybridized probe.

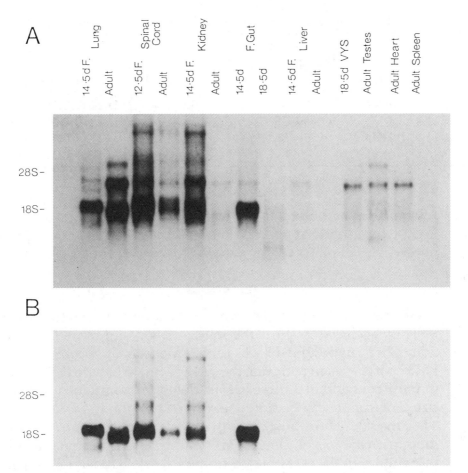

Fig. 1. Example of a Northern result using a homeobox probe on mouse embryonic tissues. Lanes contain 1–2 µg of poly A⁺ RNA from the tissues indicated at the top of each lane. **(A)** Results with washing at 80°C in 0.1× SSC, 0.5% SDS. Some crosshybridization is seen with other of the homeobox family, and this is removed when the same filter is washed using the RNase treatment method **(B)**. Note that many bands remain unchanged and that these represent transcripts of a single gene. However, bands resulting from closely related genes are removed in this high-stringency treatment. Probe: P^{32}- single-stranded Hox-2.1 RNA generated by SP6 in vitro transcription of a plasmid (1).

10. Wash the filter in 700 mL of 0.1× SSC, 0.5% SDS at 70–80°C for 1 h; repeat twice. It is helpful to use a Geiger counter to check background. Further washes may be necessary.
11. Remove the filter from the wash buffer and wrap in plastic film while moist. Expose to autoradiography at –70°C with an intensifying screen and Kodak XAR-5 film (see Notes 20–22).

Table 1
Hybridization and Washing Conditions for DNA and RNA

Probe	Filter	Hybridization temperature, °C%	Formamide in hybridization	Wash conditions
RNA	RNA	60–65	60	0.1× SSC, 0.5% SDS, 75°C
DNA	RNA	50–55	50	0.1× SSC, 0.5% SDS, 65°C
RNA	DNA	50–55	50	0.1× SSC, 0.5% SDS, 65°C
DNA	DNA	42	50	0.1× SSC, 0.5% SDS, 55°C

12. After analysis of the results, the filters are stripped for reuse by washing in 70% formamide at 80–90°C for 10–15 min (this can be repeated if necessary). The filter can be exposed to ensure probe removal.

4. Notes

1. Avoid foaming as much as possible. It is important that the sample be well-homogenized to shear the nuclear DNA, and more homogenization buffer can be added if the sample is extremely viscous.
2. It is important when removing the supernatant to be sure that the sample is not viscous and that there are no clumps of nonhomogenized material. The sample can be stored for several months at this stage.
3. Wipe the sides of the tube dry with a sterile tissue to remove as much of the supernatant as possible. This reduces any DNA contamination of the sample. In the case of large samples, it may be advisable to perform a second LiCl-urea wash to completely remove the DNA.
4. If the RNA pellet is slow to dissolve, add phenol-chloroform and vortex or place on a shaker until it dissolves.
5. If a large number of samples are being read, it is convenient to use sterile disposable UV cuvets, which minimizes crosscontamination between RNA samples and reduces the handling time of the RNA. Adjust the vol to the desired concentration and store at –20°C. This is a pure preparation of total RNA that can be used directly for many assays (S1 nuclease protection, RNase protection, and Northern) or can be used for the preparation of poly A+ RNA.
6. If, in the final ethanol precipitation steps, contaminating DNA is present, it may be removed by redissolving the RNA in TE and 2M LiCl prior to incubating overnight at 4°C. This reprecipitates the RNA, leaving the DNA in solution. The RNA is harvested by centrifugation, dissolved in TE, and reprecipitated with ethanol as above. This is generally not necessary, but improves in handling large samples when the DNA has

not been completely sheared or removed by the LiCl-urea washes. It is important to remove as much of the DNA as possible, because contaminating DNA drastically slows the flow rates of the oligo dT columns in the isolation of poly A^+ RNA.

7. If small amounts of RNA (<100 μg) are being used, nonspecific binding is reduced by adding 2 mL of binding buffer containing 5 μg/mL yeast tRNA. Allow to run through and rinse with 5 mL of binding buffer.

8. The oligo dT columns may be stored after successive rinses with 5mL of TES followed by 5 mL of 0.1*N* NaOH. The column is left at room temperature for 10–15 min to destroy any remaining traces of RNA. Then it is refilled with 0.1*N* NaOH, and the top and bottom are capped. The columns can be stored at 4°C indefinitely and reused repeatedly without future RNA loss or contamination. Storage in NaOH can result, after long periods, in some degradation of the glass-fiber filter at the bottom of the column.

9. The percentage of the gel varies with need, but for separation of 1.5–8kb RNAs, 1.4% is ideal.

10. Best results (sharp bands) are obtained using this high voltage and short running time, rather than running the gel overnight at lower voltage.

11. The pH of the buffer can change during the run, so it is advisable to recirculate the buffer with a pump or to mix the buffer several times during the run. Higher voltages can be used to shorten the length of the run if a recirculating pump is used. The pH can easily be checked with strips of pH paper.

12. The prehybridization and hybridization buffers can be made up and stored for long periods at 4°C.

13. All the details for the transfer of nucleic acids to GeneScreen®, UV-crosslinking, and hybridization work equally well for DNA and RNA. The only difference is the selection of hybridization temperatures, which depend on the nucleic acid linked to the membrane and in the probe. *See* Table 1 for alternative conditions for DNA.

14. It is important to use a 254-nm-wavelength bulb without the polarizing filter. Attempts to crosslink the samples on a standard transilluminator (normally set at 305 nm) usually do not work. The polarizing filters usually exclude too much energy, preventing effective crosslinking.

15. Many hand-held UV lamp units will work if the protective cover is removed. We recommend a standard 4-bulb transilluminator without the polarizing filter, mounted upside down on a stand in a protective box or cabinet to prevent the user being exposed to UV rays.

16. The dose of energy is important. Often specific distances from the source are noted in protocols; however, it is important to determine the proper distance for your own UV source. Use a stand UV safety measuring de-

vice that measures in units of $\mu W/cm^2$ at 254 nm. These devices are not expensive and are easily obtained from a scientific supplier. Find the distance from the source that registers 600 $\mu W/cm^2$; then fix the UV source to that height.

17. A commerical UV-crosslinker is now available from Stratagene (Strata-Linker™) and crosslinking to GeneScreen® is very efficient when the manufacturers instructions are followed.

18. Several workers describe UV-crosslinking with a dry filter. This can be successful and has the advantage that much shorter times are required, usually 10–30 s instead of 5 min. However, it is possible to overlink the RNA to the filter and reduce the usefulness of the RNA on the membrane. The optimum crosslinking times for the wet or dry method can be tested easily and directly. Prepare a test gel with a single large slot preparative comb, and transfer the RNA to the filter. Set up the crosslinking, but cover most of the filter with a black paper. At various time-points, gradually expose more of the filter to the UV source. This will provide a time-course of crosslinking. After hybridization of the filter, the optimum crosslinking times and length of the plateau for effective linking is read directly from the filter. This plateau is generally very broad when the filter is linked while wet, and the conditions are therefore very reproducible. On dry filters, the plateau may be only a few seconds and difficult to reproduce, which is why the wet-linking method is preferred.

19. Many types of nylon membranes have been tested, and they all work to varying extents. Charged membranes, such as GeneScreen® plus or Hybond™, do not work as efficiently as uncharged membranes. In general, the GeneScreen® membrane reproducibly produced the highest degree of RNA binding and low backgrounds.

20. It is important that the filter never becomes completely dried out, or it will not be possible to remove all of the bound probe.

21. If the background is still high or a higher degree of stringency is required because of crosshybridization, remove the filter from the plastic wrap. Wash the filter in 100 mL of 0.1× SSC and 10–30% formamide at 65°C, followed by 0.1× SSC and 0.5% SDS at 70°C for 30 min, and reexpose the filter.

22. Alternatively, background can be eliminated treating the filter with RNase *(1)*, but it may no longer be reused. To treat with RNase, place the filter in 2× SSC, 0.1 $\mu g/mL$ RNase A at room temperature for 20 min. Then wash in 500 mL 2× SSC, 0.5% SDS at 40–50°C for 30 min and reexpose the membrane. This treatment is analogous to the RNase protection assay. *See* Fig. 1 for an example of this treatment.

References

1. Krumlauf, R., Holland, P. W. H., McVey, J. H., and Hogan, B. L. M. (1987) Developmental and spatial patterns of expression of the mouse homeobox gene, Hox-2.1. *Development* **99,** 603–618.

2. Graham, A., Papalopulu, N., Lorimer, J., McVey, J. H., Tuddenham, E. G. D., and Krumlauf, R. (1988) Characterisation of a murine homeobox gene, Hox-2.6, related to the *Drosophila Deformed* gene. *Genes and Development* **2,** 1424–1438.

3. Graham, A., Papalopulu, N., and Krumlauf, R. (1989) The murine and *Drosophila* homeobox gene complexes have common features of organisation and expression. *Cell* **57,** 367–378.

4. Auffray, C. and Rougeon, F. (1980) Purification of mouse immunoglobulin heavy-chain RNAs from total myeloma tumor RNA. *Eur. J. Biochem.* **107,** 303–324.

5. Krumlauf, R., Hammer, R., Tilghman, S. M., and Brinster, R. (1985) Developmental regulation of alpha-fetoprotein in transgenic mice. *Mol. Cell Biol.* **5,** 163–168.

6. Aviv, H. and Leder, P. (1972) Purification of biologically active globin mRNA by chromatography on oligothymidylic acid-cellulose. *Proc. Natl. Acad. Sci. USA* **69,** 1408–1412.

7. Maniatis, T., Fritsch, E. F., and Sambrook, J. (1982) *Molecular Cloning: A Laboratory Manual* (Cold Spring Harbor Laboratory Press, Cold Spring Harbor, New York), pp. 202–204 and 383–387.

8. Southern, E. (1975) Detection of specific sequences among DNA fragments separated by cell electrophoresis. *J. Mol. Biol.* **98,** 503–512.

9. Krumlauf, R. (1989) GeneScreen® hybridisation transfer membrane: UV crosslinking protocols. *Dupont Manufacturers Instruction Booklet,* pm0014a (Du Pont, Wilmington, DE).

10. Wahal, G. M., Stern, M., and Stark, G. R. (1979) Efficient transfer of large DNA fragments from agarose gels to diazobenzloxymethal-paper and rapid hybridisation by using dextran sulfate. *Proc. Natl. Acad. Sci. USA* **76,** 3683–3688.

SECTION 6
NUCLEAR RUN-ON ASSAY
FOR NEWLY INITIATED TRANSCRIPTION COMPLEXES

CHAPTER 25

Analysis of Transcriptional Initiation in Isolated Nuclei

David Stott

1. Introduction

The level of expression of a given gene in a particular cell type is reflected by the concentration of the resultant messenger RNA. This is subject to regulation during a number of processes, including synthesis, processing, export from nucleus to cytoplasm, and degradation. Clearly, the rate of production of nascent transcripts, reflecting the rate of initiation of RNA polymerase at the promoter, is of primary importance. The nuclear run-on assay described here allows labeling of nascent transcripts as they are synthesized, thus allowing measurement of the density of transcription complexes on a gene, which is dependent on the rate of initiation of RNA polymerase at the promoter *(1)*. The essential steps involved in the procedure are outlined in Fig. 1.

In order to achieve incorporation of radiolabeled ribonucleosides during transcription, it is first necessary to isolate nuclei with transcription complexes still engaged. A brief period of further transcription (run-on) in the presence of labeled precursors incorporates radioactivity into specific sequences at a level corresponding to the density of transcription complexes. The abundance of the newly synthesized transcripts can then be measured

From: *Methods in Molecular Biology, Vol. 7: Gene Transfer and Expression Protocols*
Edited by: E. J. Murray © 1991 The Humana Press Inc., Clifton, NJ

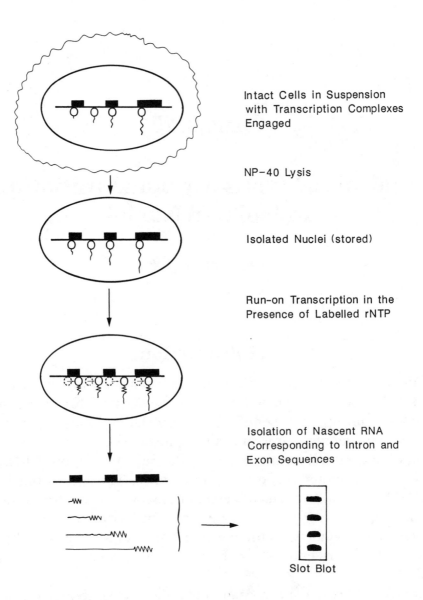

Intact Cells in Suspension
with Transcription Complexes
Engaged

NP–40 Lysis

Isolated Nuclei (stored)

Run-on Transcription in the
Presence of Labelled rNTP

Isolation of Nascent RNA
Corresponding to Intron and
Exon Sequences

Slot Blot

Unprocessed Radiolabelled RNA Hybridised to Immobilised
Complementary Sequences

O   Transcription Complex

⌇   Nascent RNA

⨼   Radiolabelled RNA Synthesized During Run-on

▬   Exons

Fig. 1. Flow diagram indicating the various steps in production and use of radio-labeled nuclear RNA.

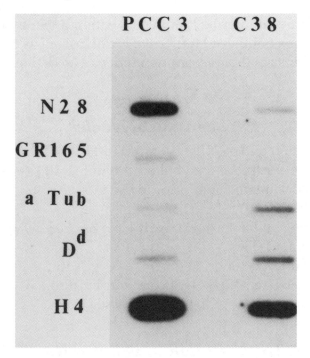

Fig. 2. Slot-blots hybridized to labeled nuclear RNA from either PCC3 cells (an embryonal carcinoma cell line) or clone 38 cells (an SV40 transformed fibroblast line). N28 is a genomic clone and GR165 is a cDNA clone from a gene that is transcribed at high levels in the PCC3 cells, but is virtually silent in the clone 38 cells; a Tub is an a tubulin cDNA, D^d is a class 1 major histocampatibility genomic clone, and H4 is a histone H4 cDNA clone.

by hybridization to immobilized complementary sequences. The choice of immobilized sequence is based on the transcription unit under study. For a unique gene, cDNA sequences can be used. However, since the labeled RNA remains unprocessed, genomic sequences (including introns) are often preferable because of the increased variation between intron sequences compared to that between exon sequences of related genes. Figure 2 shows the result of an experiment in which RNA synthesized by isolated nuclei was hybridized to cloned sequences immobilized on a slot-blot.

This technique is usually applied when comparing the rate of transcription of the same gene in different cell types. It is also of use in determining the type of RNA polymerase involved in transcription of a particular gene by virtue of their different α-amanitin sensitivities. In addition, the direction of transcription of an uncharacterized gene can be determined using immobilized single-stranded RNA sequences. Finally, radiolabeled nascent RNA allows the detection of transcribed sequences within a genomic clone when used as a probe on a Southern blot. Since intron as well as exon sequences are labeled, the limits of the transcription unit can be defined (*see* Note 1).

2. Materials

2.1. Isolation of Nuclei

1. Nuclear isolation buffer (NIB): 10 mM Tris-HCl, pH 7.4; 10 mM NaCl; 5 mM MgCl$_2$. Autoclave and add dithiothreitol (DTT) (to 1 mM) from a 1M frozen stock immediately prior to use.
2. Nonidet P-40 (NP-40).
3. Nuclei-freezing buffer: 50 mM Tris-HCl, pH 8.5; 50% w/v glycerol; 5 mM MgCl$_2$; 0.1 mM EDTA.
4. Phosphate-buffered saline (PBSA): 8.09 g NaCl, 0.29 g KCl, 0.29 g KH$_2$PO$_4$, and 1.16 g N2$_2$HPO$_4$ dissolved in 1 L distilled water.
5. Dounce homogenize with loose-fitting pestle.
6. Hemocytometer.

2.2. Transcription in Isolated Nuclei

1. 5× Run-on buffer (ROB): 25 mM Tris-HCl, pH 8; 12.5 mM MgCl$_2$; 750 mM KCl; 1.25 mM each rATP, rGTP, and rCTP. Store at –20°C.
2. ^{32}p UTP: 3000 Ci/mmol (aq). Store at –20°C.
3. RNAse-free DNAse: 12 mg/mL. Store at –20°C.
4. RNAse-free proteinase K: 20 mg/mL. Store at –20°C.
5. MgCl$_2$ and CaCl$_2$: Each 1M. Autoclave.
6. 5× SET: 5% SDS; 25 mM EDTA; 50 mM Tris-HCl, pH 7.4.
7. Phenol/chloroform: phenol saturated with 10 mM Tris-HCl, pH 7.4; chloroform; isoamyl alcohol; 25:24:1. Store at 4°C under 10 mM Tris-HCl, pH 7.4.
8. 100% ethanol.
9. 8M ammonium acetate. Filter; do not autoclave.
10. Denhardt's solution: 1% Ficoll; 1% polyvinylpyrollidone; 1% BSA. Store at –20°C.
11. NRO hybridization buffer: 10 mM Tris-HCl, pH 7.4; 0.2% SDS; 10 mM EDTA; 300 mM NaCl; 1× Denhardt's solution; 200 µg/mL *E. coli* tRNA; 200 µg/mL poly adenine. Store at –20°C.
12. 10% trichloroacetic acid.
13. Salmon-sperm DNA: Sonicate to 0.5 kb average length and make up to 0.5 mg/mL in 20 mM EDTA. Store at 4°C.

14. α-amanitin, 1 mg/mL: (NOTE: This compound is extremely toxic and must be used with caution.)
15. Glass-fiber disk filter (Whatman GF/C).

2.3. Slot-Blot Filter Preparation

1. Nitrocellulose filters (e.g., Schleider and Schuell BA 85 or Amersham Hybond-N).
2. Ammonium acetate, 4M and 1M solutions: Filter; do not autoclave.
3. 2× SSC: 0.3M NaCl; 30 mM sodium citrate, pH 7.0.

3. Methods

3.1. Isolation of Nuclei

3.1.1. From Tissue Culture Cells

1. Grow 5–10 14-cm dishes to about 70% confluence. Depending on cell type, this will yield 10^8–10^9 cells. Wash the cells in PBSA and harvest with trypsin. It is important to generate a single cell suspension at this stage. Pellet the cells as for passaging, e.g., by spinning for 5 min at 1000–1500 rpm in a bench-top centrifuge.
2. Resuspend in 20 mL ice-cold NIB (add DTT just prior to use). Again, ensure a single cell suspension is produced and repellet the cells as above, but at 0°C. Ensure all following steps are performed at 0°C; work in a cold room if possible.
3. Resuspend gently in ice-cold NIB plus 0.5% NP-40. Incubate for 10 min on ice. This step causes lysis of the plasma membrane, leaving the nucleus intact.
4. Pellet the nuclei by centrifuging at 2000 rpm at 0°C for 5 min in a bench-top centrifuge. The nuclei will pellet more slowly than intact cells and need to be centrifuged more rapidly. However, if the nuclei are spun too hard, they become difficult to resuspend, and many are lost as a result of lysis at later steps. Aim for a sloppy pellet from which the supernatant has to be removed by aspiration with a pipet.
5. Wash the nuclei two or three times in ice-cold NIB by resuspending gently and centrifuging as above. Count a small aliquot prior to the final spin (dilute× 100 in NIB and count in a hemocytometer).
6. Resuspend at 10^8 nuclei/mL in freezing buffer and pipet 210-μL aliquots into prechilled Eppendorf tubes. Store at –70°C. Nuclei preparations last at least 6 mo.

3.1.2. From Whole Tissues

1. Wash tissues in ice-cold PBSA and mince finely with scissors. Wash the pieces several times in ice-cold PBSA.
2. Dissociate the cells in a prechilled glass homogenizer with a loose-fitting pestle. The time taken to produce a single cell suspension varies with different tissues. For soft tissues, such as liver and spleen, 10 strokes are usually sufficient. Check the suspension in a hemocytometer.
3. Pellet the suspension and resuspend in ice-cold NIB. Continue as from step 2, in Section 3.1.1.

3.2. Synthesis of Radiolabeled Nascent RNA

1. Defrost the nuclei at room temperature and transfer to ice when melted. Add 25 µL (250 µCi) of ^{32}P UTP plus 60 µL of 5× ROB. Add α-amanitin if required (*see* Note 2). Mix gently with a pipet tip and incubate at 30°C for 10 min.
2. Digest DNA by adding 2 µL of 1 M MgCl$_2$; 1 µL of 1 M CaCl$_2$; 2 µL of RNAse-free DNAse. Incubate at 37°C for 45 min.
3. Digest protein by adding 75 µL of 5× SET, 5 µL of RNAse-free proteinase K. Incubate at 37°C for 45 min.
4. Add 400 µL phenol:chloroform. Ensure tubes are securely capped and vortex well (about 1 min). Spin for 20 min at full speed in a microfuge.
5. Recover 350 µL of the aqueous phase and add 150 µL of 8 M ammonium acetate plus 1mL EtOH. Mix well and leave at –20°C for 1 h to overnight.
6. Spin for 10 min in a microfuge, and then remove and discard the supernatant. Wash the pellet with 70% EtOH, and dry briefly on the bench. The pellet contains around 100 µCi of ^{32}P, so vacuum drying is inadvisable as well as unnecessary.
7. Dissolve the pellet in 100 µL of H$_2$O by incubating in a boiling water-bath for 3 min. Vortex well and check that the pellet is dissolved by spinning briefly in a microfuge and transferring the supernatant to a fresh tube. At least 80% of the counts should be in the supernatant. If not, repeat the boiling step (*see* Notes 3 and 4).
8. Take 1 µL (1%) of the radiolabeled RNA and precipitate by adding 100 µL of 0.5 mg/mL salmon sperm DNA plus 5 mL of 10% TCA. Incubate for 15 min on ice and filter onto a glass-fiber disk (Whatman GF/C). Count in a scintillation counter and calculate the total precipitable counts, which should be between 10^7 and 5×10^8 cpm. Store the remaining labeled RNA at –20°C.

3.3. Hybridization of Labeled Nascent Transcripts to Immobilized Sequences

The simplest method to analyze the level of transcripts corresponding to a known sequence is to hybridize the labeled nuclear RNA to fragments of cloned sequences immobilized on a slot-blot.

Alternatively, single-stranded RNA produced from phage promoters contained within such vectors as Bluescript or SP6 can be used to determine the transcriptional orientation of the cloned sequence. In addition, Southern blots of genomic subclones can be probed with nuclear run-on RNA to label transcribed sequences and determine the limits of a transcription unit (*see* Note 1).

3.4. Slot-Blot Preparation

It is not necessary to use purified fragments of cloned DNA, although a control slot with the vector alone should be included. Calculate the mass of DNA required to give 500 ng of the transcribed sequence, i.e., for a 4-kb plasmid including a 1-kb insert, use 2 μg of DNA/slot. The protocol allows the production of two filters, which permits a comparison of the transcription by two sets of nuclei (*see* Note 5).

1. Make up DNA to 50 μL in H_2O; add 3 μL of 5 M NaOH.
2. Incubate in boiling water-bath for 10 min and cool on ice for 5 min.
3. Add 50 μL of 4 M ammonium acetate, vortex, and apply 50 μL/slot to a nitrocellulose filter (*see* Note 6) prewetted with H_2O and assembled in a slot-blot apparatus (e.g., Schleider and Schuell minifold II) according to the manufacturer's instructions.
4. Wash through twice with approx 50 μL/slot of 1 M ammonium acetate.
5. Recover the filter and rinse in 2× SSC for 5 min. Air-dry and bake at 80°C for 1–2 h.
6. Prehybridize in NRO hybridization buffer at 65°C in a shaking water-bath for 4 h or overnight.
7. Incubate radiolabeled nuclear run-on RNA prep in a boiling water-bath for 3 min. Dilute to 10^6 cpm/mL in NRO hybridization buffer and apply to filters. Hybridize for 36 h at 65°C.
8. Wash twice (15 min each time) in 2× SSC and 0.1% SDS at room temperature, and then wash at high stringency (0.2× SSC and 0.1% SDS at 65°C) for 1 h.
9. Blot the filters dry on absorbent paper and wrap in plastic wrap prior to exposing to X-ray film at –70°C with an intensifying screen. Required exposure times vary from a few hours to two weeks, depending on the length of the immobilized fragment and the rate of transcription.

4. Notes

1. Although the usual application of this technique is to compare the rate of transcription of a particular sequence in nuclei isolated from different cells, it is also useful in other circumstances. In particular, the newly transcribed RNA includes intron as well as exon sequences. Hence, the extent of a transcription unit can be determined by hybridizing the nuclear run-on product to a Southern blot of a genomic clone. Fragments that hybridize are included in the transcription unit; those that do not hybridize lie outside it. Obviously, as more than one transcription unit may be included within a large (e.g., cosmid or λ) clone, such mapping must be of sufficiently high resolution to avoid mistaking a second gene for a continuation of the gene under examination.

   A further application is to compare polymerase density at different points within a transcription unit. If hybridization to two subclones of equal length from the 5' and 3' regions of the same transcription unit is compared, then any differences found suggest attenuation or initiation of polymerase within the transcription unit.

2. If a distinction between RNA polymerases is required, add α-amanitin prior to initiating synthesis. RNA polymerase II is inhibited by 2 μg/mL and RNA polymerase III by 400 μg/mL α-amanitin. RNA polymerase I is not sensitive to α-amanitin.

3. The incorporation of radioactive UTP into nascent RNA will vary between different batches of nuclei. In order to achieve high rates of incorporation, the nuclei must be kept ice-cold throughout the preparation procedure and, after defrosting, until the radioactive precursor is added. A single cell suspension is a prerequisite for even cell lysis, and subsequent treatments should be as gentle as possible to avoid lysis and subsequent loss of nuclei. It should be noted that the freezing process lyses the majority of the nuclei, so aliquots should be used as they are and not pelleted and resuspended after defrosting. All usual precautions for working with RNA should be observed. RNAse inhibitors can be added to the synthesis reaction, but this is not generally necessary.

4. Large RNA pellets can be very difficult to dissolve completely. If a large amount of undissolved radioactive material remains after resuspending the pellet (Section 3.2., step 7), repeat the boiling step and try to suspend the RNA by pipeting and vortexing. However, avoid using incompletely dissolved labeled RNA in hybridizations. If the entire pellet will not dissolve, spin it out and use the supernatant transferred to a fresh tube.

5. When comparing labeled nuclear RNA from different cell types (for example, to determine whether the transcription of a particular gene varies from one cell type to another), a control sequence that is anticipated to be transcribed at similar rates in the two cell types is required. The choice of such a control is not obvious. In general, a good approach is to use a panel of ubiquitously expressed genes, such as tubulin, actin, or histones, and housekeeping genes, such as hypoxanthine phosphoribosyltransferase (HPRT), and to compare the signal from the sequence under study to each of these.

6. Avoid using nylon filters. Under the hybridization conditions described, some batches of nylon filters give unacceptably high background. This is probably a result of nonspecific hybridization of short probe fragments to the filter.

References

1. Groudine, M., Peretz, M., and Weintraub, M. (1981) Transcriptional regulation of hemoglobin switching in the chicken embryo. *Mol. Cell Biol.* **1,** 281–288.

CHAPTER 26

Immunoperoxidase Staining of Gene Products in Cultured Cells Using Monoclonal Antibodies

Roger Morris

1. Introduction

Antibodies, in general, provide the most sensitive and specific methods for detecting the protein products of genes. Immunoperoxidase techniques described here detect 10^3–10^5 molecules/cell (depending on whether the protein is dispersed within the cell or concentrated at high density in a particular compartment); with various enhancement methods, this can be improved more than tenfold. Immunohistochemistry is particularly suitable for analyzing transfection in vitro, because it examines individual cells; methods based on analysis of bulk RNA (e.g., S1 nuclease protection [*see* Chapter 21, this volume]) or protein (e.g., immunoblotting) are considerably less sensitive when only a small proportion of cells are transfected. Immunoperoxidase reactions are generally more sensitive than immunofluorescence (Chapter 27) and immunogold methods and require no special optics to observe. Also, the reaction product is stable for years. On the other hand, immunofluorescence is easier to perform than immunoperoxidase, the conjugated antibody is generally more stable and so more reliable, and the fluorescence signal is easier to demonstrate in black-and-white photography. If a good fluorescence microscope is available and the signal is expected to be reasonably strong, then immunofluorescence is the method of choice.

Unlike other reagents described in these volumes, antibodies do not have a standard set of properties. They differ over a 10^2 range in their kinet-

From: *Methods in Molecular Biology, Vol. 7: Gene Transfer and Expression Protocols*
Edited by: E. J. Murray © 1991 The Humana Press Inc., Clifton, NJ

ics of binding and over a 10^6 range in their dissociation kinetics. Alteration of a single chemical moiety in the site to which they bind can lower their affinity by 10^6, although larger substitutions (for example, of one or two amino acids) are often needed to produce a change of this magnitude. Impressive as this specificity is, increasing the valency of interaction of an antibody with an immobilized antigen, such as the one we are dealing with in this chapter, can increase the affinity by 10^6, effectively changing the specificity of the reagent *(1)*. It is therefore impossible to give protocols that produce optimum results in all cases unless the user has some understanding of the principles governing antibody–antigen interactions.

This chapter therefore starts with a brief summary of the main parameters affecting antibody binding. This is followed by individual protocols, which should be taken as guides and adapted to your own requirements. If difficulties occur, the reader may find the recent book by Harlow and Lane *(2)* useful. One point should be stressed at the outset. Antibodies are remarkably specific, robust, and forgiving reagents. In most cases, you will obtain successful immunoperoxidase staining with very few problems.

1.1. Factors Governing the Use of Antibodies

1.1.1. Effect of Antigen Conformation and Fixation

Antibodies bind to just one conformation of their antigenic determinant, which usually consists of 3–5 amino acids lying sequentially along the polypeptide chain *(3)*. A major factor in determining how quickly an antibody binds is the probability of that section of the protein assuming the required conformation, which obviously must then be accessible to antibody. Once the antibody has bound, it "freezes" the conformation of this part of the protein, and even very rare forms of proteins are stabilized when so bound *(4,5)*. Yet, in order to visualize an antigen within a cell, it is necessary that the antigen be immobilized (fixed) in its proper location so that antibodies can diffuse into it. Fixation inevitably constrains and alters conformation. This in turn affects the choice of fixative used, temperature, and time of incubation.

Precipitating fixatives (notably organic solvents) leave the protein microenvironment maximally flexible; therefore, in general, they are the first choice. They have the additional advantage that they solubilize or otherwise destroy the membrane barriers, thereby permitting penetration of antibody, and a separate permeabilization step is not required. Chemically crosslinking fixatives (notably aldehydes) were developed to preserve ultra-structure as seen in the electron microscope, but there are four conditions in which they are preferable to precipitating fixatives in a light microscope analysis:

1. If the protein antigen is soluble (cytosolic), and especially if it is small (mol wt <30 kDa), then chemical crosslinking may be necessary to fix it effectively.
2. If the antigenic determinant is hidden within the protein (as with some antipeptide antibodies), then it will be necessary to denature the cells; this will solubilize them if some degree of chemical crosslinking has not been achieved.
3. Antibodies to relatively small (mol wt < 10^4 kDa) entities, such as peptides, can be raised only by coupling them to a much larger molecule, such as a protein. When this is done, the chemical crosslinking can become part of the antigenic site, and the affinity for the crosslinked group is therefore much higher than for the native group *(6)*. If the crosslinking agent used in raising the antibody can also be used as a fixative, do so.
4. The antigenicity of some proteins is remarkably resistant to aldehydes, therefore using these as fixatives gives much superior morphological preservation and the option of observing the reaction product in the electron microscope.

It should be noted that some antigenic determinants are formed by amino acids from nonsequential positions in the polypeptide chain, which are brought together by the three-dimensional folding of the protein *(3)*. These are probably best fixed by crosslinking agents and best detected with polyclonal antibodies, among which some clones will exist that recognize the fixed conformation.

1.1.2. Effect of Temperature on Kinetics and Affinity of Antibody Binding

In the few cases in which it has been examined, raising the temperature from 4 to 24°C increases the kinetics of binding by about twofold, and of dissociation by more than tenfold, causing an overall drop in affinity of about 10-fold *(1,7)*. It is generally preferable to use long incubation times at 4°C (e.g., overnight with the first antibody and at least 2–3 h with the second). A convenient variation is to set up the dishes with the first antibody at room temperature, which gives faster initial binding, and, after 1–2 h, transfer them to the cold for subsequent washes and incubations. Incubating at 37°C enables one to cut incubation times to 20–30 min, but will need higher concentrations of antibody, which may give a higher background. Incubations at 37°C can be essential when dealing with antipeptide antibodies. The greater conformational flexibility at the higher temperature may be necessary to enable the protein to adopt transiently the particular conformation recognized by your antibody. In such cases, relatively long incubations (several hours to overnight) at the high temperature, followed by cold washes and a cold incubation with the secondary antibody, will probably be optimal. (In practice, the need to keep cells adherent to the culture dish during immunohistochemical staining may compel adjustments to antibody concentrations.)

1.1.3. How Valency Affects Affinity

When binding to an immobilized ligand, such as antigen fixed in cells (or on paper in immunoblotting, on plastic in ELISA assays, and so forth), with each increase in valency of binding the affinity increases up to 10^3-fold *(1,7,8)*. This increase in affinity is the result of a dramatic effect on the dissociation kinetics. It can be readily appreciated that if antibody is bound to a cell by two binding sites, transient dissociation of either binding site does not lead to dissociation of the antibody from the cell; that can occur only when both sites dissociate simultaneously. IgG, being dimeric, can bind two antigenic determinants; IgM can bind to three sites on a surface, the other two potential binding sites being sterically constrained to the fluid phase. On the other hand, when binding to solubilized monomeric antigen (e.g., radioimmunoassays, immunoaffinity purification), no such increase in affinity occurs on multiple binding. This effect is behind much of the apparently anomolous behavior of antibodies in different assays, especially with IgM antibodies that may have little intrinsic affinity for a moiety (e.g., K_d of $10^{-2}M$) yet react with high affinity to it ($K_d = 10^{-8}M$) when presented in a polymeric array. All cases of which I am aware of unexpected cross reactivity of a monoclonal with a totally unrelated antigen have occurred with IgM antibodies binding to polymers, such as intermediate filaments. More positively, building up a high local concentration of antigen (e.g., by use of inhibitors of transport or by allowing surface antigens on living cells to patch and cap) will enhance the antigen in two ways—one's ability to see it there is more to see and the antibody will bind with a higher affinity.

1.1.4. pH, Ionic Strength, and Denaturing Conditions

Antibodies can dissociate from their antigen at a pH only 2 U away from neutrality (the pH optima of horseradish peroxidase [HRP] and alkaline phosphatase, both commonly used as marker enzymes in immunohistochemistry, are 5.2 and 9.6, respectively). The majority of antibodies will have dissociated at pHs <3 or >11. Specific antibody binding is relatively insensitive to ionic strength and composition for normal ions, although nonspecific (background) binding would be expected to increase at very low ionic strength. Chaotropic ions and denaturing detergents dissociate most antibody–antigen complexes, so, if their use is necessary (normally only with some antipeptide antibodies) to expose the antigenic site, quickly wash them from the cells before applying antibody.

1.1.5. Choice of Peroxidase Method

Immunohistochemistry works on a simple principle: add the primary antibody to the cells and it binds to its antigen; unbound antibody is then washed away and a secondary, labeled antiimmunoglobulin antibody added, which binds to the first antibody. After further washing, for immunoperoxidase procedures, the cells are incubated with HRP substrates whose reaction product is an insoluble and colored precipitate.

There are three main methods of linking HRP to the secondary antibody. The simplest to use, in which HRP is chemically coupled to the antibody, is described here. Two other main forms are also available, in which the HRP is either bound as an antigen (the peroxidase–antiperoxidase method, PAP), or linked to avidin, which binds to biotin-labeled secondary antibody (avidin–biotin complex, ABC). For an assessment of the relative merits of each, *see* Note 1.

2. Materials

1. Phosphate-buffered saline (PBS), (/L): NaCl (8.090 g), KCl (0.290 g), KH_2PO_4 (0.290 g), and Na_2HPO_4 (1.160 g dissolved in enough water to make 800 mL and mixed before use with 200 mL of water containing $CaCl_2•2H_2O$ (0.190 g) plus $MgCl_2•6H_2O$ (0.190 g). (Virtually any ionic buffer at pH 7 will do; if your laboratory has a standard formulation, use it.)
2. Gelatin-subbed glass slides: Wash slides, either (a) by overnight incubation in warm strong detergent (e.g., 10% Decon; 1 h if sonication is used; rinse first with running tap water for several h and then through at least three changes of distilled water); or (b) by incubation for several hours in 0.2 *M* HCl in 96% ethanol, followed by multiple changes of distilled water. To sub the slides, dip them in chrom alum gelatin (dissolve 2.3 g gelatin in 500 mL water by stirring at 80°C, when dissolved, add 0.25 g chrom alum, cool, and filter), drain off liquid, and air-dry for several hours. Store dry at 4°C. Poly-L-lysine at 50 µg/mL (simply immerse slides for 20 min), can be substituted for gelatin. Alternatively, slides can be dried after washing; dipped into a 2% solution of Tespa (3-aminopropyltriethoxysilane) for 10 s, washed twice with acetone, then with water, and dried at 42°C.
3. Paraformaldehyde: Use the highest-purity paraformaldehyde (EM grade) available. For 100 mL of 1% paraformaldehyde,
   a. Add 1 g of paraformaldehyde to 40 mL of water, warm to 60°C with stirring, in a fume hood; and add 50 µL of 1 *M* NaOH. The paraformaldehyde dissolves in minutes.

b. Add 50 mL of 0.2M phosphate buffer, pH 7.4 (/L, 3.588 g of NaH$_2$PO$_4$•2H$_2$O plus 10.934 g Na$_2$HPO$_4$).

c. Add 0.54 g glucose plus 0.4 mL of 0.5% CaCl$_2$.

d. Make up to 100 mL with water; filter before use.

The solution should be made up fresh every few days; for critical experiments make up fresh on the day.

4. Ethanolamine–saponin solution: For 1 L, dissolve 9.2 mL of ethanolamine in 900 mL of water and adjust the pH to 8.5 with concentrated HCl. Add 0.2 g saponin; when dissolved, make up to 1 L with water. The solution is stable for months at 4°C.

5. 10× Peroxidase enzymatic development buffer: Dissolve 80 g of NaH$_2$PO$_4$ plus 3.8 g imidazole in 1 L of water, and adjust the pH to 6.0 with phosphate (acid) or imidazole (base) as necessary. The solution is stable indefinitely at room temperature.

6. Diaminobenzidine tetrahydrochloride (DAB).

7. Hydrogen peroxide (30%).

8. Silver–gold enhancement buffers: Make up the following stock solutions:

a. Dissolve 50 g of Na$_2$CO$_3$ (anhyd) in 1.2 L of water (renew weekly).

b. Dissolve NH$_4$NO$_3$ (2.0 g), AgNO$_3$ (2.0 g), and SiO$_2$• 12WO$_3$ •26H$_2$O (tungstosilicic acid) (10.0 g) in 1 L of water in the order given (renew monthly).

c. Dissolve NH$_4$NO$_3$ (2.0 g), AgNO$_3$ (2.0 g) SiO$_2$•12WO$_3$•26H$_2$O (10.0 g), and 35% formaldehyde solution (7.3 g) in 1 L of water (renew monthly).

Just before use, make up the developer thus: to 10 mL of solution (a) add, with stirring, 5 mL of solution (b), and then, *slowly*, 5 mL of solution (c).

3. Methods

The flow diagram (Fig. 1) should be consulted as a guide to which methods you may need to use.

3.1. Preparation of Cells for Immunolabeling

3.1.1. Suspension Culture (Nonadherent Cells)

1. Wash the cells by centrifugation three times in PBS.

2. Resuspend cells at appropriate density (which can be determined only by trial and error, since it will depend on the size of the cells), so that when smeared they will lie densely on a slide, but not overlap.

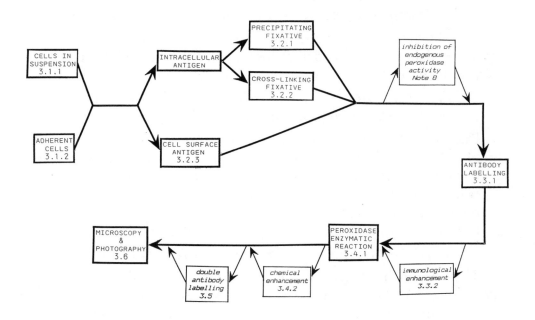

Fig. 1. Scheme showing steps in immunoperoxidase staining, paragraph numbers indicate the sections of text where the step is covered; nonroutine methods are given in italics.

3. Apply one drop to a washed and subbed glass slide, and smoothly draw a second slide along the first, forming an angle of approx 60°, to produce a smear.
4. Place the smeared slide in front of a fan to facilitate drying. If the cells are to be fixed chemically or in methanol, 10 min of drying is sufficient. If cells are to be fixed in acetone place them in a dessicator for several hours to completely dry them.

3.1.2. Adherent Cells (see Note 2)

The simplest procedure is to grow cells in 35- or 60-mm culture dishes, on which they are directly stained. If you have smaller numbers of cells, or find it more convenient to do so, cells can be grown on coverslips (e.g., plastic, Biorad Microscience Division; cells have a bad habit of coming off glass coverslips during staining) or multicompartment plastic slides (e.g., Labtek® from Miles Scientific). Wash the cells gently in three changes of PBS followed by the fixative.

3.2. Antigen Preparation

3.2.1. Intracellular Molecules: Fixation and Permeabilization of Cells with a Precipitating Fixative, Methanol (see Note 3)

Place the culture dish on ice, add methanol (prechilled to 4°C) and gently swirl around the plate. Decant, add fresh methanol, and leave for 10 min. Decant again, and wash cells in three changes of PBS. Use immediately (*see* Note 4).

3.2.2. Intracellular Molecules: Fixation and Permeabilization of Cells with a Crosslinking Fixative, Paraformaldehyde

1. Place the culture dish on ice, add 1% paraformaldehyde solution in phosphate buffer (pH 7.4) precooled to 4°C, and leave for 10 min (*see* Note 5).
2. Decant paraformaldehyde. Wash with 0.153 M ethanolamine–Cl (pH 8.5) containing 0.02% saponin, and add more ethanolamine/saponin; leave for 10 min (*see* Note 6).
3. Decant; perform three 1-min washes with PBS (*see* Note 7).

3.2.3. Cell-Surface and Extracellular Matrix Proteins

These normally require neither fixation nor permeabilization. If possible, immunolabel surface molecules on living cells, labeling for 30–60 min at room temperature using serum-free medium. Any antigen redistribution occasioned by antibody crosslinking (patching and capping) will merely enhance visibility of the signal (do not try longer incubations, which could cause antigen internalization). Should the cells need to be fixed, use paraformaldehyde or other chemical crosslinkers; organic solvents destroy the plasma membrane, and the immunoreaction can be difficult to interpret. If the cells have been stained live, they can then be fixed with paraformaldehyde (for at least an hour) without diminishing peroxidase activity. Label cells in suspension while they are in suspension (use two centrifugation washes after each antibody incubation), and then smear them on a glass slide. Air-dry; then add directly to the peroxidase substrate solution.

3.3. Antibody Labeling

3.3.1. Standard Immunolabeling Procedure (see Note 8)

1. For cells on culture dishes, mark on the bottom of the dish a circle slightly larger than that covered by the coverslip you will use to see staining. With the tip of a tissue paper, wipe clean and dry the part of the dish outside this circle.
2. Add the first antibody at the appropriate dilution (*see* Note 9) in PBS containing 1% bovine serum albumin (BSA) (0.02% NaN_3 optional), in a volume sufficient to cover your marked area (usually 50–250 µL). Incubate for the required time at the appropriate temperature (*see* Section 1.1.2., and Note 10).

3. Wash the cells three times in PBS (10 s, 2 min, and 10 min): again wipe the perimeter of the plate dry.

4. Add the HRP-coupled anti-Ig in PBS with 0.25% BSA (no azide), and incubate as before (*see* Section 1.1.2., and Notes 11–14).

5. Wash the cells four times with PBS over 15–30 min. If the cells have been incubated at 4°C, bring them to room temperature for the enzyme reaction.

3.3.2. Immunological Enhancement (see Notes 12 and 15)

Because anti-Ig antibodies bind to more than one site on Ig, one way of increasing the signal is to use a triple layer of antibodies (e.g., mouse IgG monoclonal, rabbit antimouse IgG, HRP- coupled sheep antirabbit IgG). A second way (exemplified by the PAP method) utilizes the fact that the second antibody, although bivalent (all second antibodies should be IgG), will have bound to the primary antibody at only one of its sites if there is a low density of primary antibody binding. Hence, if you add normal Ig of the same species as your primary antibody, it will bind to the vacant site on the secondary antibody. In turn, it will bind more molecules of the same secondary antibody. Thus, if your primary antibody is a rat IgG, follow it with HRP-coupled antirat IgG, then rat IgG at 10 µg/mL (If normal rat serum, in which the concentration of IgG will be approx 10 mg/mL, is used, dilute it 1:1000), and then HRP-coupled antirat IgG.

3.4. Formation of Visible Peroxidase Reaction Product, and Chemical Enhancement

3.4.1. Diaminobenzidine (DAB) Reaction (see Note 16)

1. Dilute 10× peroxidase enzymatic development buffer to working dilution at room temperature and light-shield it with foil.

2. Dissolve diaminobenzidine tetrahydrochloride to 1 mg/mL, add 1 µL of 30% H_2O_2/10 mL of buffer, and filter the solution.

3. Add the solution to cells and incubate at room temperature for 3–10 min. Stop the reaction by washing repeatedly in PBS when the desired degree of brown precipitate has formed or if a general background staining starts to develop.

4. Dispose of DAB solution by adding Chloros or other strong oxidizing agent; wash glassware in same.

5. If further procedures are not planned (chemical enhancement, Section 3.4.2.; double labeling, Section 3.5.; or counterstaining of nuclei, Note 20), decant PBS, add a drop of a water-soluble moutant (e.g., Hydromount), apply a coverslip (by allowing one corner to contact the drop of moutant and gently lowering the coverslip so that the drop expands evenly on the surface), leave 30 min to set, and view under the microscope (*see* Note 17).

3.4.2. Chemical Enhancement Using
Silver–Gold Development (see Note 18)

1. Wash cells with multiple changes of distilled water for 1–2 h.
2. Cover with 0.1% gold chloride for 5 min.
3. Wash for a total of 5 min with multiple changes of distilled water.
4. Place in neutralized 2.5% sodium sulfide for 5 min (neutralize to pH 7.4 with 1 *M* HCl; use in fume hood).
5. Wash for a total of 5 min with multiple changes of distilled water.
6. Place in developer made up immediately before use. Gently swirl the developer continuously over the cells to ensure uniform staining. Intensification occurs over a 3- to 10-min period and is seen as the brown DAB reaction product turning black.
7. Stop the reaction by washing cells with 1% acetic acid for 1 min.
8. Fix with 1% thiosulfate for 5 min.
9. Wash with multiple changes of distilled water (5 min each). Counterstain if desired (*see* Note 19), and apply a coverslip.

3.5. Double Antibody Labeling

Labeling cells with two (or more) antibodies is very simple with immunoperoxidase procedures. The peroxidase reaction appears to destroy the antigenicity of proteins within its immediate molecular environment so that the monoclonal and second antibody are no longer able to bind, or be bound by, subsequent additions of antibodies. Second antigens (e.g., defining cell type) located within the same cell can be readily stained. Thus the cells can be put through multiple cycles of staining, using DAB and blue tetramethylbenzidine *(9)*, or other colored substrates *(10,11)*, at the different stages. Alkaline phosphatase-labeled antibodies can also be used simultaneously with peroxidase labeling *(12)* or fluorescent-labeled antibodies used after peroxidase staining.

3.6. Microscopy and Photography

The DAB reaction product is brown, ranging from light tan for weak staining to dark brown for intense labeling. When viewed under phase or interference contrast optics, it appears darker; at higher power (40× or better objective) it will appear to lie on a slightly different plane to the sample. Very weak staining is best viewed under dark-field optics, since the DAB reaction product is very effective at scattering light (the signal becomes specks of bright light against a dark background).

For color photography, use no filters. For black-and-white photography, however, blue filters can be used with normal bright-field illumination to intensify the signal (Fig 2). A light-blue filter (e.g., BG38, from Leitz, Zeiss and others) gives a mild degree of enhancement and tends to sharpen the

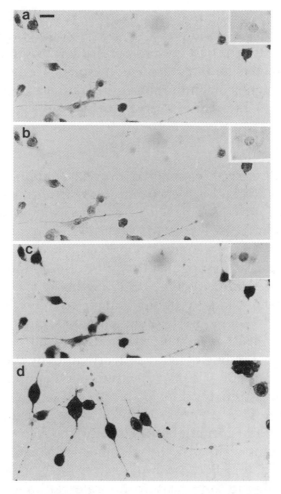

Fig. 2. Photography and silver enhancement of immunoperoxidase staining. A single field of DAB-stained cells photographed (**a**) with normal optics, no filter; (**b**) with a light-blue filter (BG38) in the incident light beam; (**c**) with a dark-blue filter (BG12) (inset in each shows a single control cell stained with an irrelevant primary antibody and the same secondary antibody; scale bar [**a**] is 20 μm). Panel (**d**) shows a companion plate that, after DAB staining, was lightly enhanced with silver–gold development. Substantial darkening of the DAB reaction product is obtained with the dark-blue filter, although at the expense of resolution. Silver enhancement gives an even darker reaction product, precisely localized and readily photographed, so that the fine varicose fibers of the cells are readily seen. (Cells are subclones of NG115–401L rodent neural cells transfected with human Thy-1/ neomycin 1132 clones selected first for G418 resistance, and then for cell-surface expression of Thy-1 glycoprotein. By immunofluorescence for human Thy-1, the cell bodies of this clone are detectable, but the fine processes cannot be seen. Cells were grown on 35-mm tissue-culture dishes, incubated for 3 h at 4°C with a 1:50 dilution of tissue-culture supernatant of a mouse antihuman Thy-1 monoclonal antibody (gift of R. Dawson and M. Ritter), and washed three times in PBS. They then were fixed 10 min in 1% paraformaldehyde, quenched 30 min in 0.153M ethanolamine, and incubated overnight in Dako HRP-rabbit antimouse IgG (1:50) before demonstrating the peroxidase reaction with DAB.)

image; a dark-blue (BG12; Kodak™ Wratten™ gelatin filter 47B is a cheap and effective alternative) will give a strong photographic image from quite weak staining. Phase contrast is most useful at low magnifications (objective 16× or less) at which color filters are least useful; it is usually disappointing in photography at higher magnifications. A dark field gives the greatest augmentation of signal, but requires very clean optics for good photography.

4. Notes

1. HRP is usually directly coupled to secondary antibodies by reduction of Schiff bases formed between oxidized sugar residues on the HRP and antibody NH_2 groups *(13)*. Such conjugates should be stable for 2–5 yr at −20°C and at least 1 yr at 4°C. It would appear that the coupling is slowly reversible, and some commercial reagents deteriorate quickly after purchase, suggesting that they were already too old when sold. In the peroxidase–antiperoxidase (PAP) method, the HRP is noncovalently linked as part of a large antibody–antigen complex. Basically, if the primary antibody is a mouse Ig, then a mouse antiperoxidase antibody is reacted with HRP. A bivalent antimouse IgG antibody is then used to form a bridge, binding both the primary antibody and the HRP-containing mouse antibody (Fig. 3). The third main approach uses the highly specific and rapid binding of biotin by avidin (or the less basic streptavidin). The secondary antibody and avidin are biotinylated, with tetravalent avidin forming a bridge between the two. (Direct avidin–HRP conjugates, coupled by the same procedure as is used for antibodies, are also available). Because avidin is very basic, it can show high background binding to some cells or substrates, although this often can be avoided by using a higher dilution, so that there remains only sufficient avidin to bind specifically. Both this and the PAP method require an extra incubation compared to direct HRP conjugates. There are many claims in the literature that the avidin-biotin and PAP complex methods are considerably more sensitive than the direct conjugates, although this is not necessarily so. The main variable is the quality of the secondary antibody, which depends on the skill (and luck) of the person producing it. The best examples of each type of coupling method produce comparable results. In choosing a secondary antibody, if possible take the advice of someone who routinely does immunohistochemical staining, or buy from one of the established specialist antibody suppliers.

2. Preferably, cells should be in a near-confluent state for ease of inspection of labeled cells. The main problem is that of keeping the cells adherent throughout antibody incubations, since cells vary greatly in adherence. Some cells growing directly on tissue-culture plastic adhere

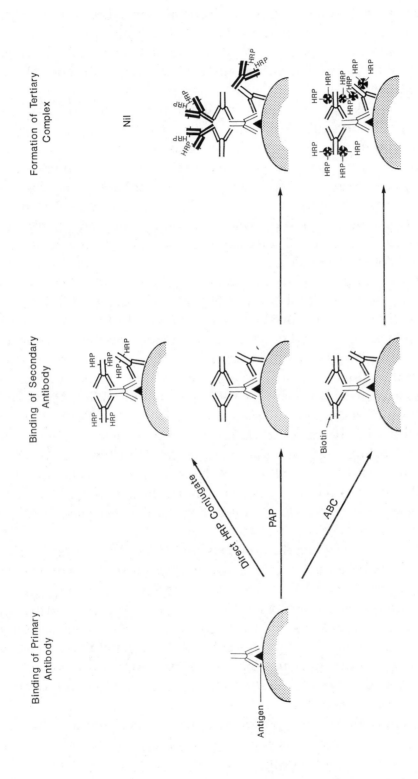

Fig. 3. Scheme showing the accumulation of HRP enzyme around an antigen during immunoperoxidase labeling using directly conjugated secondary antibody (upper), peroxidase–antiperoxidase (PAP) (middle), and avidin–biotin complexes (ABC) (lower) to bind to the primary antibody.

beautifully; others may need polylysine or protein subbing of the slides. If aldehyde fixatives are used, they will chemically crosslink the cells to the substratum. Collagen gels should be avoided, since antibodies penetrate them and give high backgrounds unless long wash times (1–2 h) are used.

3. Where available protocol for fixing the molecule while preserving its reaction with the antibody already exists, use it . If the procedure was developed with cells in culture, it can be used directly. If it was developed to see the molecule in whole tissue, you can generally use the same fixative, but for much shorter times (10–60 min) for a monolayer of cells. If such information is not available, look for control cells that express the molecule, and on which fixation and antibody staining can be optimized. If no better model system exists, try fixing and staining immunoblotted material.

    Methanol is a good all round fixative to start with, although mixtures of cold acetone/methanol (1:1), acetic acid/96% ethanol (5:95), or even 70% ethanol have all proved optimal in different situations. They do not attack plastic and can be used in this procedure. For sections smeared on glass slides, acetone can also be used. It can give better results than methanol fixation; additionally, slides are dried and can be stored at 4°C without losing reaction with many (but not all) antibodies. Place slides in a beaker of fresh analytical-grade acetone for 10 min. Remove, air-dry under a fan for 10 min, and then dry in a dessicator for 2–4 h. For immunolabeling, the primary antibody is added directly to the dry slide.

4. Cells can be air-dried directly from 100% methanol, and even stored dry at 4°C before immunohistochemical staining. Such drying will diminish the degree of preservation of morphology, and sometimes of antigenicity, but can help cells adhere to the plate.

5. Paraformaldehyde generally preserves antigenicity better than glutaraldehyde, both because it is less reactive and because it forms only reversible crosslinks (unless left to react for over 24 h), leaving a greater degree of conformational flexibility. This procedure gives very mild fixation, and will both fix and retain the antigenicity of most molecules. Should your protein be small and water-soluble, it may be useful to add 0 .1–0. 5% glutaraldehyde for better fixation. If the antigen is minimally destroyed by aldehydes, the fixation may be done at room temperature and for longer times.

6. The ethanolamine simply provides a source of —NH$_2$ groups to quench excess reactive aldehydes. Glycine, lysine, or any other convenient supply in your laboratory would do as well. An alternative method of

quenching is to use 1% NaBH$_4$ in PBS for 30 min, which would produce a smaller change in the properties of the fixed tissue and is reported to help preserve antigenicity *(14)*. The saponin renders plasma membranes permeable by complexing cholesterol and leaving membrane structure intact (as assessed ultrastructurally) *(15,16)*. Triton X-100 at 0.1–0.2%, or other similar nonionic detergent, will also render membranes permeable and is suitable for light microscopy.

7. This note is for those having real problems with fixation. Glutaraldehyde and paraformaldehyde react with similar groups, although glutaraldehyde is more reactive and immediately forms irreversible linkages *(see* refs. in *[17])*. Both fixatives react primarily with uncharged amino groups. The amino terminal NH$_2$ group is usually uncharged at pHs >7; side-chain NH$_2$, at pHs >8.5. Thus, by varying the pH, the extent and type of reaction can be controlled. This can be used productively in fixation. Attempts to direct the crosslinking reagent to side chains other than lysine have a checkered history. Willingham and Yamada *(18)* describe a combined glutaraldehyde/carbodiimide fixative that should also react with –COOH groups and was developed specifically for EM immunohistochemical use with cultured cells. The most frequently used alternative fixative is the paraformaldehyde–periodate–lysine fixative of McClean and Nakane *(19)*, which preserves antigenicity and morphology in a wide variety of cases. It was designed to crosslink via sugar residues, the periodate oxidizing vicinal—OH groups to aldehydes with which the lysine should form Schiff bases. However, this does not occur *(20)*: the lysine reacts with the paraformaldehyde before it is put near the cells, causing the pH of the fixative to drop. These reversible, reactive polymer chains, with their reactivity restricted by the low pH, do provide a useful immunohistochemical fixative.

8. In two situations, suppression of endogenous peroxidase activity may have to be undertaken prior to antibody staining. A short time (2–4 d) after transfection, some cells have abundant phacocytic vescicles in their cytoplasm, reflecting the shock procedure used to transfect. These can contain endogenous peroxidase activity, which will turn brown in the peroxidase substrate solution. Similarly, some cell types (notably hemoglobin-containing cells) naturally have endogenous peroxidase activity. If this activity needs to be suppressed, incubate your cells in 0.5% H$_2$O$_2$ in PBS for 10–30 min (depending on the extent of activity that must be suppressed).

9. Dilution and storage of primary antibodies. If appropriate dilutions have not already been established, then you will find most monoclonal super-

natants (in which the antibody will be present in the range of 1–10 µg/mL) will be optimal at dilutions in the range of 1:2 to 1:50 (1:10 is rarely wrong, although some monoclonals titrate out to beyond 1:1000). The higher the dilution, the more low-affinity crossreactions are excluded, the lower the background, and the slower the kinetics of binding. Ascitic fluid preparations of antibody contain 100–1000-fold-higher concentrations of antibody, and should be diluted accordingly. Antibody should be diluted in PBS containing a "carrier" protein to stop adsorption of the very low concentration of antibody to the plastic. For this, BSA is suggested; defatted dried milk also works extremely well, and many protocols use 1% serum from the species in which the secondary antibody is raised (since the labeled antibody will not bind to proteins from its own species). Indeed, it is often recommended that the cells be preincubated in such serum before adding the primary antibody, to keep the background down. I do not find this necessary if the aldehydes have been chemically quenched. Regarding the storage of antibodies, the only general recommendation is to avoid repeated freezing and thawing, which aggregates antibodies. I have monoclonal antibodies that have been stable at 4°C for 10 yr, and others that have lost activity within a few weeks. Aliquot your antibody into reasonable amounts in polypropylene microfuge tubes, snap-freeze them, thaw them rapidly, and keep the working dilutions at 4°C (again stored in polypropylene microfuge tubes, with carrier protein and 0.02% NaN_3 as a bacteriostatic). If the antibody is stable for months at 4°C, it is better to mail it as a solution at room temperature than to freeze-dry it, which promotes aggregation.

10. It is very important that the drop of antibody not dry out during incubations to avoid unusable background staining. For long incubations, simple humid chambers can be made by placing culture dishes inside larger, moist-filter-paper-containing dishes or sealed boxes. Ensure that the surface is level. If you are going to do a lot of immunolabeling, it is useful to make sealed humid boxes with a surface known to be level, on which your dishes, slides, or coverslips can rest.

11. Dilution and storage of your secondary HRP-coupled antibody will normally be recommended by the manufacturer. An immunoaffinity-purified antibody should be used at about 1–10 µg/mL for complete reaction within an hour at 4°C. Azide inhibits peroxidase, so it should not be added as a bacteriostatic to secondary antibody solutions. In addition, low dilutions of HRP conjugates lose activity, and so a working dilution should be made up fresh each day.

To use peroxidase–antiperoxidase (PAP) conjugates, staining with primary and secondary (in this case, unconjugated) antibodies is done as in Section 3.3.1. The PAP complex is normally made up during the second incubation, according to the manufacturer's instructions, and added as a third labeling step. Similarly, with biotin–avidin or streptavidin conjugates, staining with primary and secondary (biotinylated) antibodies is done as before. The avidin–biotinylated HRP complex is made up during the second incubation (once made, it is quite stable at 4°C unless microbial growth occurs). Follow precisely the manufacturer's recommendation for the ratio of HRP to avidin, since it is crucial that the enzyme bind to only some of the four available sites on the avidin. The actual amount used can often be decreased, benefiting background staining, especially if the total concentration of antigen involved is low.

12. The qualities that make a good secondary antibody are complex, and, because of the heterogeneity of immunoglobulin structure (differences in class [IgG, IgM, and so on], subclass, and light chain type), an optimal detection system for one monoclonal antibody is not necessarily optimal for a second. In general, match your secondary antibody in class and species to your monoclonal (thus use an antimouse IgG reagent to detect a mouse IgG monoclonal), although antibodies raised to one class will normally show substantial crossreaction with another. Indeed, antimouse Ig antibodies will normally show at least 50% crossreaction with rat Ig, and can bind to Ig from more distant species, including calf (possibly present in your cultures as newborn calf serum). Any IgG monoclonal will be of a specific subclass (IgG1, 2a, 2b, 3, or 4), and anti-subclass–specific antibodies are available. However, it is generally preferable to use an anti-IgG reagent, rather than a subclass-specific one, since it will bind to more sites on your first antibody and give a stronger signal.

Most secondary antibodies will bind two molecules per molecule of primary antibody, and ratios nearer 6:1 can be achieved. The degree to which the antibody has been conjugated (either directly with HRP, or with biotin), also varies, and the range of signal augmentation (molecules of HRP per molecule of primary antibody) can vary from two- to 20-fold. Unfortunately, this information is given neither in catalogs, nor in the literature, when the sensitivity of various methods is compared. The simplest and most common way of isolating the secondary antibody for labeling is to isolate the total IgG fraction from the serum. Of this, only 1–10% will be anti-Ig antibodies, the remainder being antibodies to the donor animal's pathogens, which can potentially contribute to a high background. Specific anti-Ig antibodies can be affinity-purified, a property that is stated in catalogs and that should ensure that at least 80% of the labeled protein is active antibody. The secondary antibody can, further, be papain-digested and the $F(ab)'_2$ fragment isolated. This lacks the Fc portion of the antibody, which binds (in an antigen-nonspecific fashion) to surface receptors on many cells involved in initiating the immune response. This can therefore give anomolous binding, although in practice, Fc binding is usually a problem only in dealing with lymphocytes or associated cells. A good immunoaffinity-purified $F(ab)'_2$ secondary antibody is the best possible reagent, although some firms have had problems with this much protein chemistry and their reagents have not been stable.

13. Immunoglobulin present in culture serum can occasionally persist through washing of the cells and then bind secondary antibody. (This should occur only if your cells have Fc receptors for immunoglobulin.) If so, during your first incubation, also incubate your secondary antibody with 1% serum of the species used in the culture (e.g., calf). Just before adding the secondary antibody, spin it in a microfuge for 10 min, and that proportion of the antibodies that crossreact with the serum immunoglobulin will be blocked.

14. Controls: Always have a batch of untransfected cells carried through, and always have cells (both transfected and control) incubated with the second antibody alone. If you are looking at transient transfection, have pseudotransfected cells as controls if possible, since they will show the same intracellular reactions (e.g., peroxidase-containing lysosomes) as the transfected calls. More sophisticated antibody controls are often undertaken (e.g., substituting for the primary antibody another that has the same Ig class and subclass, but that detects an unrelated antigen; inhibition of primary-antibody activity by purified antigen), but none is foolproof. The best guarantees of specificity are to use antibodies at high dilution, and ultimately to test specificity by an independent method, such as immunoblotting or immunoprecipitation.

15. Enhancement procedures: The immunological methods should at least double your signal, and more so if the augmentation factor of the secondary antibodies is higher than two. Chemical enhancement (Section 3.4.2.) must be of the order of tenfold. Maximal optical enhancement (Section 3.6.), obtainable with dark-field optics, can produce a convincing photograph of a signal that is barely visible under normal optics. The lower limit of detection available with peroxidase methodology depends only on the dissociation kinetics of your antibody and your back-

ground. Note that the nonoptical methods of enhancing your signal work well in other techniques, such as immunoblotting.

16. For the peroxidase reaction, imidazole acts as a cofactor and extends the optimal pH range of peroxidase to near neutrality. DAB should be treated as a suspect carcinogen (although all attempts of which I am aware to demonstrate its carcinogenic properties in experimental animals have proved negative [21]). Therefore, wear gloves, work in a fume hood, and wash in Chloros everything that has touched DAB. On buying DAB, add water to make up a solution of approx 100 mg/mL, aliquot it (e.g., 0.5 mL), freeze and store at –20°C in the dark. The concentration need not be exact; the DAB is in excess, and if you are going to silver/gold-enhance the reaction product, use half or a quarter this concentration of DAB, which will reduce the background. DAB decomposes in light; a 1 mg/mL solution should be colorless, but will normally be a light plum color, which will darken if exposed to light. It should contain no particulate matter; if it does, filter it, check your glassware for residual detergent, or change your supplier. If room temperature is rather cold (or you are in a hurry), warm the buffer. An alternative to DAB is tetramethylbenzidine, which, instead of giving a fine brown precipitate, gives large blue crystals. It is more sensitive than DAB, although at the expense of resolution, and offers a different-colored reaction product should you want to do double labeling *(9–11)*.

17. If you have glass slides, then xylene-based moutants can also be used. A convenient, stable, plastic-compatible moutant can be made by dissolving 50 g of polyvinyl pyrrolidone in 5 mL of H_2O, with stirring (overnight), and adding 2 mL glycerol and a small crystal of thymol (bacteriostatic; 0.05% NaN_3 should do). The moutant is viscous enough for the cells to be viewed immediately, and it will become hard overnight.

18. Cells should be fixed before attempting this procedure; if live cells have been labeled, fix them with paraformaldehyde before the DAB reaction. This enhancement procedure will convert light-tan-colored DAB reaction product to an unmistakable black, make otherwise invisible staining visible, and should not be attempted if your staining is already a definite brown. It is imperative that your background be perfectly clear. If your staining is weak and you want to use this method of enhancement, reduce antibody and DAB concentrations, and use longer antibody incubation and final wash times to ensure that the background is nil. Commercial silver enhancement methods are available, but this procedure is much better and cheaper than any I have tested.

19. Histological counterstains can be useful in displaying cell morphology and, in some cases, identifying cell types. DAB labeling is compatible with a wide range of such stains, although some procedures use solvents that are not compatible with tissue-culture plastic, or that are water soluble. A simple hematoxylin stain, which labels nuclei blue (a color that can be suppressed during photography with blue filters, which additionally enhance the brown DAB reaction product) can be made by dissolving 2.0 g of hematoxylin (anhydrous, CI No. 75290) in 730 mL of distilled H_2O + 250 mL ethylene glycol; add 200 mg sodium iodate, 17.6 g $Al_2(SO_4)_3 \cdot 18H_2O$, and 20 mL glacial acetic acid. The stain can be used immediately, although it achieves optimal activity after "ripening" for a few weeks; it is stable for years. To stain, wash cells twice with tap water and add hematoxylin solution. Leave for 1–2 min (depending on the intensity of blue required), wash twice with tap water, add 1% $MgSO_4$ + 0.2% $NaHCO_3$ in tap water, and, after 1 min, wash again with tap water and apply a coverslip (22).

References

1. Karush, F. (1978) The affinity of antibody: Range, variability, and the role of multivalence, in *Comprehensive Immunology*, vol. 5 *Immunoglobulins* (Litman, G. W. and Good, R. A., eds.) Plenum, New York and London, pp. 85–116.
2. Harlow, E. and Lane. D. (1988) *Antibodies: A Laboratory Manual* (Cold Spring Harbor Laboratory, Cold Spring Harbor, NY).
3. Alzari, P. M., Lascombe, M. B., and Poljak, R. J. (1988) Three-dimensional structure of antibodies. *Annu. Rev. Immunol.* **6,** 555–580.
4. Crumpton, M. J. (1974) Protein antigens: The molecular basis of antigenicity and immunogenicity, in *The Antigens*, vol. 2 (Sela, M., ed.) Academic, New York, pp. 1–78.
5. Tainer, J. A., Getzoff, E. D., Paterson, Y., Olson, A. J., and Lerner, R. A. (1985) The atomic mobility component of protein antigenicity. *Annu. Rev. Immunol.* **3,** 501–535.
6. Milstein, C., Wright. B., and Cuello, A. C. (1983) The discrepancy between the crossreactivity of a monoclonal antibody to serotonin and its immunohistochemical specificity. *Mol. Immunol.* **20,** 113–123.
7. Mason, D. W. and Williams, A. F. (1980) The kinetics of antibody binding to membrane antigens in solution and at the cell surface. *Biochem. J.* **187,** 1–20.
8. Dower, S. K., Titus, J. A., and Segal, D. M. (1984) The binding of multivalent ligands to cell surface receptors, in *Cell Surface Dynamics* (Perelson, A., ed.) Dekker, New York, pp. 277–328.
9. Carson, K. A. and Mesulam, M.-M. (1982) Electron microscopic demonstration of neural connections using horseradish peroxidase: A comparison of the tetramethylbenzidine procedure with seven other histochemical methods. *J. Histochem. Cytochem.* **30,** 425–435.
10. Trojanowski, J. Q., Obrocka. M. A., and Lee, V. M. Y. (1983) A comparison of eight different chromagen protocols for the demonstration of immunoreactive neurofilaments or glial filaments in rat cerebellum using the peroxidase-antiperoxidase method and monoclonal antibodies. *J. Histochem. Cytochem.* **31,** 1217–1223.

11. Scopsi, L. and Larsson, L. I. (1986) Increased sensitivity in peroxidase immunocytochemistry. A comparative study of a number of peroxidase visualisation methods employing a model system. *Histochemistry* **84,** 221–230.

12. Mason, D. Y. and Sammons, R. (1978) Alkaline phosphatase and peroxidase for double immunoenzymatic labelling of cellular constituents. *J. Clin. Pathol.* **31,** 454–460.

13. Wilson, M. B. and Nakane, P. K. (1978) Recent developments in the periodate method of conjugating horseradish peroxidase (HRPO) to antibodies, in *Immunofluorescence and Related Staining Techniques* (Knapp,W., Holubar, K. and Wick, G., eds.) Elsevier/North Holland Biomedical, New York, pp. 215–224.

14. Eldred, W. D., Zucker, C., Karten, H. J., and Yazulla, S. (1983) Comparison of fixation and penetration enhancement techniques for use in ultrastructural immunocytochemistry. *J. Histochem. Cytochem.* **31,** 285–292.

15. Bohn, W. (1978) A fixation method for improved antibody penetration in electron microscopical immunoperoxidase studies. *J. Histochem. Cytochem.* **26,** 293–297.

16. Willingham, M. C., Yamada, S., and Pastan, I. (1978) Ultrastructural antibody localization of alpha$_2$-macroglobulin in membrane-limited vesicles in cultured cells. *Proc. Natl. Acad. Sci. USA* **75,** 4359–4363.

17. Morris, R. J. and Barber, P. C. (1983) Fixation of Thy-1 in nervous tissue for immunohistochemistry: A quantitative assessment of the effect of different fixation conditions upon retention of antigenicity and the cross-linking of Thy-1. *J. Histochem. Cytochem.* **31,** 263–274.

18. Willingham, M. C. and Yamada, S. S. (1979) Development of a new primary fixative for electron microscopic immunocytochemical localisation of intracellular antigens in cultured cells. *J. Histochem. Cytochem.* **27,** 947–960.

19. McClean. I. W. and Nakane, P. K. (1974) Periodate–lysine–paraformaldehyde fixative, a new fixative for immunoelectron microscopy. *J. Histochem. Cytochem.* **22,** 1077–1083.

20. Hickson, D. C., Yep, J. N., Glenney, J. K., Hayes. T., and Waldborg, E. F. (1981) Evaluation of periodate/lysine/paraformaldehyde fixation as a method for cross-linking plasma membrane glycoproteins. *J. Histochem. Cytochem.* **29,** 561–566.

21. Weisburger, E. K., Russfield, A. B., Homburger, F., Weisburger, J. H., Boger, E., van Dongen, C. G., and Chu. K. C. (1978) Testing of 21 environmental aromatic amines or derivatives for long-term toxicity or carcinogenicity. *J. Environ. Pathol. Toxicol.* **2,** 325–356.

22. Gill, G. W., Frost, J. K., and Miller, K. A. (1974) A new formula for a half-oxidized hematoxylin solution that neither overstains nor requires differentiation. *Acta Cyto. (Baltimore)* **18,** 300–311.

CHAPTER 27

The Use of Flow Cytometry to Detect Transfected Gene Products

Raymond Bujdoso, David Sargan, Keith Ballingall, and Andrew Sanderson

1. Introduction

Flow cytometry and fluorescence-activated cell sorting (FACS) are techniques of great power used to screen cells rapidly for expression of particular gene products. These techniques have been of general utility in identifying and selecting populations of cells of defined characteristics from body fluids and other natural sources. More recently they have received extensive attention as methods for screening cell-surface expressed gene products in transfected cells. These methods rely on the indirect coupling of detector molecules, usually fluorochromes, to specific molecules on the target cells. This may occur through conjugation of the fluorochrome to the ligand of a receptor, or, as is more generally the case, through the use of fluorochrome-conjugated antibodies specific for the transfected gene product. Cells displaying specific surface fluorescence following exposure to a flurochrome conjugate may subsequently be positively selected (or excluded) by FACS. Since cells are sorted individually, FACS is an ideal technique for picking up very rare events and for finding very minor subpopulations. In theory at least, the experimenter may recover a single cell of the desired phenotype from a relatively large population. However, the examination of single cells

From: *Methods in Molecular Biology, Vol. 7: Gene Transfer and Expression Protocols*
Edited by: E. J. Murray © 1991 The Humana Press Inc., Clifton, NJ

makes the technique relatively slow (sorting approx 10^3 cells/s). Therefore, populations to be examined are limited to a few hundred thousand cells. For this reason, FACS has proved most useful in the selection of stable transfectants, for which positive cells can be expanded by further rounds of cell growth prior to analysis. In practice, several rounds of cell sorting and expansion are often required to obtain a clean population.

Transfected cells screened by FACS are usually used for one of two purposes: (a) for cloning of a novel gene by transfection of target cells with an expression library, or (b) for reverse genetic studies, in which a cell line expressing a gene of interest is produced by transfection with a DNA molecule that has already been cloned. In the former case, expression of the target gene will be a rare event because of the high complexity of the transfecting DNA population. It is therefore essential that all cells assayed by FACS are transfectants and that cells expressing the gene are recognized. Only a few cell types have proved capable of these high transfection rates. In general, rodent cells have proved superior to cells from other species. In addition, the cell type selected as a target must be capable of being suspended for FACS analysis without treatments that might damage proteins on the cell membrane. For this reason, suspension culture cells are the most conveniently used. In most published work, the mouse L-cell has been used as the target cell.

In order to ensure that all cells examined by FACS are transfectants, a cotransfection with a selectable marker is used. This may take the form of the *neo* gene, conferring resistance to the antibiotic G418, supplied either within the vector used for library synthesis or as a contransfected plasmid. Any of the other selection systems referred to elsewhere in this book may also be used. Cells are then grown in selective media prior to FACS selection of positives. DNA for these transfections may be supplied either as linearized cosmid clones or, more simply, as high-mol-wt DNA purified from a cell type known to express the gene of interest. In either case, the endogenous promoters are relied on to ensure expression. Alternatively, a full-length cDNA library may be generated in a vector in which it is under the control of an efficient promoter and linearized DNA from this library used in the transfections.

For reverse genetic studies, a high efficiency of stable transfection is not so essential, and the choice of cell type is dictated by the biological imperatives of the functional studies required. Here again, though, a selection for transfection is generally used prior to any FACS step.

Fluorescence detection in flow cytometry relies on the fluorochrome-conjugated antibody binding to cells expressing the transfected gene product. For this to occur, the antibody binding site (the epitope) must be present in the transfected gene product. In transfections, this places obvious limitations on the nature of the supplied DNA. In contrast to the assay of transfected cells by the use of nucleic acid hybridization techniques, for FACS, the transfected DNA must encode the antigenic epitope, together with enough additional structural sequence to give the correct folding of this part of the protein. It also must be capable of high levels of expression and correct processing; thus, a powerful promoter must sometimes be supplied. However, these limitations apply to most other methods of assay of transfected cells, such as enzymatic assay, ^{125}I-labeled ligand binding, or other single-component changes of phenotype. Most of these methods require much more elaborate assay techniques, involving multiple rounds of pool screening to isolate individual transformed cells.

Difficulties of flow-cytometric assay of the transfection technique are not always predictable. Antibody interaction with cell-surface proteins can cause their clearance from the membrane by activation and internalization. Some cell-surface receptor molecules are functional only when coexpressed and forming a complex with other proteins. This may cause a difficulty if a labeled ligand, rather than an antibody, is used to assay for presence of the gene product. However, despite the potential problems, these methods have been used to detect transfected genes products, such as the receptors for hormones, growth factors, and ferritin, as well as a large number of other cell-surface proteins.

Methods for transfection and for recovery of the transfected DNA are discussed elsewhere in this book. Here we present suitable methods for flow-cytometric analysis and fluorescence-activated cell sorting.

1.1. Principles of Flow Cytometry

Flow cytometry is the analysis of scattered and fluorescent light from cells in suspension that pass through a beam of laser light. A schematic diagram illustrating the main features of a flow cytometer and cell sorter is shown in Fig. 1. Cells for analysis enter a flow chamber that is perfused with sheath fluid. The laminar flow of the sheath fluid directs cells to the center of a liquid jet. The frequency of cells entering the liquid jet is regulated by the difference in pressure on both sample and sheath fluid, and by the cell concentration of the sample. The result is a sequential flow of individual cells within a jet of fluid that has a diameter of 50–100 μm as it leaves the nozzle of the flow chamber. This jet of fluid then passes through laser light, an intense beam of focused monochromatic light. As a consequence of cells intersecting the laser beam, light is scattered at various angles to the original axis of its travel and fluorescent molecules on the surface of cells are excited and fluoresce.

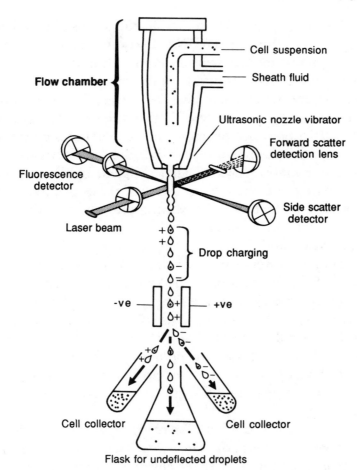

Fig. 1. A diagrammatic representation of the main features of a fluorescence activated cell sorter (FACS). *See text* for details.

1.1.1. Scattered Light

Scattered light is related to a variety of cellular parameters, including cell size, shape, granularity, and refractive index. Two types of scattered light are routinely detected in flow cytometry. The first of these is forward scatter (FSC), which represents the light scattered at low angles (0–10°) to the original axis of travel of the laser beam. At these small angles, scatter light is most proportional to cell size. Second, there is side scatter (SSC), which is light scattered at relatively wide angles (70–110°) to the laser beam axis. At these angles, this parameter relates best to the granularity and internal complexity of cells. Scattered laser light is detected by sensors that exclude uninterrupted laser light. The electronic signals generated by the detectors are amplified and presented on a visual display unit as a "dot plot" or following pulse height analysis, as a histogram of the number of cells with a particular scatter intensity. Figure 2a(i) shows the SSC and FSC profile of unfractionated afferent lymph monouclear cells. The particles with low scatter intensity represent dead cells and cellular debris. Platelets, as well as red blood cells, are also found in this region. Particles to the right of the low-scatter material are viable mononuclear cells. Two distinct populations are present: a dense grouping of low SSC and medium FSC, which represent lymphocytes, and a group of cells with high SSC and FSC, which are dendritic cells. A particular set of events may be analyzed separately within this heterogeneous mixture by electronically placing upper and lower "gates" on their scatter profile. Figure 2a(ii) shows the scatter profile following "live gating." The material of low scatter profile is now excluded from the analysis to allow subsequent measurements to be made on viable cells. Figure 2a(iii) shows the scatter profile that results from "gating" on only the high SSC and FSC cells. This allows information from dendritic cells to be collected without the need for cell fractionation procedures to exclude lymphocytes from the analysis.

1.1.2. Fluorescent Light

This light is generated by excitation of fluorescent molecules carried by fluorochrome-conjugated cells as they pass through the beam of laser light. Fluorescent light is collected at 90° to the laser beam and reflected to a detector that allows fluorescent light from one fluorochrome to enter and excludes all other light. In two-color fluorescence, a dichroic mirror used as a beam splitter directs the light of different wavelengths to the appropriate sensor. Fluorescent light is usually several orders of magnitude lower in intensity than scattered light and requires considerable amplification. The fluorescent signals are displayed in the same manner as scattered light. Depending on the difference in intensity between dull and brightly stained cells, the fluorescence scale of the displayed data may be linear or logarithmic. The cytometer fluorescence-detection system is designed to yield fluorescence signals proportional to the amount of dye associated with each cell. The size of the electronic signal produced by a cell is, then, a quantitative measure of the amount of fluorescent dye associated with the cell; in the case of cell-surface fluorescence, this will be proportional to the number of molecules identified by the fluorescent reagent. Figure 3 shows the fluorescence profiles of afferent dendritic cells measured by flow cytometry following indirect immunofluorescence staining. Cells were reacted with mouse antisheep monoclonal antibodies and subsequently reacted with fluorochrome-conjugated rabbit antimouse immunoglobulin. Figure 3i shows the background fluorescence profile of dendritic cells reacted with the fluorochrome conjugate in the absence of prior staining with any monoclonal antibody. This represents the background level or nonspecific level of fluorescence from the fluorochrome-conjugated reagent. Any fluorescence of greater intensity than the set marker

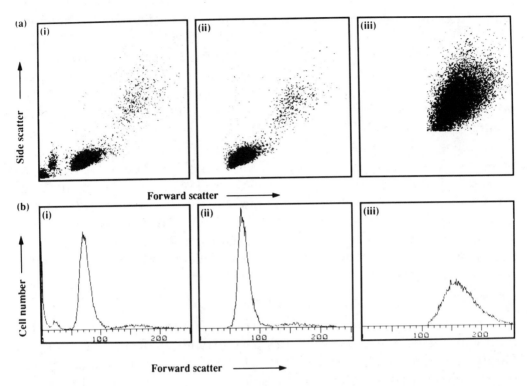

Fig. 2. (*a*) Scatter profile and (*b*) forward scatter histogram of afferent lymph monouclear cells. The "ungated" FSC and SSC profile of afferent cells is shown in **2a(i)**. By "gating out" low-scatter material, which represents dead cells and particulate matter (**a[ii]2**) data may be collected from viable lymphocytes (dense body) and dendritic cells (dispersed body). By gating on only the dendritic cells (**a[iii]**), lymphocytes may be excluded from the analysis. In each analysis, 10^4 events were collected, hence the increase in representation of dendritic cells in **a(iii)**. In **b**, the FSC histogram of each of the corresponding ungated or gated populations is shown. Cells were analyzed on a Becton Dickinson FACScan™ machine using a Consort 30 program.

(indicated by the arrow) when a monoclonal antibody is included in the staining protocol is to be judged as positive or specific fluorescence. This indicates cell-surface expression of the molecule identified by the monoclonal antibody. The overlay histogram in Fig. 3ii shows the variation in intensity of surface fluorescence, and, therefore, the level of expression of different molecules, following reaction of the dendritic cells with various monoclonal antibodies. LFA-3 and MHC Class II molecules are clearly expressed by all the dendritic cells, since the fluorescent profiles for the corresponding monoclonal antibodies are well to the left of the set marker. Anti-CD4 staining is a unimodal marginal positive, and expression of CD4 by these cells would require confirmation by another form of analysis, such as detection of CD4 mRNA.

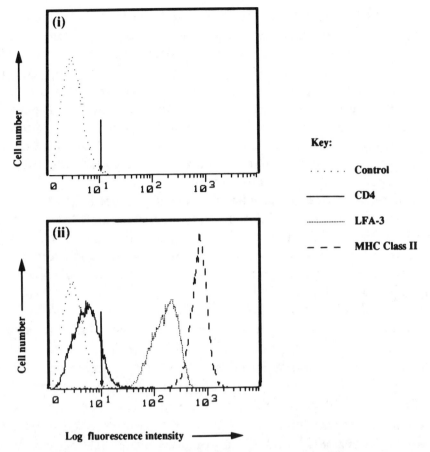

Fig. 3. Immunofluorescent profiles of afferent dendritic cells stained with various monoclonal antibodies. Purified dendritic cells were stained by indirect immunofluorescence using mouse antisheep monoclonal antibodies. Washed cells were reacted with either anti-CD4, anti-LFA-3, or anti-MHC Class II monoclonal antibody, or phosphate-buffered saline (control) followed by (Fab)$_2$ rabbit antimouse immunoglobulin-FITC. Cells were analyzed on a Becton Dickinson FACScan™ machine using a Consort 30 program with a log scale for fluorescence intensity.

1.1.3. Fluorescent Activated Cell Sorting (FACS)

In sorting, individual cells with the desired scatter or fluorescence profile may be purified. To achieve this, the liquid jet is separated into droplets at a point beyond its intersection with the laser beam, where cells are analyzed. The formation of droplets occurs by vibrating the nozzle of the flow chamber with ultrasonic sound at a frequency close to the natural break-up frequency of the liquid jet (approx 40,000 cycles/s). At the break-up point, droplets contain a single cell or no cell at all. A voltage is applied to the drops, which charges them or leaves them neutral. The drops then pass in single file through an electric field generated between two charged plates. The drop containing the selected cell will be deflected right or left, depending on the charge it has been given. Uncharged drops are collected in a central reservoir. Two populations of cells can be collected simultaneously by applying a positive charge to drops containing one population and a negative charge to drops containing the second. Since the point of analysis is some distance from the point of drop formation, there is a delay between the time of analysis and that of drop charging. It is critical for successful sorting that the selected cell is contained within a drop of the correct charge. Routinely, three consecutive drops are charged to ensure that the selected cell will be deflected into the correct receiving vessel. However, at high rates of sorting (>3,000 cells/s), there is a high chance that an undesired cell will be contained within one of the three drops. In this situation, the charge on all three drops can be neutralized and the drops unsorted. Alternatively, the charge may be left as it was originally, resulting in a sorted population contaminated with unselected cells. In general, more pure populations are collected at slower rates of sorting, but at the cost of a low yield of cells.

An example of detection by surface fluorescence followed by FACS to enrich populations of cells expressing particular transfected gene products is shown by the series of histograms in Fig. 4. These show a sequential series of sorts to produce an ovine MHC class II expressing L cell line. Cells were cotransfected with linearized cosmid cloned ovine MHC class II α and β genes, along with the HSV-tk gene, and were selected in HAT for 2–3 wk. The surviving colonies were pooled before analysis. Cells were stained with a cocktail of mouse antisheep MHC Class II monoclonal antibodies followed by a rabbit antimouse immunoglobulin-FITC. Figure 4i shows the staining profile of L cells transfected with the HSV-tk gene alone. This represents the background fluorescence staining of L cells with the antimouse immunoglobulin FITC reagent. Cells expressing a higher fluorescence intensity than the set marker are to be judged as expressing ovine MHC Class II molecules. Figure 4ii shows the staining of cells transfected with HSV-tk and the cosmid cloned MHC class II genes. A small percentage of cells (2.3%) lie to the right of the fluorescent marker; these represent L cells expressing ovine MHC class II molecules on their cell surface. These cells were positively selected by FACS and then expanded in number and reanalyzed. The analysis of the first sort is shown in Fig. 4iii, which shows that 19% of L cells now express ovine MHC class II genes. These cells were subjected to a second sort and the cells were again expanded. The fluorescence profile of this second sort is shown in Fig. 4iv, which shows >90% of the cells expressing the transfected gene products.

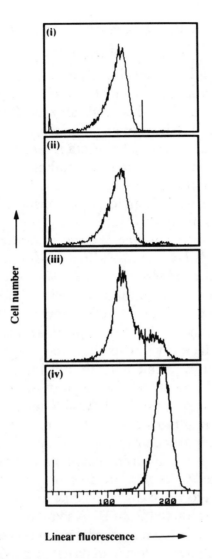

Fig. 4. Fluorescence profiles of L-cells transfected with sheep MHC Class II genes and stained with mouse antisheep MHC Class II monoclonal antibodies. Mouse L-cells were transfected with the HSV-tk gene along with sheep MHC Class α and β genes. Cells were selected in HAT, and all the surviving colonies were pooled before analysis. Cells were stained with a mixture of mouse antisheep MHC Class II monoclonal antibodies followed by rabbit antimouse immunoglobulin-FITC. Cells were analyzed and sorted on a Becton Dickinson FACS IV machine using a linear scale for fluorescence intensity. **(i)** Control L-cells transfected with HSV-tk gene alone. **(ii)** Fluorescence analysis of primary transfectants containing HSV-tk and sheep MHC CLass II α and β genes. Cells to the right of the set gate were positively sorted and expanded. **(iii)** Fluorescence analysis of cells after the first sorting. The positive-staining cells were sorted and expanded. **(iv)** Fluorescence analysis of cells after the second sorting.

1.2. Choice of Reagents

1.2.1. Antibodies

The antibody reagents used for immunofluorescent staining may be monoclonal or polyclonal. Monoclonal antibodies recognize a single epitope within a molecule, and do so with a single affinity. Polyclonal antisera recognize several epitopes within the protein molecule, each with a different affinity. On this basis, the use of polyclonal antisera is more likely to result in higher staining than the use of monoclonal antibodies. However, because of the sensitivity of the FACS, it is necessary to purify the specific antibodies from polyclonal antiserum to avoid high levels of nonspecific staining. This is best achieved by affinity chromatography, using the specific antigen as the immunoadsorbent. In the absence of large amounts of soluble antigen for this purification, as might be the case with a cell-surface protein, monoclonal antibodies would be the reagent of choice. Monoclonal antibody (MAb) is present at relatively high concentration in ascites fluid (milligram amounts), which generally needs only to be diluted for indirect fluorescence. For direct fluorescence, though, the MAb must be purified from ascites fluid; this can be accomplished satisfactorily by caprylic acid fractionation followed by ion-exchange HPLC. Affinity problem's with individual MAbs can be overcome by using a mixture of MAbs, all directed against the same molecule, but each reactive with a different epitope. It is advisable to use more than one MAb, if available, when screening transfected cells, since the transfected gene product may be deficient in particular epitopes compared to the native molecule. This may arise through variation in polypeptide sequence or glycosylation differences between cell types. For the detection of cell-surface immunofluorescence, MAbs raised to the native molecule are preferable to those raised to synthetic peptides predicted from DNA sequence data. Antibodies raised to peptides may react with full-length protein in a Western Blot analysis, but do not always react with the molecule in its native configuration. The isotype of the particular antibody used in the fluorescence assay may affect the level of nonspecific staining seen. The degree of nonspecific staining associated with different isotypes of antibody is of the order $IgG_2 > IgG_1 > IgM$. This nonspecific binding is attributable mainly to antibody binding to cellular Fc receptors. The effect can be reduced by using $F(ab')_2$ preparations of antibody.

1.2.2. Fluorochromes

The choice of fluorochrome will depend on a variety of parameters, including the laser and optical system within the flow cytometer. The system for excitation of fluorescent molecules can be a dual- or single-laser system. Dual-laser systems may utilize different fluorescent dyes with widely separated excitation wavelengths, whereas single-laser systems are restricted to dyes excited by the same wavelength. However, with the appropriate choice of fluorochromes, both systems can measure simultaneous two-color fluorescence.

A suitable fluorochrome should not only be exicted and detected by the flow cytometer, but also have a high quantum efficiency, be relatively easy to conjugate to antibodies without loss of specificity of either reagent, show little nonspecific staining, and lend itself to simultaneous use with other fluorochromes without impeding the excitation of emission spectra of the other fluorochrome. Two fluorochromes that meet these requirements are fluorescein isothiocyanate (FITC), which emits a yellow green fluorescence at an emission max. of 525 nm, and R-phycoerythrin, a phycobiliprotein, which fluoresces red at an emission max. of 578 nm. Both can be excited by argonion laser light at 488 nm and may be used for two-color fluorescence on a single-laser cytometer. Other commonly used fluorochromes are derivatives of rhodamine: tetramethylrhodamine isothiocyanate (TRITC) and X-rhodamine isothiocyanate (X-RITC). These emit yellow to red fluorescence and may also be used with FITC in dual-color fluorescence. However, these reagents display high levels of background staining.

The ease with which FITC may be conjugated to antibody has made it the principal fluorochrome in immunofluorescence assays. Other less chemically reactive fluorochromes may, by using bifunctional crosslinking reagents, such as N-succinimidyl 3-(2-pyridyldithio) propionate (SPDP) be coupled to antibodies. Alternatively, a convenient conjugation system is based on the specific reaction between biotin and avidin. Biotin is relatively easy to attach to antibodies, which may then be reacted with commercially available preparations of avidin–fluorochrome conjugates.

1.3. Immunofluorescent Staining of Cells

It is important to ensure that cells subjected to flow cytometry and FACS are well dispersed, with no aggregates or clumps present. Clumping of cells may lead to errors in analysis and clogging of the flow-chamber nozzle. Cells are washed in ice-cold medium to prevent modulation and internalization of surface molecules and then reacted with specific antibody. The amount of antibody bound to cells may be determined by direct fluorescence, in which the fluorescent label is attached directly to the specific antibody. This is the simplest and most rapid form of immunofluorescence assay, and allows th quantification of binding sites. However, with direct fluorescence, all the antibodies to be used must be conjugated with the fluorochrome. Alternatively, indirect immunofluorescence may be used if the specific antibody is detected by a second reagent that is itself fluorescently labeled. This assay requires one step more than the direct assay (and therefore requires more time), but it has the advantage of providing an amplification step that allows greater sensitivity. Following staining, cells should be stored in the dark at

4°C and analyzed as soon as possible. Cells to be analyzed and not sorted may be stored for 24 h if previously fixed with freshly prepared 1% paraformaldehyde. A common source of increased background staining in fluorescence assays is dead cells within the sample preparation. In some cases it is possible to remove nonviable cells from the sample prior to analysis. This can be achieved by centrifugation of cells over a medium of suitable density, which allows dead cells and debris to pellet and viable cells to be retained at the interface. Alternatively, nonviable cells may be discriminated by fluorescent staining. Propidium iodide (PI) binds to cellular DNA and double-stranded RNA in dead cells and is excluded at the plasma membrane of viable cells. It is excited by light at 488 nm and emits at 600 nm and can be used with FITC on a single-laser system. A third method of excluding dead cells from the analysis is based on their scatter profile. Because dead cells and debris have low FSC and SSC profiles, they can be efficiently "gated out" (*see* Fig. 2), allowing only the fluorescence signal from viable cells to be collected. When a new population of cells is examined for the first time, it is useful to stain with PI to verify the scatter profile of viable cells.

2. Materials

2.1. Isolation of Monoclonal Antibody from Ascites Fluid

For the preparation of antibody for conjugation with fluorescein isothiocyanate (FITC) or Biotin, *see* Note 1.

2.1.1. Affinity Chromatography on Immunoglobulin Antiimmunoglobulin Columns

1. Antimouse immunoglobulin raised to either unfractionated mouse immunoglobulin or antisera specific for the isotype of antibody to be fractionated.
2. Affigel or CNBr-activated Sepharose.
3. $0.1 M$ glycine, pH 4.0.
4. Phosphate-buffered saline (PBS).
5. Ascites fluid containing relevant antibody, cleared of any insoluble material by 0.22-μm filtration.
6. 1.0M Tris-HCl, pH 8.0.
7. $0.001 M$ HCl.
8. $0.1 M$ NaHCO$_3$, $0.5 M$ NaCl, pH 8.3.
9. $0.1 M$ sodium acetate containing $0.5 M$ NaCl, pH 4.0.
10. $0.1 M$ Tris-HCl containing $0.5 M$ NaCl, pH 8.0.
11. $1 M$ ethanolamine HCl, pH 8.0.
12. 0.1% sodium azide in PBS.

2.1.2. By Caprylic Acid Fractionation

1. Ascites fluid containing relevant antibody cleared of any insoluble material by 0.22-μm filtration.
2. 0.06 M sodium acetate buffer, pH 4.
3. Caprylic (octanoic) acid.
4. TSK DEAE-5PW (7.5 × 0.75 cm) HPLC column (Anachem).
5. 20 m M Tris-HCl, pH 7.7.
6. 0.5 M NaCl in 20 m M Tris-HCl, pH 7.7.
7. PBS.

2.2. Fluorescein Isothiocyanate (FITC) Conjugation to Antibody (Direct Fluorescence)

1. 0.2 M sodium bicarbonate buffer, pH 9.5.
2. FITC (Sigma).
3. Dimethyl sulfoxide (DMSO, Sigma).
4. Ice-cold PBS containing 1 mg/mL bovine serum albumin (BSA, Grade V, Sigma).

2.3. Biotin Conjugation to Antibody (Indirect Fluorescence)

1. 0.2 M sodium bicarbonate buffer, pH 9.5.
2. Biotin (Biotin-amidocaproate *N*-hydroxysuccinimide ester) (Sigma).
3. Dimethyl sulfoxide (DMSO, Sigma).
4. Ice-cold PBS containing 1 mg/mL bovine serum albumin (BSA, Grade V, Sigma).

2.4. Live/Dead Staining

1. Propidium iodide (Sigma).
2. PBS.

3. Methods

3.1. Isolation of Monoclonal Antibody from Ascites Fluid

3.1.1. Affinity Chromatography on Immunoglobulin Antiimmunoglobulin Columns

1. Purchase or prepare a monoclonal or polyclonal antibody to mouse immunoglobulin, and couple this to a column matrix, such as Affigel (Bio-Rad) or CNBr-activated Sepharose (Pharmacia), according to the supplier's instructions (*see* Note 2).

2. Wash the column with 0.1 M glycine (pH 4) and then wash extensively with PBS.

3. Cycle clarified ascites into the column over several hours, and then wash the column with PBS.

4. Elute bound antibody with 0.1 M glycine (pH 4) and collect 1-mL fractions into tubes containing 0.1 mL of 1 M Tris-HCl (pH 8).

5. Measure the optical density of each fraction, pool those with the highest concentration of protein, dialyze into PBS, and store in aliquots at –20°C.

6. Analyze a sample of fractionated antibody by SDS-PAGE.

7. Wash the column with 0.1 M glycine (pH 4) and then extensively wash PBS and store at 4°C in buffer containing 0.1% sodium azide.

3.1.2. Caprylic Acid Precipitation (see Note 3)

1. To 1 vol of ascitic fluid, add 2 vol of 0.06 M sodium acetate buffer, pH 4.0.

2. Add caprylic (octanoic) acid (37.5 µL/mL of undiluted ascitic fluid) dropwise with vigorous stirring.

3. Mix at room temperature for 30 min.

4. Microfuge for 3 min to remove precipitate, and retain supernatant containing purified antibody. If the supernatant does not clarify upon repeated microfuging, proceed with the dialysis (below) and microfuge again.

5. Dialyze purified antibody against 20 m M Tris-HCl (pH 7.7) and load (up to 25 mg) onto a preequilibrated analytical TSK DEAE-5PW (7.5 × 0.75 cm) HPLC column. Elute with a gradient of 0–0.5 M NaCl at a flow rate of 1 mL/min over 60 min. IgG antibody elutes as the major protein peak before the albumin peak.

6. Analyze fractions of purified antibody by SDS-PAGE, pool the most pure, dialyze into PBS, and store in aliquots at –20°C.

3.2. FITC Conjugation to Antibody

1. Dialyze antibody into 0.2 M sodium bicarbonate buffer, pH 9.5, adjusting the antibody concentration to 1–2 mg/mL in this buffer.

2. Add FITC (dissolved in DMSO) to give a final concentration of 1% (w/w).

3. Mix immediately, followed by end-over-end mixing at room temperature for 1 h or at 4°C overnight.

4. Dialyze the reaction mixture against PBS, and store the fluorescein conjugate in aliquots at –20°C.

3.3. Biotinylation of Antibody

1. Dialyze antibody into 0.2 *M* bicarbonate buffer, pH 8.5; then adjust the protein concentration to 1 mg/mL.
2. Prepare biotin ester at 1mg/mL in DMSO just prior to use; then add to antibody to give a biotin/protein ratio of 75 µg/mg.
3. Mix immediately, followed by end-over-end mixing at room temperature for 4h.
4. Dialyze the reaction mixture against PBS and store the biotinylated reagent in aliquots at –20°C.

3.4. Immunofluorescent Staining of Cells

3.4.1. Direct Staining

1. Cells are washed three times in ice-cold PBS supplemented with 1 mg/mL BSA (PBS-BSA) and adjusted to 1×10^7/mL.
2. Aliquot $1-2 \times 10^6$ washed cells into a small centrifuge tube, pellet cells by centrifugation at 300*g* for 3 min, and discard the supernatant; then resuspend the cells by flicking the bottom of the tubes.
3. Add 50 µL of the appropriate dilution of directly conjugated antibody and incubate the cells for 30 min on ice (*see* Note 4).
4. Resuspend cells by flicking the bottom of the tubes, add 0.75 mL ice-cold PBS-BSA, and centrifuge at 300*g* for 3 min. Discard the supernatant and repeat the washing three times.
5. Finally, resuspend the cells in 1 mL of buffer for analysis (*see* Note 5).

3.4.2. Indirect Staining

1. Follow steps 1 and 2 of Section 3.4.1.
2. Add 50µL of the appropriate dilution of primary antibody, and incubate the cells for 30 min on ice (*see* Note 4).
3. Resuspend cells by flicking the bottom of the tubes, add 0.75 mL ice-cold PBS-BSA, and centrifuge at 300*g* for 3 min. Discard the supernatant and repeat the washing three times.
4. Add 50 µL of an appropriate dilution of the second conjugated reagent and incubate the cells on ice for 30 min.
5. Resuspend cells by flicking the bottom of the tubes, add 0.75 mL ice-cold PBS-BSA, and centrifuge at 300*g* for 3 min. Discard the supernatant and repeat the washing three times. Finally, resuspend the cells in 1 mL of PBS-BSA for analysis (*see* Note 6).

3.5. Live and Dead Staining

1. Prepare a solution of propidium iodide (PI) at 2 mg/mL in PBS. Store in aliquots at –20°C.
2. After the final wash of cells in the staining procedure, add PI solution to give a final concentration of 20 µg/mL. Since free PI does not fluoresce, cells need not be washed prior to analysis.
3. Exclude positive PI staining cells from the analysis by setting the appropriate gate.

4. Notes

1. Sterile solutions of antibodies and medium are required for staining and sorting cells that will subsequently be expanded by in vitro tissue culture. All solutions for sterile FACS work should be 0.22-µm-filtered before use. Antibodies should be stored at –20°C without any preservative. Reagents to be used solely for staining and analysis of cells can be stored at 4°C in buffer containing 0.1% sodium azide.
2. The method of affinity chromatography on immunoglobulin antiimmunoglobulin columns for the fractionation of immunoglobulin in Section 3.1.1. refers to the preparation of mouse immunoglobulin, since the majority of monoclonal antibodies in use are of mouse origin. However, the method is applicable to the preparation of antibody from other species, providing a suitable antiimmunoglobulin reagent can be aquired.
3. The fractionation of ascites fluid by caprylic acid precipitation, described in Section 3.1.2., is a quick method for the isolation of antibody from ascites, although the method is not suitable for fractionation with antibodies of the IgM isotype.
4. The optimum working dilution of both fluoresceinated and biotinylated reagent conjugate antibody will need to be determined. Conjugated reagents should be microfuged for 10 min before use to remove any insoluble material.
5. Controls for direct staining should include unstained cells as well as cells stained with directly conjugated antibody of irrelevant specificity but of the same isotype as the test antibody.
6. Controls for indirect staining should include unstained cells, cells stained with the fluorochrome conjugate alone, and cells stained with a MAb of irrelevant specificity but of the same isotype as the test MAb with the fluorochrome conjugate.

Further Reading

1. Herzenberg, L. A., Sweet, R. G., and Herzenberg, L. A. (1976) Fluorescence-activated cell sorting. *Sci. Am.* **234,** 108.
2. Weir, D. M. (ed.) (1986) *Handbook of Experimental Immunology,* vol. 1, *Immunochemistry* (Blackwell Scientific, Oxford).
3. Scher, I. and Mage, M. G. (1984) Cellular identification and separation, in *Fundamental Immunology* (W. E. Paul, ed.), Raven, New York, p. 767.
4. Leiserson, W. (1985) Fluorescence cell sorter techniques in immunology, in *Immunological Methods,* vol. III (Lefkovits, I. and Pernis, B., eds.), Academic, New York, p. 289.

SECTION 8
SOUTHERN BLOT ANALYSIS
OF TRANSFECTED CELL LINES

CHAPTER 28

Determination of Foreign Gene Copy Number in Stably Transfected Cell Lines by Southern Transfer Analysis

Ronald M. Fourney, Rémy Aubin,
Kevin D. Dietrich, and Malcolm C. Paterson

1. Introduction

The quantitative appraisal of the number of foreign gene copies integrated within the genomes of stably transfected cells is most conveniently performed using the strategy known as Southern blotting *(1,2)*. First introduced by E. M. Southern in 1975 *(2)* the basic protocol involves the following steps: Size-fractionated DNA is first transferred from a gel matrix to a solid support under conditions that prevent self-annealing. The DNA molecules are then immobilized (covalently linked to the support) and processed for hybridization to a radiolabeled probe that has a nucleotide sequence complementing that of the target sequence to be detected. The blot is then washed extensively to remove unreacted probe molecules, and the hybrids formed between the probe and target sequences are revealed by autoradiography. The relative intensity of each autoradiographic signal will reflect the amount of hybridized material present. Quantification may be performed visually, by scanning laser densitometry, or, if the hybrids are sufficiently radioactive, by liquid scintillation counting.

From: *Methods in Molecular Biology, Vol. 7: Gene Transfer and Expression Protocols*
Edited by: E. J. Murray © 1991 The Humana Press Inc., Clifton, NJ

In this chapter, Southern analysis is considered in four components:

1. A rapid method for the isolation of high-mol-wt genomic DNA is offered *(3)*. A significant feature of the technique is that in the presence of urea and *N*-laurylsarcosine, cell lysis and the removal of cellular RNA and protein by enzymatic means can be carried out within a 4-h period in the same buffer. As a result of the time saved, high-purity genomic DNA (which is recovered by phenol extraction and ethanol precipitation) can be obtained from multiple samples in a single day.

2. A procedure for generating Southern blots under alkaline conditions is described *(3,4)*. This particular variation of the original method of Southern *(2)* exploits the chemical properties of a charge-modified nylon 66 membrane (BioTrace RP; Gelman Sciences, Ann Arbor, MI) and the use of $0.4 N$ NaOH as the transfer buffer to ensure the elution of fully denatured DNA from the gel matrix and allow the molecules to be covalently attached to the nylon membrane during the transfer process.

3. The preparation of high-specific-activity [^{32}P]-labeled probes by random hexadeoxyribonucleotide primer synthesis using DNA fragments contained in low-melting-point agarose is presented *(5)*.

4. Conditions for the hybridization, autoradiography, and quantification of the blots are outlined.

2. Materials

Prepare all stock solutions and buffers using "nanopure" (double-distilled and deionized) water and chemicals of the highest purity available (i.e., certified as Molecular Biology Grade).

2.1. For the Rapid Isolation of High-Molecular-Weight Genomic DNA

1. Rapid extraction (REX) buffer: 1% *N*-laurylsarcosine; 10 m*M* CDTA, pH 8.0; 0.1*M* Tris-HCl, pH 8.0; 0.2*M* NaCl; 0.4*M* urea. Sterilize the solution by filtration (0.22 μm). Store at room temperature. REX buffer is stable for at least 6 mo.

2. Phosphate-buffered saline (PBS calcium/magnesium-free): To 800 mL of nanopure water, add 8.0 g NaCl, 0.2 g KCl, 1.15 g Na_2HPO_4 and 0.2 g KH_2PO_4. Adjust the pH to between 7.2 and 7.4 and complete the vol to 1 L. Sterilize in the autoclave and store at room temperature.

3. Trypsin (10× stock; 2.5% trypsin in 0.8 g/L NaCl: Prepare a 1× working solution by diluting the stock in sterile PBS *(see above)*. Store at –20°C. Repeated cycles of freezing and thawing will reduce the potency of the solution considerably.

4. RNAse A (DNAse-free): Dissolve lyophylized RNAse A to 1 mg/mL in sterile 5 m*M* Tris-HCl, pH 7.5. Hold the preparation at 80°C for 15 min to inactivate traces of deoxyribonuclease activity. Allow to cool at room temperature. Store 100-μL aliquots at –20°C in sterile microcentrifuge tubes.

5. RNAse T1: Dilute a commercially available stock of RNAse T1 to 5000 U/mL in sterile 5 m*M* Tris-HCl, pH 7.5. Store 100-μL aliquots at 4°C in sterile microcentrifuge tubes.

6. Proteinase K: Dissolve lyophylized proteinase K at 20 mg/mL in sterile water. Store 125-μL aliquots at –20°C in sterile microcentrifuge tubes.

7. REX phenol: Combine 90 mL Tris-HCl buffered phenol (pH 8.0), 90 mL chloroform/isoamyl alcohol (24:1) and 2 mL REX buffer in an amber glass bottle. Emulsify the mixture by shaking vigorously for a few minutes. Allow the phases to separate by gravity. Store in the dark at 4°C. Phenol is stable for several months.

8. REX phenol/chloroform (1:1).

9. Chloroform/isoamyl alcohol (24:1).

10. 2.5*M* sodium acetate, pH 5.5. Sterilize in the autoclave.

11. Acetate-MOPS: 100 m*M* sodium acetate, 50 m*M* MOPS (pH 8.0). Clarify the solution by filtration (0.22 μm) before sterilizing in the autoclave.

12. HPLC-grade ethanol (95%).

13. Tris-CDTA: 10 m*M* Tris-HCl, 1 m*M* CDTA (pH 8.0). Sterilize in the autoclave.

2.2. For Southern Transfer Under Alkaline Conditions

1. 10× Spermidine trihydrochloride: Prepare a 40 m*M* stock of spermidine trihydrochloride by dissolving 30.6 mg of the chemical in 3 mL of water. Sterilize by filtration (0.22 μm) and store 500-μL aliquots at –20°C in sterile microcentrifuge tubes.

2. 10× Gel loading buffer: 0.1% bromophenol blue, 10× TPE, 50% glycerol, 0.1% sodium dodecyl sulfate. Store at 4°C.

3. 10× TPE: To 800 mL water, add 108 g Tris-HCl base, 15.1 mL phosphoric acid (85% reagent; sp. gr. 1.679 g/mL) and 40 mL of 0.5*M* EDTA (pH 8.0). Complete the vol to 1 L with water. The working solution (1×) is 80 m*M* Tris-HCl phosphate, 2 m*M* EDTA (pH ~7.4).

4. Ethidium bromide (1 mg/mL in water).

5. 0.25*N* HCl.

6. 0.4*N* NaOH.

7. 20× SSC: Dissolve 175.3 g of NaCl and 88.2 g of trisodium citrate (trihy-

drate) in 800 mL water. Adjust the pH to 7.0 and complete the vol to 1 L. Clarify the solution by filtration (0.22 µm) and sterilize in the autoclave.

2.3. For the Preparation of ^{32}P-Labeled DNA Probes by Random Hexadeoxyribonucleotide Primer Synthesis

1. 10× TAE: 0.4M Tris-HCl acetate, 50 mM sodium acetate, 10 mM EDTA (pH 8.0). Clarify the buffer by filtration (0.22 µm) and sterilize in the autoclave.
2. 10× TAE sample buffer: 10× TAE, 50% glycerol, 0.1% bromophenol blue.
3. Solution O: 1.25M Tris-HCl, 0.125M MgCl$_2$ (pH 8.0). Sterilize in the autoclave and store 1-mL aliquots at –20°C.
4. Solution A: To 1 mL of Solution O, add 18 µL of 2-mercaptoethanol and 5 µL each of dATP, dTTP, and dGTP from 100 mM stocks prepared in sterile 3 mM Tris-HCl, 0.2 mM EDTA (pH 7.0). Store this solution at –20°C.
5. Solution B: 2M HEPES, pH 6.6. Sterilize by filtration and store at 4°C.
6. Solution C: Resuspend random hexadeoxyribonucleotides (pd[N]$_6$) at 90 A$_{260}$ U/mL in sterile 10 mM Tris-HCl, 1 mM EDTA (pH 8.0). Store at –20°C.
7. ABC labeling mix: Mix 100 µL of Solution A, 250 µL of Solution B, and 150 µL of Solution C in a sterile microcentrifuge tube. Store 50-µL aliquots at –20°C. ABC mix will resist several freeze–thaw cycles.
8. Sephadex G50: Swell Sephadex G50 medium beads (DNA grade) in 10 mM Tris-HCl, 100 mM NaCl, 1 mM EDTA (pH 8.0) according to the supplier's recommended protocol and sterilize in the autoclave. Store at room temperature under aseptic conditions.
9. Column buffer: 10 mM Tris-HCl, 100 mM NaCl, 1 mM EDTA, 0.2% SDS (pH 8.0). Sterilize by filtration.
10. Bovine serum albumin (BSA): 10 mg/mL Molecular Biology Grade; BRL.
11. FPLC Pure DNA Polymerase. 1 (Klenow enzyme).
12. α[^{32}P]dCTP (800 Ci/mmol).

2.4. For the Detection of Target DNA Sequences by Southern Hybridization

1. 20× SSC (*see above*).
2. 20× SSPE: Mix 210.4 g of NaCl, 27.6 g of sodium dihydrogen phosphate (NaH$_2$PO$_4$) and 7.4 g of EDTA in 800 mL of water. Adjust the pH to 7.4 and complete the vol to 1 L. Clarify the solution by filtration (0.22 µm) and sterilize in the autoclave.

3. Deionized formamide: Deionized formamide is most conveniently prepared in 250- to 500-mL lots. Add 1 g of mixed-bed ion-exchange resin (Bio-Rad AG 501-X8, 20-50 mesh) for every 10 mL of formamide. Filter the preparation through Whatman No. 1 paper and store 50-mL aliquots in the dark at –20°C. NOTE: Prepare this solution in a chemical fume hood. Wear adequate protection.

4. 100× Denhardt's solution: Mix 2 g each of Ficoll 400, polyvinyl pyrollidone (average mol wt 360,000) and bovine serum albumin (Pentax Fraction V) in 100 mL of water. Complete solubilization will take a few hours. Store 5-mL vols at –20°C.

5. 50% Dextran sulfate: Dissolve 50 g of dextran sulfate (mol wt 500,000; Pharmacia) in 100 mL of water. Low heat will assist the solubilization process. Do not autoclave or attempt to filter the preparation. Add sodium azide (0.2% [w/v] final concentration) to inhibit microbial growth and store at room temperature.

6. 10% Blotto: Suspend 10 g of nonfat dried milk powder (available at any health-food store) in 100 mL of sterile water. Add sodium azide (0.2% [w/v] final concentration) to inhibit microbial growth, and store at room temperature.

7. Nonhomologous DNA: Commercial preparations of lyophylized salmon- or herring-sperm DNA should be purified, sheared, and denatured before use. DNA (1 g) is allowed to dissolve in 100 mL of autoclaved water overnight at 4°C on a rocking platform. The solution is then sonicated on ice for 5 min, boiled for 15 min, and quenched in ice water. The preparation is then extracted once with Tris-HCl buffered phenol/ chloroform (1:1) and once with chloroform/isoamyl alcohol (24:1). The DNA is recovered by ethanol precipitation and redissolved at a final concentration of 10 mg/mL in sterile 10 mM Tris-HCl, 1 mM CDTA (pH 8.0). Store 1-mL vols at –20°C in sterile microcentrifuge tubes.

8. Prehybridization solution (adequate for a 180-cm^2 membrane): 4.7× SSPE (3.5 mL of 20× stock), 4.7× Denhardt's solution (0.7 mL of 100× stock), 0.1% SDS (0.15 mL of 10% stock), 186 µg/mL denatured nonhomologous DNA (0.28 mL of 10 mg/mL stock), 0.33% Blotto (0.5 mL of 10% stock), 46.6% deionized formamide (7 mL), and sterile water (2.87 mL).

   Since SDS will precipitate in the presence of high salt, it should be added last. Denature the nonhomologous DNA by boiling for 10 min, and then quench in ice water before adding to the prehybridization solution. Warm the prehybridization solution to 42°C just before use.

9. Hybridization solution (adequate for a 180-cm^2 membrane): 4.7× SSPE

(3.5 mL of 20× stock), 4.7× Denhardt's solution (0.7 mL of 100× stock), 0.1% SDS (0.15 mL of 10% stock), 186 µg/mL denatured nonhomologous DNA (0.28 mL of 10 mg/mL stock), 0.33% Blotto (0.5 mL of 10% stock), 46.6% deionized formamide 7 mL, 7.5% dextran sulfate (2.25 mL of 50% stock), and finally ^{32}P-labeled DNA probe up to 0.62 mL (~2 × 10^7 cpm). Nonhomologous DNA and radiolabeled probe must be heat-denatured before incorporation to the hybridization mixture. Warm the hybridization solution to 42°C just before use.

3. Methods

3.1. Rapid Isolation
of High-Molecular-Weight Genomic DNA

1. Dislodge adherent cells from the bottom of the culture vessel(s) by gentle trypsinization, as follows: Rinse the cell monolayers twice with warm calcium/magnesium-free PBS. Add warm (37°C) dilute (0.25%) trypsin to the dishes (1 mL/100-mm-diam. dish or 2 mL/150-mm-diam. dish), and distribute the solution evenly over the cells by swirling the plates. Remove excess trypsin solution by aspiration and place the dishes in the CO_2 incubator for 1–3 min. View the dishes using a phase-contrast microscope to determine the extent of trypsinization (i.e., the majority of cells should have adopted a slightly rounded morphology when ready). Dislodge the cells from the bottom of the dishes by "bumping" the latter several times against the base of the microscope. Collect the cells in cold growth medium and pellet the material by low-speed centrifigation (200*g* for 3 min at 4°C). Pool up to 10^7 cells in a single 15-mL conical cell-culture tube, and wash the pellet twice using ice-cold PBS. Process the samples immediately or store the material at –70°C. NOTE: Alternatively, adherent cells may be harvested in cold PBS (2 mL/100-mm-diam. dish or 4 mL/150-mm-diam. dish) by scraping with a rubber policeman.

2. Resuspend the cells in 0.1 mL of PBS. REX buffer containing 100 µg/mL of RNAse A and 100 U/mL RNAse T1 is warmed to 55°C and added to the sample. A 5-mL vol is convenient and adequate for up to 10^7 cells. Mix by inversion and incubate for 2 h at 55°C. The efficiency of RNAse digestion will be greatest if the sample is mixed by inversion periodically during the incubation period.

3. Add proteinase K to a final concentration of 125 µg/mL. Ensure that the enzyme is well incorporated into the lysate by inverting the tube several times. Incubate for 2 h at 55°C. Invert the tube periodically to increase the efficiency of digestion.

4. Decant the lysate carefully into a sterile 15-mL round-bottom Corex® tube. Alternatively, disposable polypropylene culture tubes (17× 100 mm) can be used. Extract the lysate once with REX phenol, twice with REX phenol/chloroform (1:1), and once with chloroform/isoamyl alcohol (24:1). Separate the aqueous from the phenolic phase by centrifugation at 5000*g* for 5 min using a Sorvall HB-4 rotor (or its equivalent). Following each extraction, transfer the upper aqueous phase (which contains the DNA) to a new tube using sterile plastic pipet micropipet 1 mL that have been truncated approx 3 mm from the tip. The larger bore diameter will reduce the risk of shearing high-mol-wt genomic DNA. Take care not to collect proteinaceous material from the interphase.

5. Transfer the last aqueous layer to a sterile 30-mL Corex® tube. Add 1/ 10 vol of 2.5*M* sodium acetate, pH 5.5, and precipitate the DNA with 2 vol of chilled (–20°C) ethanol for 30–60 min at –70°C. Collect the DNA by centrifugation at 10,000*g* for 10 min (4°C) using a Sorvall HB-4 rotor (or its equivalent).

6. Dissolve the pellet in 5 mL of Acetate-MOPS (DO NOT VORTEX) and add 10 mL of chilled ethanol. Collect the DNA by centrifugation and dry the material briefly under vacuum. Alternatively, the samples can be air-dried for several minutes at room temperature. NOTE: Overdrying genomic DNA will make it very difficult to resuspend. Allow the DNA to redissolve overnight at 4°C in 0.5–1 mL of sterile Tris-CDTA (*see* Note 1). Determine the concentration of the sample using a spectrophotometer (assume 1.0 OD$_{260}$ unit to correspond to a concentration of 50 µg genomic DNA/mL), and verify the integrity of the sample by agarose gel electrophoresis. A single band of very high mol wt DNA (i.e., >60 kb) should be obtained. Store the DNA samples at 4°C under aseptic conditions.

3.2. Southern Transfer Under Alkaline Conditions

1. Cleave 5–10 µg of genomic DNA with a single restriction enzyme or enzyme combination chosen to produce size fragments of unit length for the transfected gene. It is often advantageous not to include vector sequences. Perform the digestion in a total reaction vol of 50–65 µL according to the enzyme supplier's recommendations with the following modifications: Use a two- to threefold excess of enzyme, and increase the efficiency of digestion by adding spermidine (4 m*M* final concentration) to the mixture. Incubate the sample overnight. Stop the reaction with 1/10 vol of 10× gel loading buffer.

2. Fractionate the DNA digest by electrophoresis through a 0.8% agarose

gel (11× 14× 0.6 cm prepared in 1× TPE). For highest resolution, run
the gel at low voltage (0.7 V/cm in 1× TPE) overnight. Size standards of
linearized DNA (i.e., λ phage DNA HindIII fragments or BRL's 1-kb linear DNA ladder markers) should be run on one of the outside lanes.

3. Following electrophoresis, stain the gel for 10 min in ethidium bromide
   (1 µg/mL) (*see* Note 2). Set the gel on a transilluminator providing long-
   wave (302 nm) UV light and place a clear plastic ruler backed with mask-
   ing tape on the side of the gel. When exposed to the UV light, the tape
   will fluoresce and highlight the graduations on the ruler. Photograph
   the gel using Polaroid™ type 665 P/N film (20-s exposure for a Polaroid™
   MP-4 industrial camera equipped with a 135-mm lens and a Kodak™
   Wratten No. 9—yellow—gelatin filter).

4. Soak the gel for no more than 10 min in 0.25*N* HCl to depurinate the
   DNA. This will increase the efficiency of transfer for DNA fragments >8
   kb in length.

5. Rinse the gel with distilled water to remove excess acid. Soak the gel in
   10 m*M* Tris-HCl, pH 8.0, while setting up the capillary blotting apparatus. The configuration of this system is presented in Fig. 1.

6. Wearing latex gloves, assemble the capillary blotting system as follows:
   Rest a clean glass plate on four rubber stoppers (No. 8) at the bottom of
   a rectangular plastic or glass dish. Place two sheets of Whatman 3MM
   filter chromatography paper (cut to exceed the length of the plate by 5
   cm at each end) over the plate and saturate the paper "wick" with 0.4*N*
   NaOH. Roll a pipet over the surface to squeeze out air bubbles. Fill the
   container with 0.4*N* NaOH until the liquid reaches a level approx 1 cm
   below the plate supporting the wick. Remove the gel from the Tris buffer
   and carefully flip it over in such a manner that the bottoms of the wells
   are now facing up. Since DNA migrates along the bottoms of the lanes,
   this maneuver will increase the speed and efficiency of transfer to the
   membrane and minimize diffusion. Center the gel on the wick and use
   a pipet to remove any air bubbles. Surround the gel with strips of
   Parafilm™ or plastic food wrap so that any exposed area of the wick is
   covered. Cut a sheet of BioTrace RP charge-modified nylon membrane
   (Gelman Sciences) leaving 1-cm margins in excess of the gel dimensions. Wet the membrane briefly in distilled water and center it carefully
   over the gel. Place a single sheet of Whatman 3MM paper (cut slightly
   larger than the membrane) over the membrane and roll a pipet over the
   surface to establish tight contact between the nylon sheet and the paper
   and to remove any trapped air. Place two additional sheets of Whatman
   3MM paper over the top and add a generous supply (i.e., a 20-cm stack)

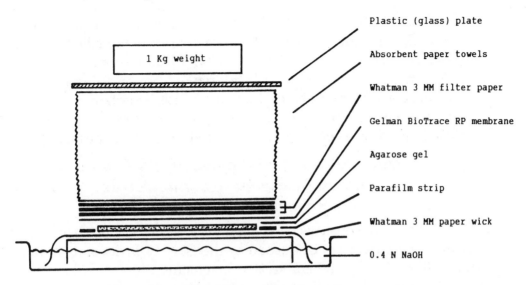

Fig. 1. Assembly of the capillary transfer apparatus.

of absorbent paper towels. Secure the stack under a glass (or plastic) plate and press a 1-kg weight (i.e., a 1-L Erlenmeyer flask filled with water) on the top.

7. Change the paper towels frequently (i.e., every 30 min) during the first 2–3 h. Transfer is usually complete within 8 h.

8. Following transfer, carefully remove the paper towels and filter paper sheets. Mark the orientation of the gel and the position of the wells with a soft (HB) lead pencil.

9. Carefully peel the membrane off the gel (*see* Note 3). Remove traces of agarose and alkali by soaking in 500 mL of 0.1× SSC/0.1% SDS warmed to 42°C. Change the solution 2–3 times during 1 h. Blot the membrane between two sheets of Whatman 3MM paper to remove excess liquid. Membranes may be air-dried and stored in heat-sealed plastic bags at this stage.

10. Alternatively large number of DNA samples can be processed simultaneously using a slot- or dot-blot filtration manifold. Assemble the apparatus according to the manufacturer's instructions and connect the manifold to a vacuum line. Wet the BioTrace RP membrane by applying between 250 and 500 µL of distilled water to each well under low to moderate suction. Using 10N NaOH, bring each genomic DNA sample to 0.4N NaOH and hold at room temperature for 5–10 min. Apply the samples to the wells under moderate suction (i.e., the liquid should be aspirated through the membrane in 10–15 s) in several loadings if nec-

essary. Load 500 µL of 0.4 *N* NaOH in each well to ensure fixation of the DNA to the nylon matrix. Turn off the vacuum, dismantle the apparatus and soak the blot in 250 mL of 0.1× SSC/0.1% SDS at room temperature for 30 min before processing for hybridization. For an accurate quantitation of gene copy number, calibrate the blot as described in the Notes Section (*see* Note 10). The DNA sequence employed for calibration should be linearized before being denatured and fixed to the membrane.

3.3. Preparation of ^{32}P-Labeled DNA Probes by Random Hexadeoxyribonucleotide Primer Synthesis

1. Cleave the vector construct containing the cloned sequence from which probe fragments are to be derived by choosing a restriction enzyme(s) that will produce unambiguous DNA fragments.
2. Add 1/10 vol of 10× TAE sample buffer and load between 2 and 5 µg of total digested DNA in each lane of a 0.8% low-melting-point agarose gel (11× 14× 0.5 cm prepared in 1× TAE). NOTE: Pour this gel at 4°C. Separate the restriction fragments by overnight electrophoresis at 4°C under low voltage (0.7 V/cm) using 1× TAE as the running buffer (*see* Notes 4 and 5).
3. Following electrophoresis, stain the gel for 10 min in ethidium bromide (1 µg/mL). Rinse the gel for 10 min in distilled water. View the restriction fragments under medium-wave (302-nm) UV light and excise the bands of interest with a scalpel. Take care to trim away any excess agarose from the slices. CAUTION: UV light is a strong mutagen. Wear a face shield and cover your forearms and hands.
4. Transfer the gel slices to a preweighed sterile polypropylene test tube (17 × 100 mm). Weigh the tube again and add 1.5 mL of sterile water for each gram of agarose. Boil the material for 10 min and dispense 32.5-µL vols (equivalent to 25–45 ng of probe DNA) in sterile 1.5-mL microcentrifuge tubes. DNA probe samples may be processed immediately or stored at –20°C. Frozen samples should be boiled for 10 min before use.
5. Place the boiled probe sample in a 37°C water bath for 30 min. Add to the tube, in sequence, 10 µL of ABC labeling mix, 2 µL of BSA (10 mg/mL), 5 µL of [α^{32}P]dCTP (800 Ci/mmol) and 2 U of FPLC pure Klenow enzyme. The final vol should be 50 µL. Incubate at 37°C for 5 h. Add another 5 U of Klenow enzyme and prolong the incubation for a further 12 h. Stop the reaction by adding 200 µL of column buffer and heat the mixture at 55°C for 15 min. This will dilute the agarose and free the

radiolabeled probe from the agarose matrix. Hold the sample at 55°C until ready to load on the Sephadex G5O column (*see below*).

6. Load the mixture on a 0.9 × 30 cm Sephadex G5O Medium column (BioRad Econo Column). Set up a continuous flow of column buffer through the column and collect ~0.2 mL fractions in sterile 1.5-mL microcentrifuge tubes. Monitor the radioactivity by Cerenkov emission. The peak of radiolabeled DNA should emerge between fractions 8 and 12, whereas unincorporated $[\alpha^{32}P]dCTP$ will be eluted beyond fraction 15. Store the probe at 4°C in a lead pig or an acrylic box designated for this purpose.

3.4. Detection of Target DNA Sequences by Southern Hybridization

3.4.1. Prehybridization

1. If the blotted membrane was air-dried, wet it in 0.1× SSC/0.1% SDS for 10 min. Blot the membrane between two sheets of Whatman 3MM paper to remove excess liquid, but do not allow to dry out. Place the membrane in a 0.1-mm-thick polyethylene bag. If multiple blots are to be probed, place each membrane in a separate bag. Heat-seal the bag except for one corner, leaving a 1-cm margin between the edge of the membrane and the sides of the bag (*see* Notes 6 and 7).

2. Prepare the prehybridization solution as described in the Materials section. Remember to heat-denature the nonhomologous DNA before adding it to the mixture. Warm the solution to 42°C and add 0.08 mL/cm² membrane surface area. Gently squeeze out any air bubbles by rolling a pipet over the surface of the bag and heat-seal the corner.

3. Place the bag in a box of water resting in a shaking water bath equilibrated at 42°C. Set the bath to shake at a speed that will allow the prehybridization solution to sweep gently over the surface of the membrane. Incubate for 4–24 h.

4. Take the bag out of the water bath. Cut a corner of the bag and drain the prehybridization solution. Remove as much of the liquid as possible by rolling a pipet over the bag. Once again, take care not to let any area of the membrane dry out.

3.4.2. Hybridization

1. Prepare the hybridization solution as described in the Materials Section. Again, remember to heat-denature the nonhomologous DNA as well as the radiolabeled probe before adding them to the mixture. Warm the solution to 42°C and add 0.08 mL/cm² of membrane surface area.

Squeeze out any air bubbles and heat-seal the corner. Verify the seal by rolling a pipet over the bag.

2. Incubate the blot in the shaking water bath at 42°C for 24–36 h.

3.4.3. Washing

1. Cut one corner of the bag and drain the hybridization solution into a vessel for the disposal of the radioisotope or into a sterile polypropylene tube if the probe is to be reused (*see* Note 8).
2. Cut the bag open and transfer the membrane to a plastic box containing no less than 500 mL of 1× SSC/0.1% SDS at room temperature. Rinse the membrane with two changes of this solution over a 20-min period, with gentle shaking. Discard the liquid in a designated sink.
3. Wash the membrane at moderate stringency for 1 h with 3 changes of 1× SSC/0.1% SDS (500 mL each) at 60°C, with shaking.
4. Wash the membrane at high stringency for 1 h with 3 changes of 1× SSC/0.1% SDS (500 mL each) at 65°C, with shaking.
5. Rinse the membrane briefly in 1× SSC/0.1% SDS at room temperature. Blot between two sheets of Whatman 3MM paper to remove excess liquid, and seal the membrane in a new polyethylene bag. CAUTION: It is imperative that the blot not be allowed to dry out if it is to be reprobed.

3.4.4. Autoradiography

1. Place the blot in a film casset (Kodak or DuPont Cronex) and expose the membrane to Kodak XAR-5 X-ray film for 2–3 d at –70°C between intensifying screens (DuPont Cronex Lightning Plus). Combining Kodak T-MATH film with Kodak Lannex Fast screens will yield comparable results overnight (*see* Note 9).
2. Develop the autoradiogram according to the film supplier's recommendation. An automated film processor is very convenient.
3. Use a laser densitometer to obtain an accurate measurement of the relative band intensities on the autoradiogram (*see* Notes 10–12).

3.4.5. Stripping

1. Remove hybridized probe by submerging the blot in a plastic tray containing no less than 1 L of 0.1× SSC/0.1% SDS warmed to 100°C. Place the tray on a shaking platform and incubate at room temperature for 30 min. Repeat this procedure once.
2. Place the blot in fresh room-temperature 0.1× SSC/0.1% SDS and shake for another 30 min.
3. Monitor the efficiency of probe removal by autoradiography over a 5-d period. Repeat the procedure if necessary.

4. Keep the blot wet and store in a sealed plastic bag at 4 or –20°C for future use. Alkaline DNA blots will resist many cycles of stripping and reprobing without significant loss of immobilized DNA.

4. Notes

1. We recommend using Tris-CDTA for the storage of genomic DNA samples. CDTA posesses a higher chelating potential than EDTA and has a slight bacteriostatic effect.
2. By including ethidium bromide (0.5–1.0 µg/mL) in the running buffer, the subsequent staining of genomic DNA gels can be avoided. This time-saving technique should not, however, be adopted for the preparation of DNA probe fragments in low-melting-point agarose gels or for obtaining mol wt. The saturating amounts of ethidium bromide will reduce the efficiency of radiolabeling and produce significant band shifting during electrophoresis.
3. Covalent binding of DNA fragments to the charge-modified nylon matrix is extremely efficient in the presence of 0.4*N* NaOH. Do not attempt to increase binding by crosslinking with UV light or baking *in vacuo*. This will cause very high backgrounds during hybridization to radiolabeled probe.
4. Bromophenol blue and xylene cyanol will inhibit the random primer DNA synthesis reaction. Therefore, if probe DNA restriction fragments are expected to comigrate with either of these compounds on the low-melting-point agarose gel, these dyes should be omitted from the 10× TAE sample buffer.
5. We do not recommend the use of TPE or Tris-HCl borate buffers for the preparation of DNA probe fragments in low-melting-point agarose gels. Both of these buffer formulations make recovery of DNA from the gel matrix very difficult and may inhibit the random primer labeling reaction significantly.
6. Generally high background, "hot-spots," and faint areas of hybridization can be avoided by paying particular attention to the following:
   a. Ensure that residual alkali and agarose have been thoroughly removed from the membrane prior to prehybridization.
   b. Never allow membranes to dry out.
   c. Do not prehybridize membranes in the presence of dextran sulfate.
   d. When conducting hybridizations in the presence of dextran sulfate, keep the radiolabeled probe concentration ≤10 ng/mL

(for a high-specific-activity probe, i.e., $>10^8$ cpm/µg, this translates to 1 or 2×10^6 cpm/mL).

   e. Use sturdy polyethylene bags to prevent collapse.

   f. Never wash more than 5 blots at a time.

7. Southern hybridizations can be performed in 1/4-in.-thick acrylic boxes equipped with a hermetic lid. This provides protection against high levels of radiation, facilitates the handling of materials, and permits the processing of several blots (up to 6 in our experience) simultaneously. Optimally, the hybridization box should be constructed to allow 1-cm margins from the edges of the blots. Care should be taken to add blots sequentially to the prehybridization and hybridization solutions in order to prevent adhesions between membranes. Solution vols should be adjusted for the number and size of blots present. The boxes either can be accommodated by a shaking water bath or may be placed on a rocking platform in a dry incubator.

8. Hybridization solution can be reused. Because the mixture contains formamide, the probe can be denatured again by heating the solution for 30 min at 70°C.

9. Static electricity can ruin an autoradiogram. To circumvent the problem, seal the blots in polyethylene bags instead of using plastic food wrap, and wipe the intensifying screens with the antistatic cleaning fluid provided by the manufacturer before exposing the film. Allow film cassets to reach room temperature before removing and developing the film.

10. The relative intensities of the autoradiographic bands will reflect the number of foreign gene copies residing in the cell's genome. To facilitate their quantification, individual blots may be calibrated by running samples of genomic DNA from the nontransfected cell line supplemented with increasing amounts of the foreign gene sequence, which translate to, for example, 0, 1, 5, 10, 25 and 50 copies/diploid genome. The standards should be cleaved with the same restriction enzyme(s) used to digest the samples of genomic DNA under study. The calibration can be verified by stripping the blot and probing for a resident single copy gene.

11. An overexposed autoradiogram leads to qualitative estimates of target gene copy number as a result of the saturation of signal intensity. To avoid this common problem, obtain several exposures from the blots.

12. Probes bearing significant homology to vector sequences will hybridize strongly to most commercially available mol-wt markers. As a result, that particular area of the blot will emit a very intense signal. Since this will pose a problem for the detection of single or low-copy-number integration events, the marker DNA lane(s) should be removed before transfer

to the nylon membrane. However, a small amount of the markers (i.e., 500 pg to 1 ng) can be run and blotted, thus providing an internal mol-wt ladder of moderate to low intensity.

References

1. Meinkoth, J. and Wahl, G. (1988) Analytical strategies for the use of DNA probes. *Anal. Biochem.* **169,** 1–25.
2. Southern, E. N. (1975) Detection of specific sequences among DNA fragments separated by gel electrophoresis. *J. Mol. Biol.* **98,** 503–517.
3. Fourney, R. M., Dietrich, R. D., and Paterson, M. C. (1989) Rapid DNA extraction and sensitive alkaline blotting protocol: Application for detection of gene rearrangement and amplification for clinical molecular diagnosis. *Disease Markers* **7,** 15–26.
4. Reed, K. C. and Mann, D. A. (1985) Rapid transfer of DNA from agarose gels to nylon membranes. *Nucleic Acids Res.* **13,** 7207–7221.
5. Feinberg, A. B. and Vogelstein, B. (1983) A technique for radiolabelling DNA restriction endonuclease fragments to high specific activity. *Anal. Biochem.* **132,** 6–13.

CHAPTER 29

Evaluation of Extrachromosomal Gene Copy Number of Transiently Transfected Cell Lines

Angus C. Wilson and Roger K. Patient

1. Introduction

The short-term expression of DNA introduced into eukaryotic cells is now widely used to investigate the biological activities of cellular and viral genes or their products. A number of different transfection methods are in common use and can be broadly divided into two categories, based on the method by which DNA is introduced (either as a complex with a carrier substance that facilitates uptake by the cell [e.g., DEAE-dextran transfection *(1,2)*, calcium phosphate coprecipitation *(3)*, or lipofection *(4)*] or by direct exposure to the cytoplasm [e.g., electroporation *(5)*, microinjection *(6)* or scrapefection *(7)*]). In each case, transfected cells can maintain a considerable number of plasmids in their nuclei for several cell cycles. Plasmids lacking functional replication origins are lost progressively in subsequent mitoses. It appears that, for at least some transfection protocols, the majority of DNA that is taken up, remains circular and extrachromosomal, and is present as chromatin *(8,9,* and Wilson and Patient, unpublished).

Transient assays are particularly attractive because they are rapid and avoid the problems produced by differences in the site of integration, copy number, and potential DNA rearrangements. Some variation may occur,

From: *Methods in Molecular Biology, Vol. 7: Gene Transfer and Expression Protocols*
Edited by: E. J. Murray © 1991 The Humana Press Inc., Clifton, NJ

however, in the quantitative uptake of DNA by individual batches of cells, particularly with techniques such as calcium phosphate coprecipitation, and it is important to control for these when comparing the activity of different plasmids. Cotransfection with a second plasmid, the activity of which can be monitored along with that of the test plasmid, is advisable, but it may be influenced by experimental conditions. For example, in a study of a potent and highly promiscuous viral transactivator protein, both the test and the reporter gene may be significantly regulated. It can be useful, therefore, to control for experimental variation by monitoring the number and form of transfected templates.

This chapter describes two relatively simple protocols to recover and analyze input DNA. The first, based on the method devised by Hirt *(10)*, is extremely rapid and is ideal for the DNA analysis of a large number of transfections. Once the cells are lysed and genomic DNA allowed to precipitate, samples can be stored for many months. This means that DNA can be collected routinely with little effort and analyzed at leisure if desired. The second method specifically recovers DNA within (or tightly associated with) the nucleus. Treatment of nuclei prepared by this protocol with nucleases such as DNase I, micrococcal nuclease, or restriction enzymes, also allows analysis of the chromatin structure of the transfected templates *(see* refs. *8,9,* for further details).

2. Materials

1. Phosphate-buffered saline: Store at 4°C (does not need to be sterile).
2. Hirt lysis buffer: 0.6% SDS, 10 mM EDTA.
3. Glycerol TKM: 50% glycerol, 50 mM Tris-HCl (pH 7.9), 100 mM KCl, 5 mM MgCl$_2$. Store at 4°C.
4. 10% Saponin: Filter-sterilize and store at 4°C.
5. Phenol: Saturate in 1 M Tris-HCl (pH 8.0), add 8-hydroxyquinoline (to 0.1%), and equilibrate with several changes of TE. Store in dark at 4°C for up to 2 mo or at –20°C for up to 1 yr. Phenol/chloroform is made at a concentration of 1:1 v/v.
6. TE: 10 mM Tris-HCl (pH 8.0), 1 mM EDTA.
7. Buffer A: 100 mM NaCl, 50 mM Tris-HCl (pH 8.0), 3 mM MgCl$_2$, 0.1 mM PMSF. Store at 4°C.
8. 10× Proteinase K/SDS: 500 µg/mL proteinase K, 0.5% SDS. Store as aliquots at –20°C.
9. 5 M NaCl.
10. Ethanol.

3. Method

3.1. Recovery of Transfected DNA (see Note 1)

3.1.1. Hirt Extraction

1. Transfer the cells into a disposable 13-mL polystyrene tube in 10 mL of culture medium. Adherent cells should be resuspended by gently scraping the flask bottom using a disposable cell scraper. Keep the cells on ice from this point. Pellet by centrifugation for 3–5 min at 1000–1500 rpm in a bench-top centrifuge at room temperature. Pour off the medium and, by vortexing, resuspend the cell pellet in the liquid clinging to the tube. Add 5 mL of ice-cold phosphate buffered saline (PBS) and repellet the cells. Resuspend once more in 1 mL of PBS and transfer to a 1.5-mL microcentrifuge tube. At this point, all the cells may be used for DNA analysis, or, if only a fraction is used, the rest may be retained for different assays, such as that for the transfected genes' products. Routinely $1–2.5 \times 10^5$ cells with a reasonable efficiency of transfection will give an adequate recovery of plasmid. The quantities described below, however, are satisfactory for the preparation of up to 1×10^6 cells, and allow all clean-up steps to be performed in the same tube. If larger numbers of cells are to be analyzed, then the vol should be increased proportionally and the sample split before ethanol precipitation (step 8).

2. Repellet the cells by centrifugation at 10,000–13,000 rpm for 20–30 s in a microcentrifuge and remove the PBS. Resuspend in the liquid trapped on the tube walls by thorough vortexing (*see* Note 2) and lyse the cells by adding 0.25 mL of Hirt lysis buffer. DO NOT PIPET OR VORTEX ONCE CELLS ARE LYSED. Incubate at room temperature (15–25°C) for 15 min.

3. Precipitate genomic DNA and cellular debris by adding 0.1 mL of $5M$ NaCl (approx $1.4M$ final concentration). Mix by gentle inversion (5– 10 times) and store at 4°C. Typically, genomic DNA is allowed to precipitate overnight, but it can usually be removed after 4 h or more.

4. Pellet genomic DNA and cell debris by centrifuging at 10,000–13,000 rpm for 10 min in a microfuge. If possible, this is best done at 4°C. Transfer the supernatant to a fresh tube, taking care not to disturb the pellet, which may not be tightly packed at the tube bottom. Alternatively, slide the genomic DNA out of the tube using a pipet tip. This may be necessary if a large number of cells have been used.

5. Add an equal vol of phenol (saturated in $1M$ Tris-HCl (pH 8.0) and equilibrated in TE), vortex, and separate the phases by centrifugation for 4 min (*see* Note 3).

6. Remove most of the phenol layer and repeat the extraction with an equal vol of phenol:chloroform (1:1).

7. Remove the organic layer and extract with an equal vol of chloroform.

8. Remove the chloroform and add 2.5 vol of prechilled (−20°C) ethanol, mix by vortexing, and allow DNA to precipitate for at least 10 min at −20°C. Samples can be stored in this form at −20°C for many months.

9. Pellet DNA by centrifugation at 10,000–13,000 rpm for 10–15 min, remove the supernatant, and wash the pellet (which should be fairly small) by vortexing in 70% ethanol. Centrifuge for 3–4 min and remove the supernatant. Dry the DNA pellet thoroughly in a vacuum desiccator before resuspending in 20 µL of TE. The DNA is now ready to be digested with restriction enzymes or size-fractionated directly.

3.1.2. Nuclei Prep by Gentle Lysis (see Note 4)

1. Collect and wash the cells as described in Section 3.1.1., step 1. Resuspend the cell pellet in 0.72 mL of ice-cold glycerol TKM lysis buffer mixed to 0.05% saponin (i.e., 5 µL of 10% saponin/mL of glycerol TKM). Mix by vortexing briefly and incubate on ice for 10 min. It may be worthwhile, particularly with a new cell type, to check that lysis has occurred. This is done by taking a very small aliquot and looking for nuclei, using a light microscope.

2. Pellet the nuclei by centrifugation for 45 s in a microcentrifuge, remove the supernatant, and resuspend by gently flicking the end of the tube (*see* Note 2). Nuclei should resuspend more readily than unlysed cells. Add 0.3 mL of ice-cold buffer A, mix, and repellet.

3. Resuspend the nuclei in 18 µL of buffer A and 2 µL of 10× proteinase K/SDS mix, and incubate overnight at 37°C.

4. Add 30 µL of 3*M* sodium acetate (pH 5.5) followed by 250 µL of TE. Then phenol-extract and precipitate DNA as described in Section 3.1.1., steps 5–8 (*see* Note 5).

3.2. DNA Analysis by Size Fractionation

Uncut or restricted samples can be seen by agarose gel electophoresis and, if necessary, transferred to nitrocellulose and hybridized to a specific radioactively labeled probe. Methods for running agarose slab gels and Southern blotting are very adequately covered elsewhere (e.g., *11,12; see also* Volumes 2 and 4, this series). An advantage of Hirt extraction (Section 3.1.1.) is that the background of contaminating genomic DNA is often so low that high-copy-number plasmids can be seen directly by staining the gel with ethidium bromide (1 µg/mL) and viewing under UV light. With Method 3.1.2., plasmids cannot be distinguished against the background smear of genomic DNA, and therefore they must be detected by hybridization to a labeled probe.

To obtain estimates of the number of plasmids recovered, it is usual to run reference samples of plasmid on the same gel. Suitable quantities might be in the range of 10 pg to 5ng. Note that plasmid dilutions should be made fresh since, in very dilute samples, significant amounts of DNA tend to stick to the sides of tubes and are consequently lost. Important limitations of this quantification method, however, are the accuracy of the control plasmid dilutions and the loading of the test samples. If precise estimates are required, then Method 3.1.2. is preferable to Method 3.1.1., because a comparison of the "smears" of digested genomic DNA is a good guide to whether equal numbers of cells are being compared. If necessary, it also is possible to probe for a single-copy host-cell gene. An alternative to using plasmid controls is loading different amounts of digested genomic DNA containing endogenous copies of the gene used in the transfection.

The hybridization reaction should be in large probe excess and autoradiographic film should be preflashed to ensure a linear reponse (*see* Note 6). The intensity of the bands on the resulting autoradiograph should be quantified by scanning densitometry of a variety of exposures of the film to ensure that exposure time is in the linear range.

There are a number of factors to consider when choosing whether or not to digest samples and if so, with which enzymes. The topological state of transfected DNA has a major influence on the level of gene expression *(13,14)*. For example, the SV40 early transcription unit is 50- to 200-fold more active on supercoiled than on linearized templates when transfected into CV-1 cells *(14)*. If the relative levels of expression of different plasmids are to be compared, then it is particularly important to correct for differences in the number of supercoiled molecules, which make up the bulk of the active population. Therefore, samples either should not be digested or, if Method 3.1.2. is used, should be digested with an enzyme that does not cut within the test plasmid (to reduce the size of high-mol-wt host genomic DNA fragments). Electrophoresis should also be carried out in the absence of ethidium bromide to best resolve supercoiled molecules from those with other topologies. For further detailed information on identification of the various topoisomers, *see* ref. *15.*

Choice of the probe for Southern blotting will depend on the particular experiment. If mixtures of several plasmids were transfected, then it may be preferable to probe with sequences that hybridize to only one particular species, hence reducing the complexity of the autoradiograph. Alternatively, if the probe contains only sequences represented equally in all the plasmids, then all templates can be monitored simultaneously. If the transfected gene is present as a host genomic copy as well, then it may be useful to choose an enzyme that will produce fragments containing homologous sequences, but of different sizes. For example, use of an enzyme that recognizes a site in the vector sequences will probably generate a fragment size different from that produced by sites flanking the endogenous genomic copy.

4. Notes

1. Both methods described here efficiently recover minichromosomal DNA from transfected vertebrate cell lines and primary cells. If the transfection efficiency is reasonably high, then only a small number of cells (e.g., 1–2.5×10^5) need to be used, leaving the rest for other forms of analysis. Conversely, the removal of genomic DNA in Method 3.1.1. allows Southern blotting of material collected from a considerable number of cells (e.g., 5×10^7 and 1×10^8). This is useful if very low levels of transfection are to be detected.

2. Inaccurate quantitation will arise for both approaches if there is incomplete cell lysis. In the case of Method 3.1.1., this is most often caused by inadequate resuspension of the cell pellet. If this occurs, then the pellet should be disrupted further using a pipet tip, although more contaminating genomic DNA will be recovered than usual. Likewise, for Method 3.1.2., near-complete lysis is desirable, and difficulty in resuspending the pellet at step 2 usually indicates the presence of many intact cells. If cells fail to lyse after 15 min, then additional saponin should be added. When working with an unfamiliar cell line, the appropriate saponin concentration needed to lyse nearly 100% of cells within 10 min on ice should be established empirically.

3. The organic extraction steps separate protein and carbohydrates from the nucleic acids. If large numbers of cells are used, then a thick boundary layer may form at the interface. Some plasmid DNA will be withheld in this layer; it is advisable to pool the phenol and phenol:chloroform phases and to back-extract them with a small vol (e.g., 100 µL) of TE. Similarly, the pellet of genomic DNA formed in Hirt extraction is known to trap some plasmid DNA (15–20% of total), though this proportion appears relatively constant between different cell types and, presumably, between preparations from different batches of the same cells *(16)*.

4. It is sometimes important to know from where in the cell transfected DNA is being recovered. Method 3.1.2. first isolates nuclei and thereby reduces the likelihood of detecting templates derived from cytoplasmic compartments. The presence of supercoiled molecules or, better still, templates in chromatin argues further for nuclear localization. A further possibility is that plasmids are bound to the cell exterior (particularly if transfected using polyanionic carriers, such as DEAE-dextran), and may never actually become internalized. To exclude this possibility, washed cells can be treated with DNase I before lysis (i.e., at step 1 of Method 3.1.2.). However, it appears that, within the first 22 h extracellular DNA is naturally degraded, presumably by nucleases present in the medium *(16)*.

5. Because total genomic DNA is recovered by this method, before gel electrophoresis it must be fragmented by either restriction enzyme digestion or sonication.

6. Flashing the film sensitizes it to low intensities of light, making it more linear *(17)*. Use an ordinary camera flash unit with a heavy white paper filter (e.g., Whatman 3MM). Flashing is done in total darkness with the film held flat against the wall with the thumb of one hand and the flash gun held in the other hand at a measured distance from the wall. Full arm span is usually about the right distance, but distance and number of filter layers should be adjusted to yield a developed fogged film of approx 0.15 A_{540}.

References

1. McCutchan, J. H. and Pagano, J. S. (1968) Enhancement of the infectivity of simian virus 40 deoxyribonucleic acid with diethyl-amino-ethyl-dextran. *J. Natl. Cancer Inst.* **41**, 351–356.

2. Lopata, M., Cleveland, D., and Sollner-Webb, B. (1984) High level transient expression of chloramphenicol acetyl transferase gene by DEAE-dextran mediated DNA transfection coupled with a dimethyl sulfoxide or glycerol shock treatment. *Nucleic Acids Res.* **2**, 5707–5717.

3. Graham, F. L. and van der Eb, A. J. (1973) A new technique for the assay of infectivity of human adenovirus 5 DNA. *Virology* **52**, 456–467.

4. Fraley, R., Subramani, P., Berg, P., and Papahadjopoulos, P. (1980) Introduction of liposome-encapsulated SV40 DNA into cells. *J. Biol. Chem.* **255**, 10431–10435.

5. Andreason, G. L. and Evans, G. A. (1988) Introduction and expression of DNA molecules in eukaryotic cells by electroporation. *BioTechniques* **6**, 650–660.

6. Capecchi, M. R. (1980) High efficiency transformation by direct microinjection of DNA into cultured mammalian cells. *Cell* **22**, 479–488.

7. Wilson, A. C. and Patient, R. K. Scrapefection—A rapid and simple method for transfecting adherent cells. Manuscript in prep.

8. Enver, T., Brewer, A. C., and Patient, R. K. (1985) Simian virus 40-mediated *cis* induction of the *Xenopus* β globin DNase I hypersensitive site. *Nature* **318**, 680–683.

9. Brewer, A. C., Enver, T., Greaves, D. R., Allan, J., and Patient, R. K. (1988) 5' structural motifs and *Xenopus* β globin gene activation. *J. Mol. Biol.* **199**, 575–585.

10. Hirt, B. (1967) Selective extraction of polyoma DNA from transfected mouse cell cultures. *J. Mol. Biol.* **26**, 365–369.

11. Ogden, R. C. and Adams, D. A. (1987) Electrophoresis in agarose and acrylamide gels, in *Methods in Enzymology*, vol. 152 (Berger, S. L. and Kimmel, A. R., eds.), Academic, New York, London, 61–90.

12. Wahl, G. M., Meinkoth, J. L., and Kimmel, A. R. (1987) Northern and Southern Blots, in *Methods in Enzymology*, vol. 152 (Berger, S. L. and Kimmel, A. R., eds.), Academic New York, London, 61–90.

13. Lehman, A. R. and Oomen, A. (1985) Effect of DNA damage on the expression of CAT after transfection. *Nucleic Acids Res.* **13**, 2087–2095.

14. Weintraub, H., Cheng, P. F., and Conrad, K. (1986) Expression of transfected DNA depends on DNA topology. *Cell* **46**, 115–122.

15. Shure, M., Pulleybank, D. E., and Vinograd, J. (1977) The problems of eukaryotic and prokaryotic DNA packaging and *in vivo* conformation posed by superhelix density heterogeneity. *Nucleic Acids Res.* **4,** 1183–1205.
16. Alwine, J. C. (1985) Transient gene expression control: Effects of transfected DNA stability and *trans*-activation by viral early proteins. *Mol. Cell. Biol.* **5,** 1034–1042.
17. Laskey, R. A. and Mills, A. D. (1975) Quantitative film detection of ^{3}H and ^{14}C in polyacrylamide gels by fluorography. *Eur. J. Biochem.* **56,** 335–341.

CHAPTER 30

Use of Dpn I Restriction Enzyme to Assess Newly Replicated Gene Copies in Amplifiable Vector Systems

Alison C. Brewer and Roger K. Patient

1. Introduction

Bacterially propagated plasmid DNA can be transfected into established eukaryotic cell lines or primary cell cultures by a variety of techniques, such as electroporation *(see* Chapter 5, this vol) *(1)*, scrape-loading *(2)*, and DEAE dextran *(see* Chapter 3) or calcium phosphate mediated gene transfer *(see* Chapter 2) *(3–5)*. At least some of the DNA introduced into the cells enters into the nucleus, where it is thought to be assembled into chromatin *(6)*, and is maintained extrachromosomally for at least 48 h. During this time, the cellular chromosomal DNA may have undergone one or more rounds of DNA replication. However, the extrachromosomal transfected DNA will not replicate unless the DNA sequences contained in the plasmid include a DNA origin of replication recognized by the host cell.

Origin sequences have so far proved difficult to identify in eukaryotic chromosomes. In contrast, viral genomes, such as SV40 and polyoma, have well-characterized origins of replication *(7)*, which, when included on DNA

From: *Methods in Molecular Biology, Vol. 7: Gene Transfer and Expression Protocols*
Edited by: E. J. Murray © 1991 The Humana Press Inc., Clifton, NJ

constructs used in transient transfection experiments, will direct replication on extrachromosomal DNA copies in the appropriate cellular environment.

It is often useful to assess whether replication has occurred in a transient transfection experiment and/or to quantify the extent of that replication. This information is important if replication affects gene expression *(8)* and can provide convincing evidence of successful transfection. Replication can be readily monitored using the methylation-sensitive restriction enzyme Dpn I.

Dpn I will digest only DNA that is bacterially methylated on both strands. Most strains of *E. coli* used to propagate plasmid DNA contain a site-specific methylase encoded by the dam gene that transfers a methyl group to the N7 position of the adenine residues in the sequence 5' GATC 3'. 5' GATC 3' is the recognition sequence of the Dpn I restriction enzyme and, provided the DNA to be used in the transfection experiment has been grown up in a dam⁺ bacterial strain, all the 5' GATC 3' sites will be fully A-methylated and will therefore all be digestible with Dpn I.

Eukaryotic cells lack these A methylation enzymes. Thus, if the transfected DNA copies undergo one or more rounds of replication, they will become first hemi- and then unmethylated at the A residues and so refractory to digestion by Dpn I. Digestion of transiently transfected DNA by Dpn I can therefore be used to quantitate replication in an amplifiable vector system.

2. Materials

1. Phosphate-buffered saline (PBS, Flow): Store and use at 4°C.
2. Glycerol TKM: 50% Glycerol, 50 mM Tris-HCl pH 7.9, 100 mM KCl, 5 mM MgCl$_2$. To ensure ice temperature, this should be stored at 4°C and incubated on ice for 30 min prior to use.
3. 10% saponin: Filter-sterilize and store at 4°C.
4. Lysis buffer is glycerol TKM containing 0.05% saponin, which is added just prior to use.
5. Buffer A: 100 mM NaCl, 50 mM Tris-HCl (pH 8.0), 3 mM MgCl$_2$. Store and use at 4°C.
6. 250 mM EDTA, pH 8.0. Stored at room temperature.
7. Proteinase K at 1 mg/mL in H$_2$O. Store at –20°C.
8. 10% SDS. Store at room temperature.
9. Phenol that has been equilibrated three times with 50 mM Tris-HCl, pH 8.0; 1 mM EDTA. Phenol/chloroform is made 1:1 v/v.
10. Restriction enzyme Dpn I. Available from many companies, but we have generally purchased it from BCL.
11. 10× Dpn I buffer. Made up to manufacturer's specifications and stored at –20°C in 1-mL aliquots.

12. 1 mg/mL BSA, made up in sterile H_2O and stored in 1-mL aliquots at –20°C.
13. TE: 10 mM Tris-HCl, pH 8.0, 1 mM EDTA. Store at 4°C.

3. Method

3.1. Isolation of Nuclei and Purification of Total Nuclear DNA (see Note 1)

1. Remove the medium from the cell culture. If the cells are growing on the surface of a flask or Petri dish, this can be done by simply pipeting away the medium. For cells growing in suspension however, the culture must first be spun down and the excess medium poured off. In a typical experiment, 5×10^6–10^7 cells are usually processed (*see* Note 2).
2. Wash the cells in 10 mL of PBS. Adherent cells can be washed in their dishes. Suspension cultures will be in the form of a pellet at this point. Disperse the pellet by gently flicking before adding the PBS. This will ensure that the cells resuspend evenly and do not clump together.
3. Harvest adherent cells by scraping off the surface of the flask or Petri dish with a disposable cell scraper. Centrifuge PBS-washed cells at 2500 rpm in a bench-top centrifuge at 4°C for 5 min.
4. Carefully pipet off excess PBS and disperse the pellet by gentle flicking before resuspending the pellet in 720 μL of ice-cold lysis buffer. Tap gently to ensure mixing.
5. Incubate on ice for 7 min (*see* Note 3).
6. Transfer to an Eppendorf tube, and spin for 15 min at 5500 rpm in a Sorvall HB4 rotor at –4°C (*see* Note 4).
7. Remove the supernatant. The nuclei should form a milky white pellet, which must be dispersed by flicking, before resuspension in 1 mL buffer A at 4°C.
8. Invert the tube several times to ensure even washing of nuclei. Spin for 5 min at 3000 rpm in a Sorvall HB4 rotor at 4°C.
9. Remove the supernatant. Disperse the pellet and resuspend it in 100 μL of buffer A (*see* Note 5). Add 5 μL of 250 mM EDTA. This will immediately inactivate all Mg^{2+}- and Ca^{2+}- dependent nucleases.
10. Add proteinase K to a final concentration of 50 μg/mL and SDS to 0.25%.
11. Incubate at 37°C overnight (*see* Note 6), then add 200 μL TE.
12. Extract once with phenol, twice with phenol/chloroform (1:1 v/v), and twice with chloroform (*see* Note 7).
13. Add sodium acetate to a concentration of 0.3M and 2.5 vol of ethanol. Mix well by inverting tube several times.
14. Precipitate the DNA by centrifugation, wash with 70%, EtOH, and dry the pellet.

3.2. Restriction of DNA by Dpn I and Another Enzyme of Choice

The isolated DNA is usually restricted first by an enzyme that linearizes the transfected plasmid. This is important since it will focus all the transfected material into one band in a subsequent autoradiogram and avoid any confusion arising from the different agarose gel mobilities of the various circular and linear forms of the plasmid. In addition, the enzyme of choice should not be sensitive to eukaryotic CpG methylation, so that the cellular genomic DNA will be cut and will therefore enter the subsequent agarose gel. If there is not a suitable enzyme available to linearize the transfected DNA, any enzyme that cuts the plasmid only a few times is appropriate.

1. Resuspend the DNA pellet (which will be approx 20–50 μg) in 80 μL sterile H_2O.
2. Add 10 μL of 10× restriction enzyme buffer (made according to the manufacturer's specifications), and 10 μL of 1 mg/mL BSA.
3. Add 50 U of restriction enzyme of choice (*see* Note 8). Tap the tube to ensure mixing.
4. Incubate overnight at an appropriate temperature (usually 37°C) (*see* Note 9).
5. The following morning, ensure that digestion has occurred by pipeting the digest up and down gently. It should no longer be unmanageably viscous. If sufficient digestion has not occurred, add another 5 U of enzyme and leave at least 4 h more. When the DNA has been cut, remove half the digest to a new tube for ethanol precipitation as in step 13, Section 3.1.).
6. Wash ethanol precipitate with 70% ethanol, and resuspend it in 40 μL H_2O.
7. Add 5 μL of 10× Dpn I buffer and 5 μL of 1 mg/mL BSA.
8. Add 5–10 U of Dpn I, mix well, and incubate at 37°C for at least 2 h (*see* Note 10).
9. Ethanol-precipitate both the digests (before and after Dpn I digestion). *See* Section 3.1., steps 13 and 14.
10. Wash in 70% ethanol and dry the pellets.
11. Resuspend in an appropriate vol of agarose gel-loading dyes.

3.3. Analysis of Replicated DNA by the Southern Blot Procedure

Fractionate the digests on an agarose gel (*see* Note 11) alongside a suitable marker, and transfer by standard procedures to nitrocellulose or a nylon membrane (*see* Chapter 28). The blot should then be hybridized to a radioactively labeled plasmid DNA probe (*see* Note 12). Subsequent autoradiography should reveal in one lane a linear band that Dpn I will have totally or partially digested into smaller bands in the next lane. The remaining linear band in the Dpn I lane represents the amount of replication that has occurred. If no linear band is visible, then no detectable replication has occurred.

This technique thus gives qualitative information as to whether replication has occurred, and comparative densitometry of the linear bands in each lane can give quantitative information as to what proportion of the nuclear-localized transfected DNA has undergone replication.

4. Notes

1. An alternative to isolating and purifying total nuclear DNA is the Hirt procedure described in Chapter 29. This additionally separates the genomic DNA from the transfected DNA. However, because it is performed on whole cells, the plasmid DNA that is recovered may not all have entered the nucleus, and so may make quantification of nuclear DNA replication more difficult.

2. The number of transfected cells used for analysis depends very much on the cell type and the transfection procedure adopted. Some cells (e.g., HeLa cells) transfect fairly efficiently, so relatively few cells are needed for Southern analysis. In addition, some methods of transfection are more efficient than others. Thus the number of cells to be analyzed in any experiment will need to be determined empirically.

3. The lysis time of the cells is cell-type-specific and should be determined empirically by monitoring the reaction under a microscope. The saponin lysis described here is very gentle and lysis of nuclei does not generally occur. Seven to 10 min is adequate for most cell types.

4. Temperature –4°C stabilizes nuclei against lysis.

5. For up to 10^7 cell nuclei, 100 µL of buffer A is usually sufficient. For a larger number of cells, a proportionally greater volume of buffer A should be used at this step.

6. The proteinase K digestion must be incubated overnight if a large number of cells (>10^6) is being processed. For smaller numbers of cells, 4–6 h may be sufficient.

7. The genomic DNA will be very viscous and difficult to manipulate with a pipet at this point. Sawing off the ends of the pipet tips may help.

8. The enzyme of choice should be an inexpensive one, since a large amount of enzyme is necessary to ensure efficient digestion of genomic DNA.

9. If small amounts of genomic DNA (1 µg or less) are being analyzed, the digestion time can be reduced to several hours if more convenient.

10. An excessive amount of enzyme is no longer necessary (as it was in step 3.2.3.), since the genomic DNA will not be digested by this enzyme.

11. Only a portion of each sample needs to be run on the gel. The important thing is that an equal proportion of the two test samples (before and after Dpn I digestion) are run alongside each other. The required proportion will depend on the efficiency of transfection of the plasmid DNA and will need to be determined empirically.

12. The choice of probe should be carefully considered. If more than one plasmid has been transfected, it may be necessary to isolate from one or another plasmid a fragment containing sequences unique to that plasmid in order to analyze its replication unambiguously.

References

1. Andreason, G. L and Evans, G. A. (1988) Introduction and expression of DNA molecules in eukaryotic cells by electroporation. *BioTechniques* **6,** 650–660.
2. Wilson, A. C. and Patient, R. K. Scrapefection—A rapid and simple method for transfecting adherent cells. Manuscript in prep.
3. McCutchan, J. H. and Pagano, J. S. (1968) Enhancement of the infectivity of simian virus 40 deoxyribonucleic acid with diethyl-amino-ethyl-dextran. *J. Natl. Cancer Inst.* **41,** 351–356.
4. Lopata, M., Cleveland, D., and Soller-Webb, B. (1984) High level transient expression of chloramphenicol acetyl transferase gene by DEAE-dextran mediated DNA transfection coupled with a dimethyl sulfoxide or glycerol shock treatment. *Nucleic Acids Res.* **12,** 5707–5717.
5. Graham, F. L. and van der Eb, A. J. (1973) A new technique for the assay of infectivity of human adenovirus 5 DNA. *Virology* **52,** 456–467.
6. Reeves, R., Gorman, C. M., and Howard, B. (1985) Minichromosome assembly of non-integrated plasmid DNA transfected into mammalian cells. *Nucleic Acids Res.* **13,** 3599–3615.
7. Hay, R. T. and Russell, W. C. (1989) Recognition mechanisms in the synthesis of animal virus DNA. *Biochem. J.* **258,** 3–16.
8. Enver, T., Brewer, A. C., and Patient, R. K. (1988) Role for DNA replication in β-globin gene activation. *Mol. Cell. Biol.* **8,** 1301–1308.

CHAPTER 31

Use of Polymerase Chain Reaction (PCR) to Detect Homologous Recombination in Transfected Cell Lines

Andreas Zimmer and Peter Gruss

1. Introduction

When DNA is introduced into eukaryotic cells, it can be integrated into the genome by homologous or illegitimate recombination *(1,2)*. Despite great efforts to gain insight into the molecular mechanisms, our understanding of the recombination process is still in its infancy. In the absence of a molecular model, predictions concerning the frequency of homologous recombination compared to illegitimate recombination cannot be precisely made. In mammalian cells, illegitimate recombination is the most predominant event (for review, *see* ref. *3*). Thus, if the integration of DNA via homologous recombination into mammalian cells is the goal of the experiment, a single homologous recombination event has to be detected among many illegitimate recombination events. Described here is a method of detecting homologous recombination events in a small subpopulation of cells by using the polymerase chain reaction (PCR), a primer-directed enzymatic amplification of specific DNA sequences. This method can be used to determine the homologous recombination frequency and to facilitate the cloning of homologously recombined cells *(4–6)*. Homologously recombined alleles are identified by their amplification products, which are generated by the PCR reaction (*see* Fig. 1). The specificity of the reaction is dependent on the two primers. One

From: *Methods in Molecular Biology, Vol. 7: Gene Transfer and Expression Protocols*
Edited by: E. J. Murray © 1991 The Humana Press Inc., Clifton, NJ

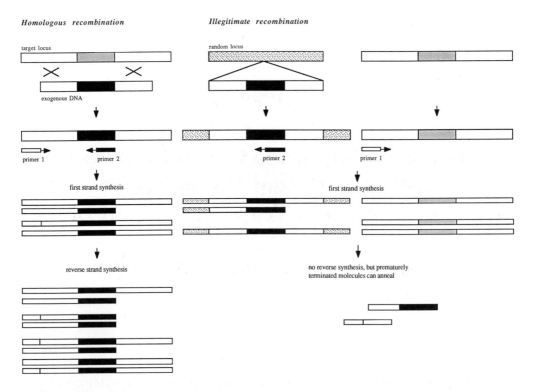

Fig. 1. Detection of homologous recombination events by PCR. Homologous recombination between a target locus and exogenous DNA yields a new recombinant molecule in which a small portion of the target locus is replaced by a heterologous sequence of the exogenous DNA. This recombination event links two priming sites for the PCR. Primer 1 primes DNA synthesis from the target sequence, outside of the region homologous to the exogenous DNA. Primer 2 is specific for the heterologous sequence residing in the exogenous DNA. These priming sites are not linked (in the same manner) after the integration of the exogenous DNA by illegitimate recombination. Yet, DNAs of a heterogeneous length are made from the target and the illegitimately recombined sequence during every PCR cycle. Those molecules that terminate in the region of homology could anneal, thus creating a recombinant molecule.

primer (primer 2 in Fig. 1) primes DNA synthesis specifically at the nonhomologous sequences of the exogenous DNA. The other primer (primer 1 in Fig. 1) is specific for the target locus, but outside of the exogenous DNA. Thus, both priming sites are physically linked in a predictable manner only after homologous recombination.

The reaction involves reiterated cycles of heat denaturation of the genomic DNA, annealing of the primers, and the extension of the annealed primers by the heat-stable *Taq* DNA polymerase *(7)*. The primers anneal to complementary DNA strands and are oriented such that the extension proceeds through the region between the primers. The extension products serve as a template in subsequent cycles, resulting in an exponential amplification of a DNA fragment that is flanked by the two primers. The extent of the amplification can be calculated with the formula $A = (X+1)^n$, in which A is the extent of the amplification, X is the mean efficiency/cycle ($0 \leq X \leq 1$), and n is the number of cycles.

Although it is possible to create an indistinguishable fragment from illegitimately, recombined DNAs during the PCR (*see* Fig. 1), the extent of this amplification is usually 4–6 orders of magnitude lower than that of homologously recombinant DNA. However, this possible artifact necessitates pilot experiments to determine the extent of the amplification and the mean efficiency for every set of primers (*see* Fig. 2).

To establish the PCR analysis, a control template that contains both priming sites is needed. This control plasmid should be used to establish the optimal conditions for the given template/primer combination. In particular, such parameters as $MgCl_2$ concentration, annealing and elongation temperature, and the elongation time should be carefully evaluated. Testing the likelihood of an artificial amplification by combining a plasmid representing the target locus with the construct used for cell transfections is also recommended.

An intrinsic problem with the PCR analysis is the fact that even small contaminations can give rise to false positive results. Therefore, including a negative control (e.g., genomic DNA from parental cells) in every analysis is highly recommended. It is not necessary to take special precautions when setting up the PCRs, e.g., placing them in laminar flow hood or a separate room. However, to avoid contamination, PCR solutions should not be used for other purposes.

2. Materials

1. TE: 10 mM Tris-HCl, pH 7.5, 1 mM EDTA.
2. 10× PCR buffer: 670 mM Tris-HCl, pH 8.3; 166 mM NH$_4$SO$_4$; 100 mM 2-mercaptoethanol; and 1.7 mg/mL BSA (Pentax fraction V) (*see* Note 1).
3. 10 µM PCR primer stock solution: Combine aliquots of primers for PCR and dilute to a concentration of 10 µM in TE (*see* Note 2).
4. 50 mM MgCl$_2$.
5. DMSO (Dimethylsulfoxide).
6. 10 mM dNTP stock solution: 10 mM dATP, 10 mM dCTP, 10 mM dGTP, 10 mM dTTP (store at –20°C).
7. *Taq*-Polymerase 2 U/µL (*see* Note 3).
8. Paraffin.

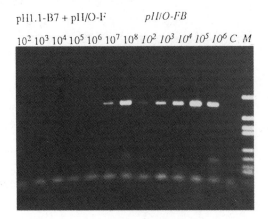

pH1.1-B7 + pH/O-F   pH/O-FB

10^2 10^3 10^4 10^5 10^6 10^7 10^8 *10^2 10^3 10^4 10^5 10^6* C M

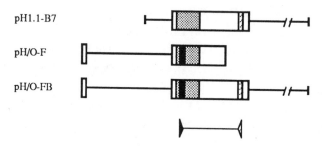

pH1.1-B7

pH/O-F

pH/O-FB

Fig. 2. Typical comparison of the amplification efficiency exemplified by a recombinant Hox 1.1 molecule with both priming sites (pH/O-FB) and that of two overlapping Hox 1.1 molecules, each containing only one priming site (pH1.1-B7; pH/O-F). From the plasmid pH/O-FB, 10^2 molecules can be amplified to yield a visible band in an ethidium bromide-stained gel after 35 PCR cycles. Of each of the mixed plasmids, pH1.1-B7 and pH/-F, 10^7 molecules, are required for the amplification of a visible band, so this event is $10^5 \times$ less efficient. C = control amplification without DNA; M = DNA marker.

9. 10× loading buffer: 0.4% bromophenol blue, 0.4% xylene cyanol, and 25% Ficoll (type 400) in H_2O.
10. 10 ng/µL of a linearized DNA (1–2 kb) in 1× loading buffer (to serve as a quantification standard).
11. Proteinase K buffer: 50 mM Tris, pH 8.0; 100 mM EDTA; 100 mM NaCl; and 1% SDS.
12. Proteinase K stock solution: 10 mg/mL, dissolved in H_2O (store at –70°C).
13. Phenol/chloroform/isoamylalcohol, 25:24:1.
14. 100% ethanol.

3. Methods

3.1. Establishing the PCR Conditions

3.1.1. Mg^{2+} Concentration

1. The PCR conditions should be established with a template that contains priming sites for both primers, reflecting the chromosomal structure after homologous recombination (*see* Note 4). Dilute the template to 100 pg/µL in TE (*see* Note 5).

2. Set up PCR mixes with different Mg^{2+} concentrations:

10 × PCR buffer	5 µL
10 µ*M* primers	2 µL
DMSO	2.5 µL
template DNA, 100 pg/µL	1 µL
10 mM dNTP	1 µL
50 m*M* MgCl$_2$	1–8 µL
Taq-polymerase, 2U/µL	1 µL
H$_2$O	to 50 µL

   Make two independent reactions for each concentration of Mg^{2+}.

3. Overlay the reaction mixes with a few drops (200 µL) of paraffin to prevent condensation.

4. Subject the reaction mixes to the following temperature cycles:

Initial denaturation	94°C, 2 min
Main cycles	50°C, 1 min (to anneal the primers)
	65°C, 1 min/100 bp product length (to activate the polymerase)
	91.5°C, 1 min (to denature the DNA); repeat 19 times
Final step	50°C, 1 min
	65°C, 1.5 min/100 bp product length

   (The PCR products can be stored in the reaction mix at room temperature.)

5. To analyze the PCR product by conventional nondenaturing agarose or acrylamide gel electrophoresis (Volume 2, this series), add 5 µL of 10× loading buffer, mix, and load directly onto the gel. It is advisable to run two gels with different amounts of the PCR mix, e.g., one gel with 5 µL and a second gel with 30 µL. Coelectrophorese a linear DNA of a size similar to that of the predicted band and of a known concentration to determine the amount of the PCR product in a semiquantitative manner.

3.1.2. Temperatures and Times

1. Dilute the template to 1 pg/µL in TE.
2. Set up PCR reactions with the Mg^{2+} concentration that gave the best results:

10× PCR buffer	5 µL
10 µM primers	2 µL
DMSO	2.5 µL
Template DNA, 1 pg/µL	10 µL
10 mM dNTP	1 µL
50 mM MgCl$_2$	optional
Taq-polymerase, 2U/µL	1 µL
H$_2$O	to 50 µL

3. Overlay with paraffin.
4. Amplify with different elongation temperatures.
   Try the following temperatures: 65, 68, 71, and 74°C.
5. Determine the best elongation temperature as described in Section 3.1.1., step 5. Electrophorese all products in only one gel.
6. Taking the highest elongation temperature that gave the best amplification, repeat the PCR reaction using different annealing temperatures. Try the following temperatures: 50, 55, 60, 65, and 70°C.
7. Electrophorese the reaction products to determine the annealing temperature that gave the best amplification result.

3.2. Determination of the Amplification Efficiency in Comparison of Homologous Recombination to Illegitimate Recombination

1. After establishing the optimal reaction conditions, one should be able to detect reliably the amplification products of 10 or 100 molecules in an ethidium bromide stained gel (*see* Note 6). Make a serial dilution of the template DNA in the range of 10^1–10^4 molecules/µL in TE.
2. Also make serial dilutions, in the range of 10^2–10^8 molecules/µL in TE, of the plasmid used for transfections and a plasmid representing the target DNA sequence.
3. Set up PCRs with increasing template-DNA concentrations in the range of 10^1–10^4 molecules.
4. Set up PCRs with increasing concentrations of a mixture of the plasmids used for transfections and representing the target sequence.
5. Amplify the DNAs under optimal conditions for 35 and 40 cycles.
6. Analyze the products by gel electrophoresis.

7. Determine the efficiency of the amplification of the template DNA (reflecting the chromosomal structure after homologous recombination) and the mixed plasmids (mimicking the chromosomal situation after an illegitimate recombination). A typical example of such an experiment is shown in Fig. 2.

3.3. Analysis of Cell Pools
for Homologous Recombination Events

1. Harvest the cells (*see* Note 7).
2. Transfer the cells into a microcentrifuge tube and pellet them by brief centrifugation. Carefully remove the supernatant. (At this stage the cells can be stored at –20°C.)
3. Add 50 μL proteinase K buffer and 1 μL proteinase K; mix by "flicking" with the fingers. Incubate at 55°C for 1–2 h.
4. Add 50 μL of phenol/chloroform/isoamylalcohol, vortex 10 s, and separate the liquid from the organic phase by a 2-min centrifugation at 13000 rpm.
5. Transfer 40 μL of the liquid phase into a new tube, leaving any interphase and organic phase behind.
6. Add 100 μL ethanol, mix, and precipitate the DNA for 10 min on dry ice.
7. Centrifuge for 10 min at 13,000 rpm in a microcentrifuge to pellet the DNA, and carefully remove the supernatant.
8. Dissolve the DNA pellet in 40 μL TE.
9. Subject the DNA to 35–40 PCR cycles with the optimal conditions.
10. Analyze the product by gel electrophoresis as described. Bands with a lower mol wt are often present; however, after homologous recombination, you should see clearly a prominent band at the expected position.
11. If necessary, analyze by Southern hybridization (*see* Chapter 28).

4. Notes

1. Store at –20°C. Make small aliquots; BSA may precipitate after repeated freezing/thawing.
2. We obtained the best results with 20- to 25-oligonucleotide primer with a 60–70% G + C content.
3. Most polymerases are supplied at higher concentrations and should be diluted in the storage buffer recommended by the manufacturers.
4. It is not always necessary to clone such a template, which probably could be generated by PCR when the plasmid used for homologous recombination and a plasmid with the target sequence are mixed, as described in Figs. 1 and 2.

5. With a mean efficiency of 50% , the extent of the amplification after 20 cycles is $A = (0.5 + 1)^{20} = 3.3 \times 10^3$. Since 30-ng DNA are easily detectable in an ethidium bromide stained gel, 10–100 pg of the control plasmid are sufficient for one reaction.

6. The number of cycles that is required to amplify the molecules to a visible band largely depends on the efficiency. You should expect an efficiency of 70–80%. If the product has a length of 1000 bp, 50-ng DNA contains 4.5×10^{10} molecules. Thus, the number of cycles to detect 10 molecules is calculated according to the formula $A = (X + 1)^n <=> 4.5 \times 10^9 = (0.7 + 1)^n <=> n = 42$.

7. For each reaction, $10^2–10^3$ individual cells of the same genotype should be used. If the pool has been derived from 10^3 individual cells, you would need $10^5–10^6$ cells for a single reaction. The pool size should be smaller than the window that was determined to discriminate reliably between homologous and illegitimate recombination events. Thus, if a homologously recombined template DNA is 10^4 times more efficiently amplified than a mixed template, the complexity of the pool should not be larger than 10^3 individual cells. One microgram of genomic DNA represents approx 3×10^4 diploid murine or human cells.

References

1. Folger, K. R., Wong, E. A., Wahl, G., and Capecchi, M. R. (1982) Patterns of integration of DNA microinjected into cultured mammalian cells: Evidence for homologous recombination between injected plasmid DNA molecules. *Mol. Cell. Biol.* **2**, 1372–1387.
2. Smithies, O., Gregg, R. G., Boggs, S. S., Koralewski, M. A., and Kucherlapati, R. S. (1985) Insertion of DNA sequences into the human chromosome β-globin locus by homologous recombination. *Nature* **317**, 230–234.
3. Kucherlapati, R. (1986) Homologous recombination in mammalian somatic cells, in *Gene Transfer* (Kucherlapati, R., ed.), Plenum, New York, London, pp. 363–381.
4. Kim, H.-S. and Smithies, O. (1988) Recombinant fragment assay for gene targetting based on the polymerase chain reaction. *Nucleic Acid Res.* **16**, 8887–8903.
5. Zimmer, A. and Gruss, P. (1989) Production of chimaeric mice containing embryonic stem cells carrying a homeobox *Hox 1.1* allele mutated by homologous recombination. *Nature* **338**, 150–153.
6. Joyner, A. L., Skarnes, W. C., and Rossant, J. (1989) Production of a mutation in mouse *En-2* gene by homologous recombination in embryonic stem cells. *Nature* **338**, 153–156.
7. Saiki, R. K., Gelfand, D. H., Stoffel, S., Scharf, S. J., Higuchi, R., Horn, G. T., Mullis, K. B., and Ehrlich, H. A. (1988) Primer-directed enzymatic amplification of DNA with a thermostable DNA polymerase. *Science* **239**, 487–491.

SECTION 9
USE OF CELL LINES FOR STUDYING
TISSUE-SPECIFIC GENE EXPRESSION

CHAPTER 32

Induction of Erythroid-Specific Expression in Murine Erythroleukemia (MEL) Cell Lines

Michael Antoniou

1. Introduction

Murine erythroleukemia (MEL) cell lines are erythroid progenitor cells derived from the spleens of susceptible mice infected with the Friend virus complex (1). These virally transformed cells are arrested at the proerythroblast stage of development and can be maintained in tissue culture indefinitely (2). Most MEL cell lines show a low (approx 1%) level of spontaneous erythroid differentiation, which is dependent on the culture conditions as well as the cell line in question (2–4). However, upon treatment with various chemical agents, MEL cells can be induced to undergo erythroid differentiation at much higher levels (30–100%). Among the most potent inducers of differentiation are polar–planar compounds (such as dimethyl sulfoxide [5] and hexamethylene bisacetamide [6]), fatty acid salts (for example, sodium butyrate [7], retinoic acid and some of its derivatives [8]) (for a comprehensive list of inducers, see ref. 9).

Erythroid differentiation of MEL cells in culture is characterized by changes that are analogous to normal red-cell maturation. These include

1. Synthesis of hemoglobin (Hb) (10);
2. An increase in the enzymes involved in heme biosynthesis (11);

From: *Methods in Molecular Biology, Vol. 7: Gene Transfer and Expression Protocols*
Edited by: E. J. Murray © 1991 The Humana Press Inc., Clifton, NJ

3. Appearance of red-cell-specific membrane proteins such as α- and β-spectrin *(12,13)*, band 3 *(14)*, and band 4 *(15);* and

4. Chromatin condensation and other morphological changes culminating in a cessation of cell division and ultimate enucleation *(16)*. Thus, MEL cells proved to be an excellent model system for studying changes in chromatin structure and coordinated gene expression associated with differentiation *(see* refs. *17–20* and refs. therein).

The most thoroughly investigated aspect of MEL cell differentiation is the increase in adult globin gene expression *(17)*. Although overall RNA synthesis and content decreases *(21)*, β^{maj} and α-globin gene transcription increases approx 30- to 40-fold after a 48–72 h exposure to inducer *(18,20)*, resulting in >10,000 copies of β^{maj} mRNA/cell after 3–4 d of differentiation *(22)*. This elevation in the amount of β^{maj} and α-globin mRNA appears to result principally from the increase in transcription of their genes *(23)*. At the time of peak globin mRNA levels, 25% of the total protein being synthesized is α- and β-globin *(10)*.

The potential of MEL cells as an erythroid expression system was first demonstrated by the introduction of the human β-globin gene into MEL cells, either in its natural chromosome environment by cell fusion *(24,25)*, or by DNA-mediated transfection *(22,26)*. The results showed correctly regulated expression of the human gene in parallel with the endogenous β^{maj} transcription unit upon induced differentiation. These initial observations resulted in transfection in MEL cells being used to localize and characterize the genetic elements responsible for the erythroid-specific expression of the human β-globin gene. Using mutant and hybrid gene constructs, it has been shown that the human β-globin gene possesses both erythroid-specific promoter elements *(27–29)* and two downstream enhancers *(27,28,30)*. The results demonstrating the presence of the enhancers are similar to those obtained in vivo with transgenic mice *(31,32)*.

It recently has been discovered that the human β-like globin gene locus or chromatin domain is flanked by powerful erythroid-specific regulatory regions *(33)*. This "dominant control region" (DCR) confers high-level, position-independent expression on a linked β-globin gene in transgenic mice. The DCR has also been shown to function in an analogous fashion in MEL cells upon induced differentiation *(34,35)*.

There is thus a striking similarity between the results obtained in vivo with transgenic mice and those obtained with MEL cells in tissue culture. This strongly suggests that MEL cells closely mimic the molecular regulatory processes associated with normal red-cell maturation. Therefore, MEL cells would appear to be a good model system in which to study erythroid-specific gene expression, despite their transformed phenotype.

A limitation of MEL cells as an erythroid model system is that they cannot be used to study the molecular mechanisms underlying the turning on and off of different globin genes ("hemoglobin switching") that occurs during embryonic development (for a review, *see* ref. *36*). However, they continue to serve as a convenient system in which to study general erythroid function. Our laboratory has used MEL cells to investigate the molecular mechanisms controlling β-globin gene expression for several years. This chapter describes the methods that we currently use to generate stable transfected populations of MEL cells, which have allowed us to assess the erythroid-expressing capability of a series of globin-gene constructs within 2–3 wk.

1.1. Maintenance of MEL Cell Lines

Many MEL cell lines have been produced with varied properties. All grow easily in standard DMEM or αMEM tissue-culture medium supplemented with 10% (v/v) fetal calf serum in a 5% CO_2 atmosphere at 37°C. Most MEL cell lines grow in suspension, although semiadherent *(37)* and adherent types *(38)* have been described. Variants with mutant phenotypes, namely TK⁻ *(38)*, HPRT*(39,40)*, and APRT⁻ *(37)* also have been generated. These mutants have proved useful in selection procedures for transformed cells *(see 22,30)*.

Our most recent work has been performed with the semiadherent APRT⁻ cell line C88, originally described by Deisseroth and Hendrick *(37)*. Stock cultures are maintained in αMEM plus 10% fetal calf serum as described above. This cell line grows rapidly, dividing every 12 h, and can grow to a high cell density (4×10^6 cells/mL). As a rule, we subculture to 5×10^4 cells/mL when a cell density of 2×10^6 cells/mL is reached. A sharp tapping of the tissue-culture flask is usually sufficient to dislodge the adherent cells, although trypsinization may also be employed. If it is desired to retain the APRT⁻ status of the cells, then the growth medium must be supplemented with 50 μg/mL diaminopurine, which kills revertants within 2–3 cell divisions. The diaminopurine is dissolved directly in the growth medium. Its poor solubility precludes the use of concentrated stock solutions.

The APRT⁻ phenotype allows selection by transfection with the wild-type APRT gene and subsequent growth in the presence of azaserine (and absence of diaminopurine) *(30)*. However, we have found that our stock of C88 MEL cells has a high reversion rate to the APRT⁺ phenotype. Thus, we have opted for alternative drug-selection procedures, described in the following Sections.

1.2. Stable Transfection of MEL Cells by Electroporation

MEL cells are very difficult to transfect efficiently. Classical $CaPO_4$–DNA-precipitate-mediated transfer results in only a few transformed colonies/10⁶ cells *(22,30)*. Recently, transfection of MEL cells by DEAE-dextran and chloro-quine treatment, allowing transient expression analysis, has been described *(41)*.

In recent years, we have found that the most convenient and reproducible method of transfecting MEL cells is by electroporation (*see* Chapter 5, this vol). This method generates large, stably transfected populations of cells (of at least 100 clones/10^6 cells used) with an average transgene copy number of 4–5. These populations have proved quite suitable for erythroid expression studies *(28,29,34,35)*. Our methods are described below and illustrated in Fig. 1.

2. Materials

2.1. Preparation of MEL Cell Plasmid DNA Mixture for Electroporation

1. MEL cells: We use the semiadherent APRT–cell line C88 maintained in αMEM supplemented with 10% fetal calf serum and antibiotics (60 μg/mL penicillin, 100 μg/mL streptomycin) plus L-glutamine (2 mM). Cells are used in logarithmic growth phase.
2. Dulbecco's PBS A: 170 mM NaCl; 3.3 mM KCl; 10 mM Na$_2$HPO$_4$; 1.8 mM KH$_2$PO$_4$, pH 7.0.
3. Electroshock buffer (ESB): 25 mM HEPES, pH 7.15; 140 mM NaCl; 0.7 mM Na$_2$HPO$_4$. Filter-sterilize and store at 4°C.
4. Plasmid DNA: Purified on CsCl gradient (*see* Chapter 1). Linearized with restriction enzyme and stored at –20°C as an ethanol precipitate until use.
5. Bio-Rad "Gene-Pulser" (Bio-Rad, South Richmond, CA) electroporation unit.
6. 70% ethanol.
7. 100 mg/mL Geneticin® (G418 sulfate): Dissolve in PBS, filter-sterilize and store at –20°C.
8. Selection medium: 800 μg/mL G418 in growth medium (*see above*, item 1).

2.2. Induction of Erythroid Differentiation of Transfected MEL Cell Populations

1. Liquid N$_2$ storage.
2. Dry ice.
3. Freezing medium: 10% DMSO (Analar grade) in growth medum. Make fresh as required.
4. Induction medium: 2% DMSO in growth medium. Make fresh as required.

2.3. Extraction of Total RNA from MEL Cells

1. Lysis buffer: 3M LiCl, 6M urea (both Analar grade) in double-distilled H$_2$O; store at 4°C.

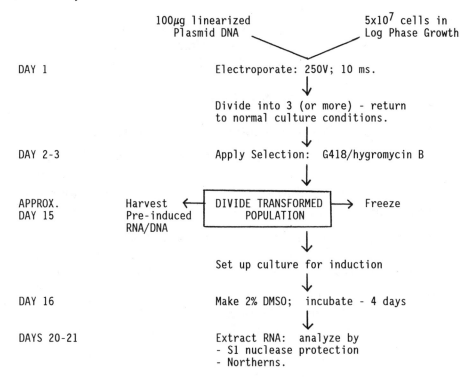

Fig. 1: Protocol for the production of stable transfected MEL cell populations.

2. Sonicator: e.g., Cole-Palmer Instruments 4710.
3. TES: 10 mM Tris-HCl, pH 7.5; 1 mM EDTA; 0.5% SDS in dd H$_2$O. Sterilize by autoclaving.
4. 3M sodium acetate, pH 5.5. Autoclave before use.
5. Phenol/chloroform (1:1 v/v) saturated with TE (*see below*, Section 2.4., item 6).
6. 100% ethanol.
7. 70% ethanol.
8. RNase-free dd H$_2$O. Autoclave prior to use.

2.4. Extraction of DNA from MEL Cells

1. Dulbecco's PBS A: *See above*, Section 2.1.2.
2. TNE: 50 mM Tris-HCl, pH 7.5; 100 mM NaCl; and 5 mM EDTA. Autoclave prior to use.
3. 20% SDS: prepare in dd H$_2$O. Do not autoclave.
4. Proteinase K: Dissolve in double-distilled H$_2$O at 10 mg/mL and store at –20°C.
5. Phenol/chloroform (1:1 v/v): *See above*, Section 2.3.5.
6. TE: 10 mM Tris-HCl, pH 7.5; 1 mM EDTA.
7. 70% ethanol.

8. DNase-free RNase A: RNase A (Sigma) dissolved in 10 m*M* Tris-HCl, pH 7.5; 15 m*M* NaCl (10 mg/mL). Heat treat at 100°C for 15–20 min to inactivate DNase. Slowly cool to room temperature and store at –20°C.

3. Methods

3.1. Preparation of Plasmid DNA (see Chapter 1)

The thorough planning of a series of gene constructs will save time at the tissue-culture stage of the experiment and generate more easily interpretable expression data. The following points should thus be considered when preparing mutants for analysis:

1. The gene of interest and the gene that codes the drug-resistance function to be used in selecting stable transformants, should ideally be present on the same plasmid molecule. We have not found cotransfection to work well with electroporation. This may be a result of the small number of plasmid molecules taken up by any given cell. If cotransfection is unavoidable, then a ratio of five parts expressing plasmid to one part drug-resistance plasmid is recommended.

2. The drug-resistance gene should be driven by a promoter without an enhancer that might also interfere with the expression of the linked gene of interest. For example, expression from the SV40 promoter-enhancer complex has been found to increase upon MEL cell differentiation (*42*). Under these circumstances, it is difficult to assess the erythroid-specific expression of a linked gene, as it is possibly being influenced by the erythroid-responsive SV40 enhancer. Thus, we have used the "neutral" thymidine kinase promoter to express the genes conferring resistance to G418 or hygromycin B (*see 28*).

3. Plasmids in either single or cotransfection experiments should be linearized, since this increases efficiency of integration into the host-cell genome. We try to select a restriction enzyme that cuts as far as possible from the genes on the plasmid molecule. The enzymatic reaction mixture is extracted with phenol:chloroform and the DNA stored as an ethanol precipitate until use.

4. As little as 10–20 µg/mL of DNA can be used during electroporation. However, since transfection efficiency has been found to improve with increasing DNA concentration (*43*), we use 50–100 µg/mL of electroporation mixture.

3.2. Preparation of MEL Cell-Plasmid DNA Mixture for Electroporation

Stock flasks of MEL cells are set up 2 d prior to electroporation. They are seeded in such a way that they will be in rapid, log-phase growth (cell density, 0.5–1 × 10^6 cells/mL) on the day of transfection. In the case of our MEL C88 cells, this means seeding at a density of 5 × 10^4 cells/mL.

Cell density in the electroporation mixture does not influence transfection efficiency to any marked degree *(43)*. A density between 10^6 and 10^8 cells/mL can be used. However, the more cells that are used, the larger the transformed population that is generated. The cells are prepared for electroporation as follows:

1. Spin out the desired number of cells (we use 3–5 × 10^7 cells for each transfection).
2. Wash in 20–50 mL of phosphate-buffered saline (PBS). Pellet and aspirate PBS.
3. Resuspend the cells in ESB at a cell density of 3–5 × 10^7 cells/0.9 mL buffer.
4. Aliquot cells (0.9 mL) into separate tubes in readiness to receive DNA.
5. Briefly spin down linearized, plasmid DNA precipitate (15 s in a microfuge). Aspirate ethanol supernatant and dissolve DNA in 100 µL of ESB without drying the pellet. The plasmid should dissolve very easily within a min.
6. Add the plasmid DNA solution to the cells at 50–100 µg/mL. Mix and allow to stand at room temperature, with occasional shaking, for 10 min prior to electroporation.
7. Transfer the MEL cell–DNA mixture to the electroporation cuvet and deliver a single pulse of 250 V, 960 µF *(see* Note 5).
8. After the electroshock pulse, leave the cells in the cuvet for 5–10 min.
9. Remove the cell suspension from the cuvet, divide equally between three (or more) 75-cm^2 flasks containing 30 mL of growth medium, and return to the 37°C incubator. The division of the electroporated mixture at this stage gives rise to independent populations of transfected cells from a single electroporation.

3.3. Selecting for Stable Transfected Cells

1. Place the cells in selection growth medium by adding G418 or hygromycin B, to 800 µg/mL 24–48 h after electroporation.
2. Set up an untransfected stock culture in selection medium in order to have a negative control.
3. The cells continue to divide rapidly for a few days before the effect of the drug becomes evident. Hence, medium changes every 48 h may be necessary initially. The cells do not seem to suffer from the overcrowded nature of the cultures at this stage as long as fresh medium is applied.
4. Cell death becomes apparent 5 d after the application of drug selection and is complete after 7 d. (At this point it already may be possible to see small clusters of transfected cells, either in suspension or attached to the plastic substratum.)

5. When the cultures are 50% confluent a few days later, carry out a further medium change and reduce the G418 concentration to 400 μg/mL *(see* Note 4).

6. The cultures are near confluency (2×10^6 cells/mL) about 14 d after the application of selection. They are now ready to be further analyzed for erythroid functions.

3.4. Inducing Erythroid Differentiation of Transfected MEL Cell Populations

The near-confluent cultures of transfected MEL cell populations are now prepared as follows for induced differentiation:

1. Freeze one-quarter of the culture in liquid nitrogen to act as a future stock. Spin the cells (about $1-2 \times 10^7$) and resuspend in 1.5 mL of 10% DMSO in growth medium. Immediately transfer to a freezing vial and place in dry ice for 1 h. The vial can then safely be immersed in liquid nitrogen for storage.

2. Process two other quarters of the culture for DNA and uninduced RNA, respectively *(see* Sections 3.5. and 3.6.). The DNA is analyzed for copy number and integrity of the transfected gene(s). The preinduced RNA sample is the control for the subsequent expression studies.

3. Prepare the final quarter of the culture for induction by diluting the cells to not more than 5×10^5/mL in a final vol of 30 mL and incubating overnight. This allows the cells to enter log-phase growth, the optimum condition from which to start erythroid differentiation *(see* Notes 1–3).

4. Induce the cultures to undergo erythroid differentiation for 4 d by adding DMSO (to 2% v/v) *(see* Note 6).

5. Perform a half-culture-volume medium change 2 d into the period of differentiation. This maintains ideal culture conditions. G418 may also be omitted at this stage.

6. Prior to harvesting the cells after 4 d of differentiation, spin down a 5- to 10-mL aliquot of the culture. A deep-red coloration of the cell pellet is indicative of satisfactory differentiation. If the cell pellet is still pale red at this stage, the incubation is continued for a further 24 h. The cells are then harvested and RNA extracted for analysis.

An example of the consistent results obtained with this method is given in Fig. 2.

A number of different methods are currently available for extracting both DNA and RNA from tissue-culture cells *(see* elsewhere in this vol.). The protocols routinely used in our laboratory, which enable rapid and consistent isolation of RNA and DNA, are given below.

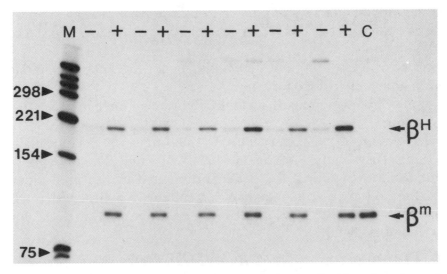

Fig. 2. Induced expression of human β-globin in MEL cells. Transfected populations of MEL C88 cells containing the human β-globin gene linked to its dominant control region (*36*) were produced as described in this chapter. Total RNA (2 µg) from preinduced (-) and 4-day induced (+) cells was then assayed for mouse (β^m) and human (β^H) β-globin sequences by S1 nuclease protection analysis (*45; see* ref. *29* for probe details). This figure shows the autoradiogram of the S1-protected products after resolution on a 6% polyacrylamide gel in the presence of 8*M* urea as denaturant. The positions of the 212 nucleotide human β-globin products and 95 nucleotide mouse β^{maj}-globin products are marked. The negative control (C) is RNA from induced, untransfected cells.

3.5. Extraction of Total RNA from MEL Cells

1. Spin down cells in a 25-mL plastic Universal tube (Sterilin), drain off the supernatant medium, and wipe the sides of the tube with clean tissue.
2. Vortex to loosen the cell pellet, add 3*M* LiCl/6*M* urea, and continue vortexing until a homogeneous cell lysate is produced. We use 5 mL of LiCl/urea per 2×10^7 cells. This may be scaled up or down, maintaining the ratio of cells to LiCl/urea as described.
3. Sonicate the cell homogenate for 1 min with a small-diameter probe (approx 3 mm). This shears the DNA and produces a nonviscous lysate.
4. Store overnight (or longer) at 4°C. This allows the RNA, which is insoluble in 3*M* LiCl, to precipitate.
5. Centrifuge in a Beckman J6-B at 3000 rpm for 30–45 min at 4°C (if vol are small, spin in a microfuge for 15–20 min).
6. Aspirate the supernatant, resuspend the RNA pellet in 1 mL of 3*M* LiCl/6*M* urea, and transfer to a microfuge tube. Spin in a microfuge for 5 min.
7. Aspirate the supernatant, dissolve the RNA pellet in 200-400 µL of TES, and add sodium acetate to a concentration of 0.3*M*.

8. Extract with an equal vol of phenol + chloroform (1:1 v/v).
9. Transfer the aqueous phase to a new microfuge tube and add 2.5 vol of 100% ethanol.
10. Store for at least 30 min at –20°C and pellet the RNA precipitate by spinning in a microfuge for 5 min.
11. Suction off the supernatant, wash the RNA pellet once in 70% ethanol, and respin.
12. Again, suction off the supernatant, so that only a wet pellet remains in the tube. Dissolve the RNA in 100–400 µL of water. The RNA goes into solution more rapidly if the pellet is disrupted by repeated pipeting. This method gives good-quality RNA, suitable for either S1 nuclease protection, RNase protection, primer extension, or Northern analysis (*see* Chapters 23–26).

3.6. Preparation of DNA from MEL Cells (see Note 8)

1. Spin down $1–2 \times 10^7$ cells and wash once in PBS. Aspirate PBS.
2. Resuspend the cells in 3–5 mL of TNE in 15-mL snap-cap polypropylene tubes.
3. Add SDS (to 1%), and proteinase K (to 0.5 mg/mL), and mix thoroughly but gently. Incubate the viscous lysate at 37°C overnight.
4. Extract the homogenate once with an equal vol of phenol-chloroform (1:1 v/v).
5. Transfer the aqueous phase to a new 25-mL plastic Universal tube and precipitate the nucleic acids by adding 2.5 vol of 100% ethanol and mixing gently by repeated end-over-end inversion of the sample. The DNA should precipitate as a single mass.
6. Spool out the DNA on the end of a Pasteur pipet or plastic pipet tip, rinse in 1–2 mL of 70% ethanol, drain, and dissolve in 2–3mL of TE in a 15-mL tube without drying the pellet.
7. Add 10 µg/mL RNase A (DNase-free) and incubate at 37°C for 15–30 min.
8. Extract once with an equal vol of phenol–chloroform, as in step 4.
9. Transfer the aqueous phase to a new tube, add sodium acetate to a concentration of 0.2*M*, and ethanol-precipitate the DNA as in step 5.
10. Spool out the DNA, rinse in 70% ethanol, drain, and dissolve in 0.5–1 mL of water.

4. Notes

1. MEL cells undergo 3–4 cycles of cell division as part of the erythroid differentiation process (*19*). MEL cell cultures should therefore be set up 1–2 d prior to the commencement of erythroid differentiation, so that they are in rapid, log-phase growth ($0.5–1 \times 10^6$ cells/mL) at the time of application of the inducer. (A confluent, slow-dividing culture will

differentiate poorly). It may be possible to obtain higher levels of differentiation for a given MEL line of interest by selecting for a rapidly dividing subpopulation or clone of cells (*see* ref. *16*).

2. The fetal calf serum to be used in the growth medium of MEL cells must be tested to ensure that (a) the cells grow at their normal rate, (b) the spontaneous rate of differentiation is not increased (it should be about 1%), and (c) normal differentiation will take place when the inducer is added. We check these parameters by growing the cells in a given batch of serum for 1 wk and then inducing a portion to differentiate. The level of β^{maj}-mRNA in preinduced and induced cells is then measured. This mRNA should be barely detectable in a 1- to 2-µg sample of total RNA from uninduced cells. An increase of 50- to 100-fold on 4 d of differentiation is deemed satisfactory (*see* Fig. 2). We have repeatedly failed to effectively grow and induce MEL cells on the various serum-free media (for example, Ultroser G, GIBCO) that recently have become available.

3. The efficacy of a given inducer to promote erythroid differentiation will vary with the cell line being used. It is thus advisable to test a range of substances for their potency. The most commonly used are 1.5–2% DMSO, 3–5 mM hexamethylene bisacetamide, and 1.5 mM sodium butyrate.

4. An initially high G418 or hygromycin B concentration (800 mg/mL) is needed in order to kill nontransfected cells in a short period of time. Once cell death is complete, a lower drug concentration (400 µg/mL) confers sufficient selective pressure to maintain the transfected population. The drug may also be omitted from medium changes performed after a transfected population has been induced to differentiate.

5. We perform electroporation with a Bio-Rad "Gene-Pulser" unit with settings of 250 V and 960 µF. The Gene-Pulser is used in conjunction with disposable cuvets with built-in aluminum electrodes as the electroporation chamber. We have found that a low voltage (250 V) and a long pulse time (12–15 ms) gives better results than the high voltage (2 KV) and microsecond pulse times originally described for MEL cells (*44*).

6. Among the changes that will be noticed 24–48 h after the addition of inducer to the MEL cells are
   a. cessation of noticeable cell division;
   b. a marked shrinkage in cell size; and
   c. a detachment of any adherent cells and dispersion of cell clusters to form a single cell suspension.

7. Strict sterile techniques must be used throughout the RNA preparation procedure in order to avoid possible RNase contamination. This is especially crucial once the RNA is out of the denaturing conditions of the LiCl/Urea solution.

8. All mixing during the preparation of DNA must be done gently (with no vortexing) in order to avoid excessive shearing of the DNA.

Acknowledgments

This work is being conducted in the Laboratory of Frank Grosveld, for whose continuing support I am very grateful. I would also like to thank Drs. Grosveld and Peter Fraser for constructive criticism of this manuscript. The patient secretarial assistance of Cora O'Carroll is greatly appreciated.

References

1. Friend, C. (1957) Cell-free transmission in adult Swiss mice of a disease having the character of a leukemia. *J. Exp. Med.* **105**, 307–318.
2. Singer, D., Cooper, M., Maniatis, G. M., Marks, P. A., and Rifkind, R. A. (1974) Erythropoietic differentiation in colonies of cells transformed by Friend virus. *Proc. Natl. Acad. Sci. USA* **71**, 2668–2670.
3. Orkin, S., Harosi, F. I., and Leder, P. (1975) Differentiation in erythroleukemic cells and their somatic hybrids. *Proc. Natl. Acad. Sci. USA* **72**, 99–102.
4. Rovera, G. and Bononuto, J. (1976) The phenotypes of variant clones of Friend mouse erythroleukemic cells resistant to dimethyl sulfoxide. *Cancer Res.* **36**, 4057–4061.
5. Friend, C., Scher, W., Holland, J. G., and Sako, T. (1971) Hemoglobin synthesis in murine virus-stimulated leukemic cells in vitro: Stimulation of erythroid differentiation by dimethyl sulfoxide. *Proc. Natl. Acad. Sci. USA* **68**, 378–382.
6. Reuben, R. C., Wife, R. L., Breslow, R., Rifkind, R. A., and Marks, P. A. (1976) A new group of potent inducers of differentiation in murine erythroleukemia cells. *Proc. Natl. Acad. Sci. USA* **73**, 862–866.
7. Leder, A. and Leder, P. (1975) Butyric acid, a potent inducer of erythroid differentiation in cultured erythroleukemic cells. *Cell* **5**, 319–322.
8. Garg, L. C. and Brown, J. C. (1983) Friend erythroleukemia cell differentiation induction by retinoids. *Differentiation* **25**, 79–83.
9. Marks, P. A. and Rifkind, R. A. (1978) Erythroleukemic differentiation. *Annu. Rev. Biochem.* **47**, 419–448.
10. Kabat, D., Sherton, C. C., Evans, L. H., Bigley, R., and Koler, R. D. (1975) Synthesis of erythrocyte-specific proteins in cultured Friend leukemia cells. *Cell* **5**, 331–338.
11. Sassa, S. (1976) Sequential induction of heme pathway enzymes during erythroid differentiation of mouse Friend leukemia virus-infected cells. *J. Exp. Med.* **143**, 305–315.
12. Eisen, H., Bach, R., and Emery, R. (1977) Induction by spectrin in erythroleukemic cells transformed by Friend virus. *Proc. Natl. Acad. Sci. USA* **74**, 3898–3902.
13. Pfeffer, S. R., Huima, T., and Redman, C. V. (1986) Biosynthesis of spectrin and its assembly into the cytoskeletal system of Friend erythroleukemia cells. *J. Cell. Biol.* **103**, 103–113.
14. Sabban, E. L., Sabatim, D. D., Marchesi, V. T., and Adesnik, M. (1980) Biosynthesis of erythrocyte membrane protein bound 3 in DMSO-induced Friend erythroleukemia cells. *J. Cell. Physiol.* **104**, 261–268.

15. Pfeffer, S. R. and Redman, C. M. (1981) Biosynthesis of mouse erythrocyte membrane proteins by Friend erythroleukemia cells. *Biochim. Biophys. Acta* **641**, 254–263.

16. Volloch, V. and Housman, D. (1982) Terminal differentiation of murine erythroleukemia cells: Physical stabilization of end-stage cells. *J. Cell. Biol.* **93**, 390–394.

17. Hofer, E., Hofer-Warbinek, R., and Darnell, J. E. (1982) Globin RNA transcription: A possible termination site and demonstration of transcriptional control correlated with altered chromatin structure. *Cell* **29**, 887–893.

18. Salditt-Georgieff, M., Sheffery, M., Krauter, K., Darnell, J. E., Rifkind, R., and Marks, P. A. (1984) Induced transcription of the mouse β-globin transcription unit in erythroleukemia cells. *J. Mol. Biol.* **172**, 437–450.

19. Cohen, R. B. and Sheffery, M. (1985) Nucleosome disruption precedes transcription and is largely limited to the transcribed domain of globin genes in murine erythroleukemia cells. *J. Mol. Biol.* **182**, 109–129.

20. Fraser, P. J. and Curtis, P. J. (1987) Specific pattern of gene expression during induction of mouse erythroleukemia cells. *Genes Dev.* **1**, 855–861.

21. Sherton, C. C. and Kabat, D. (1976) Changes in RNA and protein metabolism preceding onset of hemoglobin synthesis in cultured Friend leukemia cells. *Dev. Biol.* **48**, 118–131.

22. Wright, S., deBoer, E., Grosveld, F. G., and Flavell, R. A. (1983) Regulated expression of the human β-globin gene family in murine erythroleukemia cells. *Nature* **305**, 333–336.

23. Ganguly, S. and Skoultchi, A. I. (1985) Absolute rates of globin gene transcriptional and mRNA formation during differentiation of cultured mouse erythroleukemia cells. *J. Biol. Chem.* **260**, 12167–12173.

24. Willing, M. C., Nienhuis, A. W., and Anderson, F. (1979) Selective activation of human β- but not γ-globin gene in human fibroblast × mouse erythroleukemia cell hybrids. *Nature* **277**, 534–538.

25. Pyati, J., Kucherlapati, R. S., and Skoultchi, A. J. (1980) Activation of human β-globin genes from nonerythroid cells by fusion with murine erythroleukemia cells. *Proc. Natl. Acad. Sci. USA* **77**, 3435–3439.

26. Chao, M. V., Mellon, P., Charnay, P., Maniatis, T., and Axel, R. (1983) The regulated expression of β-globin genes introduced into mouse erythroleukemia cells. *Cell* **32**, 483–493.

27. Wright, S., Rosenthal, A., Flavell, R., and Grosveld, F. G. (1984) DNA sequences required for regulated expression of β-globin genes in murine erythroleukemia cells. *Cell* **38**, 265–273.

28. Antoniou, M., deBoer, E., Habets, G., and Grosveld, F. G. (1988) The human β-globin gene contains multiple regulatory regions: Identification of one promoter and two downstream enhancers. *EMBO J.* **7**, 377–384.

29. deBoer, E., Antoniou, M., Mignotte, V., Wall, L., and Grosveld, F. G. (1988) The human β-globin promoter: Nuclear protein factors and erythroid specific induction of transcription. *EMBO J.* **7**, 4203–4212.

30. Charnay, P., Treisman, R., Mellon, P., Chao, M., Axel, R., and Maniatis, T. (1984) Differences in human α- and β-globin gene expression in mouse erythroleukemia cells: The role of intragenic sequences. *Cell* **38**, 251–263.

31. Kollias, G., Hurst, J., deBoer, E., and Grosveld, F. G. (1987) The human β-globin gene contains a downstream developmental specific enhancer. *Nucleic Acids Res.* **15**, 5739–5747.

32. Behringer, R. R., Hammer, R. E., Brinster, R. L., Palmiter, R. D., and Townes, T. M. (1987) Two 3' sequences direct erythroid specific expression of human β-globin genes in transgenic mice. *Proc. Natl. Acad. Sci. USA* **84,** 7056–7060.

33. Grosveld, F., Blom van Assendelft, M., Greaves, D. R., and Kollias, G. (1987) Position-independent, high-level expression of the human β-globin gene in transgenic mice. *Cell* **51,** 975–985.

34. Blom van Assendelft, M., Hanscombe, O., Grosveld, F., and Greaves, D. R. (1989) The β-globin dominant control region activates homologous and heterologous promoters in a tissue-specific manner. *Cell* **56,** 969–977.

35. Talbot, D., Collis, P., Antoniou, M., Vidal, M., Grosveld, F., and Greaves, D. R. (1989) A dominant control region from the human β-globin locus conferring integration site-independent gene expression. *Nature* **388,** 352–355.

36. Collins, F. S. and Weissman, S. M. (1984) The molecular genetics of human hemoglobin. *Prog. Nucleic Acid Res. Mol. Biol.* **31,** 315–462.

37. Deisseroth, A. and Hendrick, D. (1978) Human β-globin gene expression following chromosomal dependent gene transfer into mouse erythroleukemia cells. *Cell* **15,** 55–63.

38. Spandidos, D. A. and Paul, J. (1982) Transfer of human globin genes into erythroleukemia mouse cells. *EMBO J.* **1,** 15–20.

39. Nomura, S. and Oishi, M. (1983) Indirect induction of erythroid differentiation in mouse Friend cells: Evidence for two intracellular reactions involved in the differentiation. *Proc. Natl. Acad. Sci. USA* **80,** 210–214.

40. Zavodney, P. J., Roginski, R. S., and Skoultchi, A. I. (1983) Regulated expression of human globin genes and flanking DNA in mouse erythroleukemia-human cell hybrids, in *Globin Gene Expression and Hematopoietic Differentiation* (Alan R. Liss, New York, pp. 53–62).

41. Cowie, A. and Myers, R. M. (1988) DNA sequences involved in transcriptional regulation of the mouse β-globin promoter in murine erythroleukemia cells. *Mol. Cell. Biol.* **8,** 3122–3128.

42. Rutherford, T. and Nienhuis, A. W. (1987) Human globin gene promoter sequences are sufficient for specific expression of a hybrid gene transfected into tissue culture cells. *Mol. Cell. Biol.* **7,** 398–402.

43. Chu, G., Hayakawa, H., and Berg, P. (1987) Electroporation for the efficient transfection of mammalian cells with DNA. *Nucleic Acids Res.* **15,** 1311–1326.

44. Beggs, S. S., Gregg, R. G., Borenstein, N., and Smithies, O. (1986) Efficient transformation and frequent single site, single copy insertion of DNA can be obtained in mouse erythroleukemia cells transformed by electroporation. *Exp. Haematol.* **14,** 988–994.

45. Antoniou, M., deBoer, E., and Grosveld, F. (1986) Fine mapping of genes: The determination of the transcriptional unit, in *Human Genetic Diseases—A Practical Approach* (Davies, K. E., ed.), IRL, Oxford, UK, pp. 65–84.

INDEX